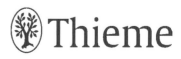

Connective Tissue Massage

Bindegewebsmassage According to Dicke

Roland Schiffter, MD
Professor of Neurology
Former Head Physician
Vivantes Auguste-Viktoria Hospital and
Vivantes-Wenckebach Hospital
Berlin, Germany

Elke Harms †
Former Practising Physical and Massage Therapist
Oldenburg, Germany

With the collaboration of Nancy Toner Weinberger,
Youngsville, NC, USA

140 illustrations

Thieme
Stuttgart • New York • Delhi • Rio

Library of Congress Cataloging-in-Publication Data

Bindegewebsmassage nach Dicke. English

Connective tissue massage: Bindegewebsmassage according to Dicke / [edited by] Roland Schiffter, Elke Harms; with contributions by Rauthgundis Gleich von Münster, Michael Weber, Mahmoud Mesrogli, Paul Hutzschenreuter, Axel Gehrke.

    p. ; cm.

"This book is an authorized translation of the 15th German edition published and copyrighted 2009 by Georg Thieme Verlag, Stuttgart. Title of the German edition: Bindegewebsmassage: Neuronale Abläufe - Befund - Praxis."

Translated from German.

ISBN 978-3-13-171431-2 (alk. paper) – ISBN 978-3-13-171441-1 (eISBN)

I. Schiffter, Roland, author. II. Harms, Elke, author. III. Title.

[DNLM: 1. Dicke, Elisabeth, 1884-1952. 2. Connective Tissue. 3. Massage. 4. Musculoskeletal Manipulations. WB 537]

RM721

615.8'22–dc23   2014005532

This book is an authorized translation of the 15th German edition published and copyrighted 2009 by Georg Thieme Verlag, Stuttgart. Title of the German edition: Bindegewebsmassage: Neuronale Abläufe – Befund – Praxis.

Translator: Terri Doerrzapf, Edenkoben, Germany

Illustrator: Gusta, Piotr, and Malgorzata, Champigny sur Marne, France

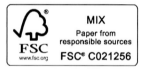

© 2014 Georg Thieme Verlag KG

Thieme Publishers Stuttgart
Rüdigerstrasse 14, 70469 Stuttgart, Germany
+49 [0]711 8931 421, customerservice@thieme.de

Thieme Publishers New York
333 Seventh Avenue, New York, NY 10001, USA
+1 800 782 3488, customerservice@thieme.com

Thieme Publishers Delhi
A-12, Second Floor, Sector-2, Noida-201301, Uttar Pradesh, India
+91 120 45 566 00, customerservice@thieme.in

Thieme Publishers Rio, Thieme Publicações Ltda.
Argentina Building, 16th floor, Ala A, 228 Praia do Botafogo
Rio de Janeiro 22250-040 Brazil
+55 21 3736-3631

Cover design: Thieme Publishing Group
Typesetting by DiTech Process Solutions Pvt. Ltd., India
Printed in China by Everbest Printing Ltd., Hong Kong

ISBN 978-3-13-171431-2

Also available as an e-book:
eISBN 978-3131714411

Important note: Medicine is an ever-changing science undergoing continual development. Research and clinical experience are continually expanding our knowledge, in particular our knowledge of proper treatment and drug therapy. Insofar as this book mentions any dosage or application, readers may rest assured that the authors, editors, and publishers have made every effort to ensure that such references are in accordance with **the state of knowledge at the time of production of the book**. Nevertheless, this does not involve, imply, or express any guarantee or responsibility on the part of the publishers in respect to any dosage instructions and forms of applications stated in the book. **Every user is requested to examine carefully** the manufacturers' leaflets accompanying each drug and to check, if necessary in consultation with a physician or specialist, whether the dosage schedules mentioned therein or the contraindications stated by the manufacturers differ from the statements made in the present book. Such examination is particularly important with drugs that are either rarely used or have been newly released on the market. Every dosage schedule or every form of application used is entirely at the user's own risk and responsibility. The authors and publishers request every user to report to the publishers any discrepancies or inaccuracies noticed. If errors in this work are found after publication, errata will be posted at www.thieme.com on the product description page.

Some of the product names, patents, and registered designs referred to in this book are in fact registered trademarks or proprietary names even though specific reference to this fact is not always made in the text. Therefore, the appearance of a name without designation as proprietary is not to be construed as a representation by the publisher that it is in the public domain.

Preface

"My Connective Tissue Massage" ("Meine Bindege-websmassage") was written by Elisabeth Dicke and first published in 1952 just a few weeks after her death. It is her life's work and explains the successful treatment method she developed while suffering from arterial circulatory disturbances in her right leg in 1929. Time and again she discovered skin zones on her own body and on patients' bodies that showed sensitive changes and, upon manual manipulation, appeared to cause reflex effects in the internal organs. She studied these observations in many patients and on this basis developed her own "systematic treatment method," for which she later found a neurophysiological explanation of the segmental "hyperalgesic zones" in Henry Head's concept. She significantly overestimated the role of the connective tissue (German: *Bindegewebe*), hence the name given to the method. My late teacher Hans Schliack, neurologist and former editor of this work, had already emphasized the significant role of neurovegetative reflexes and I further elaborated this neurophysiological effect model in the last German editions. There is no doubt that of all treatment methods applied directly to the skin, those processes caused by a reflex are the most effective.

I am very pleased that this book is now also available worldwide to my English-speaking audience. It is intended for students of physical therapy, massage therapists, but also for interested physicians. It conveys neurophysiological knowledge and manual skills, which cannot be acquired through machines or computers.

I would like to thank all the staff at Thieme Publishers for their excellent work.

I hope that this book finds a broad audience and will help to alleviate the pain of patients around the world.

Professor Roland Schiffter, MD

Contributors

Axel Gehrke, MD
Professor
Centre for Physical Medicine and Rehabilitation
Hanover Medical School
Hanover, Germany

Rauthgundis Gleich von Muenster
San Leo Bastia, Italy

Elke Harms †
Former Practising Physical and Massage Therapist
Oldenburg, Germany

Professor Paul Hutzschenreuter, MD, †

Mahmoud Mesrogli, MD
Professor
Director, Department of Gynecology and Obstetrics
Husum District Hospital
Husum, Germany

Roland Schiffter, MD
Professor of Neurology
Former Head Physician
Vivantes Auguste-Viktoria Hospital and
Vivantes-Wenckebach Hospital
Berlin, Germany

Michael Weber, MD
Professor
Department of Surgery
University Medical Center Freiburg
Freiburg, Germany

Contents

Contents

Chapter 1

Introduction

1

1 Introduction

Roland Schiffter

1.1 Origin and Development

The German physical therapist Elisabeth Dicke (1884–1952) once explained how she discovered and developed this method of treatment. The text is now legendary and worth quoting here in full:

"I discovered the method of 'massaging reflex zones in the connective tissue' when I was personally ill. In 1929, I was suffering from extremely poor circulation in the right leg. The leg was cold, the skin had a grayish-white complexion, and the toes looked as if they were being strangled by rings and were about to become necrotic. The dorsal artery of the foot was no longer palpable. The physicians told me that amputation might be needed as a final treatment option.

In this bleak situation, I tried to find a way of relieving the severe back pain I also had, which had developed after 5 months of being confined to bed. I had been working as a physical therapist for 2 years. In the lateral position, I was able to palpate some tense, 'infiltrated' tissue over the sacrum and iliac crest and found that there was increased tension in the skin and subcutaneous tissue in comparison with the left side. I tried to spread the tension using pulling strokes. The affected areas were hypersensitive, and simple fingertip strokes caused massive pain. However, the tension gradually declined; the back pain faded with the loosening strokes, and a strong sensation of warmth developed. After trying this several times, I noticed there was persistent alleviation of the symptoms.

Tingling and stinging sensations now started in the affected leg that extended down to the sole, alternating with waves of heat. The leg continued to improve. Then I started to include the regions above the right trochanter and the lateral thigh (the iliotibial tract) in the strokes. There was a noticeable 'adhesion' of the skin and subcutaneous tissue. After this treatment, the veins in the thigh became visible again and spontaneously filled with blood.

Within 3 months, the severe disease symptoms had completely disappeared. A colleague took up where I left off, providing me with treatment over a longer period. After a year, I was able to resume working as a physical therapist again.

On the basis of this experience of my own illness, I gradually developed a systematic treatment method. In the course of the disorder, several other illnesses involving the internal organs had developed, including chronic gastritis, inflammatory enlargement of the liver, symptoms of cardiac angina, and finally renal colic. I was able to treat all of these organic and functional disorders successfully with the newly developed treatment method. The gastric and cardiac symptoms, which were accompanied by shortness of breath and anxiety, improved during the treatment. The renal colic episode, during which it was not possible to contact a physician, resolved within 5 minutes, with a kidney stone and a quantity of urinary gravel being released.

The colleague treating me followed my instructions. It was possible to expand the method as it was being used. The zones capable of influencing the individual organs that I discovered on the body's surface were also found in my patients. On the basis of the empirical facts that I discovered and formulated, reflex zones of this type exist not only in the skin and skeletal muscles, but first and foremost in the subcutaneous connective tissue. In cases of functional disorders and certain organic disorders in the region of the internal organs, I identified distensions, retractions, increased tension, and intense pain—known as 'maximal points'—that had to be circumvented, as the irritation arising from them and affecting the diseased organ was too intense.

After I had developed a systematic treatment method for myself in this way, I discovered that the English physician Henry Head had already described corresponding skin areas that were related to the internal organs. This observation made it possible to place the similar treatment method that I had discovered on established foundations in pathophysiology.

In 1935, I visited Professor Veil in Jena to demonstrate my work on patients at his hospital. He recognized the value of the method and suggested I should approach a physical therapy college to evaluate it further. In 1938, I was invited to demonstrate the treatment method by Dr. Hede Teirich-Leube, director of the Physical Therapy College in Freiburg im Breisgau in the Black Forest. The method was then clinically tested for a year by Professor Kohlrausch and Dr. Teirich-Leube. My experience was confirmed. We then jointly published the results of the study in a book entitled Massage of Reflex Zones in the Connective Tissue in Patients with Rheumatic and Internal Medicine Disorders. The major focus on connective tissue led to the name 'connective tissue massage', which has since become established, although it is not quite exact."

The development of Dicke's method thus started with experience with her own body and observations of changes in the skin and subcutaneous tissue in herself and in other patients whom she was treating, as a physical therapist. She then systematically documented spontaneous courses and the ways in which changes responded to massage stimuli, and drew her own conclusions. She even believed that she had discovered segmental sensory skin areas before Henry Head noticed them. Later, she certainly studied and made use of his scientific discoveries. Today, it is possible to explain the tremendous therapeutic effects of her massage method not only on the basis of the research results published by Head and McKenzie, but also based on the extensive research conducted by K. Hansen and his student Hans Schliack (the co-editor of earlier editions of this volume on connective tissue massage). While it might be desirable to explain Dicke's connective tissue massage mainly on a neurophysiological basis, it also has to be pointed out that the connective tissue as such is much less significant than Dicke thought. Hans Schliack already noted this in the fifth (German) edition of this book in 1962, and this approach is followed and further extended in the present edition.

1.1.1 History

Massage in any form is a time-honored treatment method. The Yellow Emperor of China, Huangdi (said to have lived from 2698 to 2598 BCE, proclaimed in his medical works that massage is one of the four essential principles of medicine. Hippocrates (460 BCE), the forefather of Western medicine, recommended it for joint diseases. In ancient Greece, it was part of the care that athletes received. During the early Roman Empire, Asclepiades (c. 124–40 BCE) described the "benefits of circling manual movements" in his textbook on massage. Thermal baths in ancient Rome were equipped with massage and gym rooms. Ibn Sina, more commonly known as Avicenna (979–1037 CE), the great physician and philosopher of ancient Persia, prescribed massages for athletes "to release deposits in the muscles." The English philosopher Francis Bacon (1561–1626 CE) recommended massage and gymnastics to maintain the self-healing powers and capacities of a healthy body. Finally, a French physician, A. C. Lorry, in 1797 wrote a treatise on dermatology in which massaging the skin was recommended on the basis of the modern notion that the skin is an organ of the body and more than just its outer cover. Perhaps this can already be regarded as anticipating connective tissue massage.

1.2 Theoretical Foundations for the Mechanism of Effect

A treatment method discovered empirically and tested in practice needs to be comprehensible, plausible, and also scientifically explicable if at all possible. This is certainly the case to some degree for connective tissue massage, although it is not immediately understandable why pulling and grasping of skin should have a functionally beneficial effect on organs and tissue in other regions. However, age-old experiences in traditional medicine have long suggested that such interrelations exist.

The antispasmodic effect of placing a hot-water bottle on the abdomen to relieve painful spasms in the stomach, intestines or bladder, the soothing effect caused by a

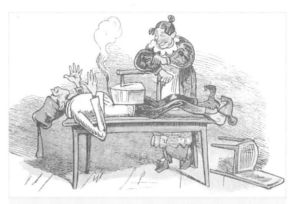

Fig. 1.1 Tailor Buck, in Wilhelm Busch's *Max and Moritz*

mother's soft, warm hand on the tummy of a baby suffering from colic, or even the iron placed by "Mrs. Buck" on her husband's chilled, wet belly in Wilhelm Busch's *Max and Moritz* (▶ Fig. 1.1) are just a few examples.

The distant effect of local stimuli applied to the skin—such as massage, heat applications, mustard plasters, and acupuncture—suggests that there must be a neural reflex mechanism involved. In addition to the local effects caused by what are known as axon reflexes, segmental spinal reflexes and global reflex interconnections that have generalized effects are also particular possibilities. This is discussed in more detail below.

In principle, connective-tissue massage can be expected to have the following effects, and these can also be rationally explained:
- Connective tissue massage may have an immediate local effect on the small subcutaneous vessels, which is regularly experienced as intense reddening of the skin (due to vascular dilation), which influences the local blood supply in the skin and also affects the hemodynamics of the whole circulatory system. Reflex mechanisms and the release of tissue hormones and various substances with cellular and tissue effects play an important role here.
- Mainly via segment reflexes, it can trigger functional changes (including an antispasmodic effect) in distant organs.
- Through the ascending sensory stimuli that it creates, it can trigger autonomic and psychological whole-body responses in the central nervous system, which can have a healing effect (with projection of the sensory pathways into the reticular formation in the brain and directly into the limbic system and cerebrum).

To begin with, however, some preliminary remarks on the anatomy and physiology of the connective tissue itself are needed. The connective tissue in the hypodermis (subcutaneous tissue) is the focus of interest here.

1.2.1 Anatomy, Physiology, and Pathophysiology of the Connective Tissue

As mentioned above, it is more the neuronal mechanisms —that is, reflex mechanisms—that are important for the effectiveness of connective tissue massage, and not so much any components that can be found in the connective tissue itself. Nevertheless, these anatomical and physiological facts also have to be described and considered in addition to the nerves.

As can be seen in ▶ Fig. 1.2, human skin is divided into an upper layer (the epidermis), the dermis (corium) underneath it, and below that the subcutaneous tissue (hypodermis), usually thicker. It is probably the subcutaneous tissue that plays the most important role in connective tissue massage, as the receptors and free nerve endings are located in it. The epidermis comprises stratified squamous cells, which are constantly being regenerated from the lowest layers and keratinize in the uppermost layers.

The important subcutaneous tissue lies underneath the relatively thin dermis, which is of no significance for massage effects.

Blood vessels, receptors, nerves, and nerve endings are located in loose tissue in the subcutaneous tissue, which is described in more detail below.

Elisabeth Dicke chose to call her method "connective tissue massage" because the traction effects caused by the massage mainly take place in the loose connective tissue in the subcutaneous layer.

In humans, the connective tissue makes up about 16% of body weight and contains about 23% of the total body water; it extends through the subcutaneous tissue as well as the sheaths surrounding muscles, tendons, and ligaments. It is located in the vessel walls and nerve sheaths as well as in the intercellular supporting structures of the internal organs. Loose and dense connective tissue

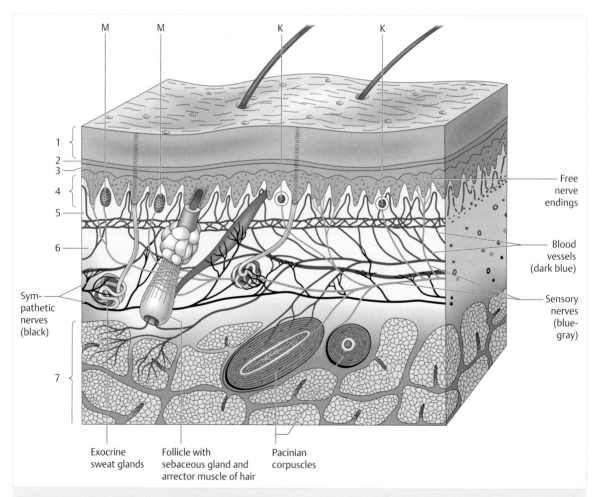

Fig. 1.2 Sectional view of the skin and receptors. M, Meissner corpuscles; K, Krause end bulb; 1, epidermis (stratum corneum, corneal layer); 2, epidermis (stratum lucidum); 3, epidermis (stratum granulosum); 4, dermis (stratum papillare); 5, dermis (stratum reticulare); 6, dermis (layer of sweat glands and hair roots); 7, subcutaneous adipose tissue.

(supporting tissue) provides stability as well as elasticity in various degrees for all physical movements. Various fiber structures, cells, and more complex organ structures such as vessels and nerves, which all have highly differentiated functions, are located in connective tissue.

▶ **Cells in connective tissue.** Cells known as fibroblasts and fibrocytes are the mother cells that form these fiber structures.
- Histiocytes are "resting wandering cells" that are mobilized in response to stimuli such as inflammation and absorb the waste products of various diseases processes to render them harmless.
- Mast cells are located above all in the vicinity of small vessels. They play a role in the dilation of capillaries and in coagulation processes.
- Plasma cells (antibody formation), lymphocytes, monocytes, and leukocytes have important functions in immune defense and in organizing inflammatory processes.
- Reticular cells form cellular networks and also have immune defense functions.
- The amorphous ground substance in the connective tissue, which binds water, should also be mentioned. Water binding is essential for the state of tension in tissue—its turgor.

▶ **Fibers in connective tissue.** A distinction is made between collagenous, reticular, and elastic fibers. They form the basic structure of all supporting and connective tissue. Collagenous fibers form a gluelike substance in the bone which gives strength to the tissue.

Reticular fibers have a latticed structure and form the framework of basal membranes. They coat muscle fibers, glandular acini, fat cells, etc.

The elastic fibers are most likely formed by fibroblasts. They can be stretched up to two and a half times their length and return to their original form. They are found in all types of elastic tissue—for example, in the lungs and blood vessels, as well as in the skin and membranous coverings of organs.

Tendons and ligaments consist of nearly parallel collagen fibers arranged in the direction of traction, which provide resistance against tension.

The elastic fibers of the connective tissue are often parallel to the collagen fibers, so that elasticity and tensile strength are achieved. The formation of certain patterns is also important here for the individual functions of the tissue.

In the subcutaneous tissue, the connective-tissue structures combine with fat cells as well as with the organ structures and cells described above. Adipose tissue (fatty tissue) is malleable, has cushioning properties, and is also held in shape by collagen fibrils and elastic fibrils. The adipose tissue thus has mechanical functions as well as its familiar energy storage functions. Brown adipose tissue (brown fat) in particular is thought to provide cushioning in the joints, soles, and various other parts of the body.

There is a wealth of further details about connective tissues extending to the various specific organ regions, but these details are less important in connection with the effectiveness of connective tissue massage.

Summary

On the one hand, connective tissue has filling and supporting properties, as well as vital metabolic functions, and it plays an important role in inflammatory and immunological defense processes. Connective tissue is also significantly involved in the healing of injuries, wounds, etc., and responds actively to various hormonal influences, toxins, and a wide variety of harmful substances.

1.2.2 Neuroanatomical and Neurophysiological Principles

The effects of connective tissue massage are primarily mediated through the nervous system. As suggested above, there are local, segmental, and global reflex mechanisms that are responsible for this, but broader psychosomatic and psychological effects are also involved.

In connective tissue massage, pulling, adhering, and hook techniques, as well as circling or linear strokes of the hand, always represent sensory stimuli to the skin that lead to excitations of the nervous receptors and nerve endings. These excitations are transmitted via the sensory nerves (afferent nerves) to the spinal cord and brain, where segmental reflexes and global reflex responses, as well as changes of mental state, are triggered that subsequently lead to muscle relaxation or tension, vascular dilation or constriction, increased peristalsis, and many other effects through the returning motor and autonomic pathways and nerves (efferent nerves). This may also help to block pain stimuli at the level of the spinal cord (posterior root entry zone). In the skin, the stimuli cause local reddening (due to vascular dilation) and other changes of state, which are either caused by the controversial "axon reflexes" or more likely by the release of tissue hormones and neurotransmitters from the sensory and sympathetic nerve endings (prostaglandins and other substances).

Significant anatomical structures for these effects thus include the receptors, the sensory, motor, and autonomic nerves (sympathetic and parasympathetic nerves), the spinal cord, and the brain with their cellular and neural pathways. Sensory nerves are simply the receiving processes (dendrites) of the spinal ganglia cells, whereas motor nerves are the neurites of the anterior horn cells of the spinal cord.

By contrast, the motor pathways in the brain and spinal cord (pyramidal pathway) are the neurites of the cortical motor cells in the motor cerebral cortex. The ascending sensory pathways represent the processes of spinal cord cells from the segmental levels and the spinal ganglia.

Autonomic nerve stimuli originate in the brain and brainstem, in particular in the hypothalamus, travel down the spinal cord, and then pass together with the peripheral nerves to the internal organs, vessels, glands, gastrointestinal tract, urinary tract, etc., and also to the skin and the sweat glands. The task of the sympathetic nerves is to prepare the body for high-stress events such as the fight-or-flight response. Stimulating the sympathetic nervous system therefore increases the heart rate and cardiac output as well as blood pressure and respiratory rate. Sweating is also initiated. In addition, muscle tension in the striated muscles is always increased during this process, and psychologically there is also corresponding tension in the form of readiness to fight or aggressiveness.

In general, the exact opposite happens when there is a heightened parasympathetic nervous system—that is, a reduction in heart rate, blood pressure, and respiratory rate and depth. Instead, there is increased peristalsis, glandular secretion, digestive activity, urination, and defecation. The muscles lose tension and the mind is at rest and relaxed. These structures are interconnected with each other in close and complex ways and more or less involuntarily control living processes, depending on requirements, in a delicate balance. Connective tissue massage can also influence and facilitate these mechanisms.

Injury to or transection of peripheral nerves can in principle be repaired by the growth of new processes from the axons, provided the corresponding cell is still intact. In the central neural pathways of the spinal cord and brain, however, this is virtually impossible, or only possible to a very limited extent. Exercise to train replacement circuits is necessary here.

Sensory System

The sensory or afferent nervous system ensures that stimuli from connective-tissue massage, or administered in other ways, are transported from the skin to the spinal cord and brain. Important nervous structures in the skin itself, and above all in the subcutaneous tissue, need to be described here in detail (▸ Fig. 1.2):

- Free nerve endings. These are low in myelin content and branch freely into the epidermis or form small networks known as the Merkel cell–neurite complex, or contact certain tactile cells on the nerve roots of the hair, or also branch into a finely ramified endings. These free nerve endings transmit pain and touch stimuli.
- Myelinated receptor organs in the subcutaneous tissue:
  - Pacinian corpuscles. These are mechanoreceptors that are highly sensitive, especially for the perception of pressure and touch and for the perception of vibration and tickling stimuli.
  - Meissner corpuscles, which lie close to the epidermis, are only found on hairless skin. They are therefore mainly found on the lips, eyelids, tongue, fingertips, and genitals. They are also very sensitive tactile receptors.
  - The Krause end bulbs are primarily found in mucosa.
  - The network of nerve endings of hair shafts also transmit touch sensations.

Eighty percent of the nerve fibers have a thin myelin coat—that is, they have little or no myelin and therefore have a slower conduction velocity (1 to 2 m/s). Twenty percent of them are thick and contain myelin, and therefore have a high conduction velocity (10 to 60 m/s).

In summary, the primary functions of the myelinated receptors include the perception of pressure, vibration, and touch, and they have fast-conducting A fibers. By contrast, the unmyelinated nerve ends respond more to pressure, heat, cold, and acute initial pain (the first pain sensation) with fast conduction. The completely free nerve endings have a slow conduction velocity and are sensitive to touch, heat, cold, and itching, as well as to agonizing blunt pain (the second pain sensation or C-fiber pain). According to recent studies in Sweden, the C fibers are thought to respond particularly sensitively to slow movements (massage) on the skin.

All impulses from these structures—including stimuli from connective tissue massage—are transmitted via the peripheral nerves and the posterior nerve roots into the spinal cord. In the entry zone of the posterior nerve roots, the stimuli are filtered and selected in such a way that some of the impulses trigger a reflex, some ascend to the brain and consciousness, and some are deleted. It is mainly irrelevant, repeated stimuli that are deleted. These reflex stimuli can be transmitted via motor nerves to the muscles or via autonomic nerves to the visceral organs such as vessels, glands, etc.

Free nerve endings and the receptors described above can be found not only in the subcutaneous tissue but also in the mucosa, the serous membranes of the viscera, the muscles, and the vascular walls, as well as in the periosteum and perichondrium and in practically all connective tissue structures. They are thus the recipients of the stimuli triggered by connective tissue massage. Their impulses also pass into the spinal cord via the posterior nerve roots, where they are conducted along with all the other sensory stimuli through the anterolateral column, which is responsible for conducting pain and temperature stimuli, as well as urges to defecate and urinate. The impulses also pass through the posterior bundle (responsible for touch and highly differentiated sensory stimuli, as well as vibration and what is known as deep sensibility or the kinesthetic sense) up to the brain (▸ Fig. 1.3).

The clinically most important sensory quality is **pain**. The receptors for pain are also known as nociceptors (from Latin *noxa*, hurt, pain, injury). Almost all tissues in

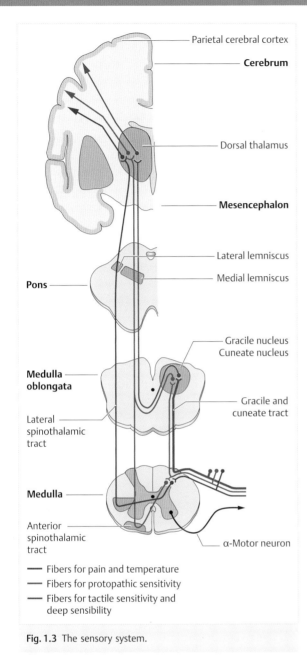

Fig. 1.3 The sensory system.

Labels on figure:
Parietal cerebral cortex
Cerebrum
Dorsal thalamus
Mesencephalon
Lateral lemniscus
Medial lemniscus
Pons
Gracile nucleus
Cuneate nucleus
Medulla oblongata
Gracile and cuneate tract
Lateral spinothalamic tract
Medulla
Anterior spinothalamic tract
α-Motor neuron

— Fibers for pain and temperature
— Fibers for protopathic sensitivity
— Fibers for tactile sensitivity and deep sensibility

Due to its alerting effect and the initiation of an elevated sympathetic tone, pain triggers flight reflexes, as the pain conduction is also projected into the brainstem (reticular formation) as well as into the hypothalamus and finally also into the limbic system, where it causes discomfort and anxiety.

The pain is then conducted into the cerebrum, where a rational response with defense strategies and a rational analysis of the pain becomes possible.

For connective tissue massage, it is important to realize that segmental reflex muscle tension can itself cause pain—thus creating a vicious circle that needs to be interrupted, partly using the massage.

Motor System

Much has already been said above about the motor system. ▶ Fig. 1.4 provides an overview of the whole system. In general, a distinction needs to be made between the central and the peripheral motor system. The difference is extremely important, as they involve two fundamentally different patterns of paralysis.

Lesions in the originating motor cells in the cerebral cortex or its processes—that is, the pyramidal pathway in the brain and spinal cord—cause paralysis states such as hemiplegia, paraplegia, and quadriplegia, with increasing intensification of the muscle tone (spasm), enhancement (i.e., disinhibition) of stretch reflexes, and positive Babinski sign (dorsal flexion of the great toe after sensory stimulus of the sole and foot).

Injuries to the peripheral neurons—that is, the anterior horn cells or their processes in the anterior nerve roots, the nerve plexus, and the individual nerves, also trigger paralysis, but with a flaccid muscle tone, absent muscle stretch reflexes, and rapidly progressing muscle atrophy.

The physical exercises and physical therapy required for the treatment of central (i.e., spastic) and peripheral (i.e., flaccid) atrophying paralysis are very different for fundamental reasons. In cases of central spastic paralysis, an attempt is made to release the spasms in addition to providing motor training. When peripheral flaccid paralysis is being treated, greater emphasis is given to muscle training and therapy for concomitant vasomotor disturbances—that is, circulatory disturbances.

Autonomic Nervous System

The functions of the autonomic nervous system are largely, but not completely, involuntary and thus "autonomic." They affect the control and monitoring of the "internal organs," in particular of heart strength and heart rate, blood pressure and blood distribution, respiration, heat regulation, gastrointestinal activity, urination, sexuality, and glandular secretion. In the skin, the most important receptor organ for connective tissue massage, secretion of sweat and the development of goose bumps

the human body contain these pain receptors (the exceptions being osseous tissue, intervertebral disks, and the brain itself).

Pain is a signaling system that is old in terms of evolutionary history, which is used to prevent physical harm through fast reflexes and alerts. It triggers protective reflexes (e.g., the sudden pulling away of the leg when injury to the foot is caused by stepping on a piece of broken glass) that pass through the spinal cord, and also segmental muscle contractions to "immobilize" a painful area—for example, the scoliotic slanted posture of the lumbar spine or the "relieving posture" seen in patients with slipped disks.

Pyramidal pathway

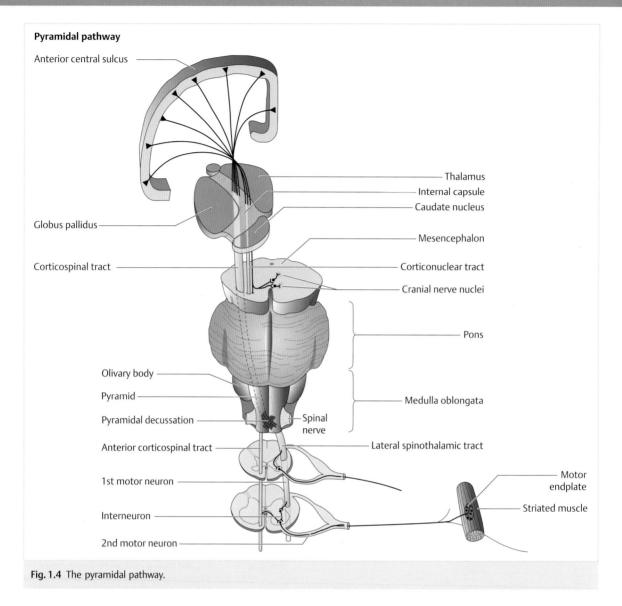

Anterior central sulcus

Thalamus

Internal capsule

Caudate nucleus

Globus pallidus

Mesencephalon

Corticospinal tract

Corticonuclear tract

Cranial nerve nuclei

Pons

Olivary body

Pyramid

Pyramidal decussation

Spinal nerve

Medulla oblongata

Anterior corticospinal tract

Lateral spinothalamic tract

1st motor neuron

Motor endplate

Interneuron

Striated muscle

2nd motor neuron

Fig. 1.4 The pyramidal pathway.

(the raising of hair or piloerection) also occur. The whole system is divided into three subsystems:

- The sympathetic system
- The parasympathetic system
- The intramural system (in the wall structures of hollow organs)

These three elements are in a finely tuned, mobile dynamic balance that is adjusted according to life requirements and the performance needed.

The central sympathetic and parasympathetic pathways mainly originate in the hypothalamus, which in turn is also subordinated to the regulating influence of the limbic system (for drives, affects, and moods) and of the cerebrum (for targeted rational thought and action, and considered decision-making). The posterior cell groups in the hypothalamus, which is located deep within the brain, send sympathetic pathways to the lower brainstem and spinal cord, while the anterior cell groups send parasympathetic pathways to them. The parasympathetic impulses are transmitted from the brainstem via the appropriate cranial nerves to the organs, with the vagus nerve having the most extensive supply area and playing a predominant role. The parasympathetic nerves for the urinary, rectal, and genital systems originate at the sacral bone part of the spinal cord (▶ Fig. 1.5, ▶ Fig. 1.6).

The sympathetic fibers for the organs leave the spinal cord through the anterior motor nerve roots between the last cervical segment (C8) and the second lumbar segment (L2), extend to what is known as the sympathetic trunk lateral to the whole spinal column, are further divided there to supply the body, and then course together with the blood vessels to the internal organs and with the sensory nerves to the skin. In the skin, they supply the

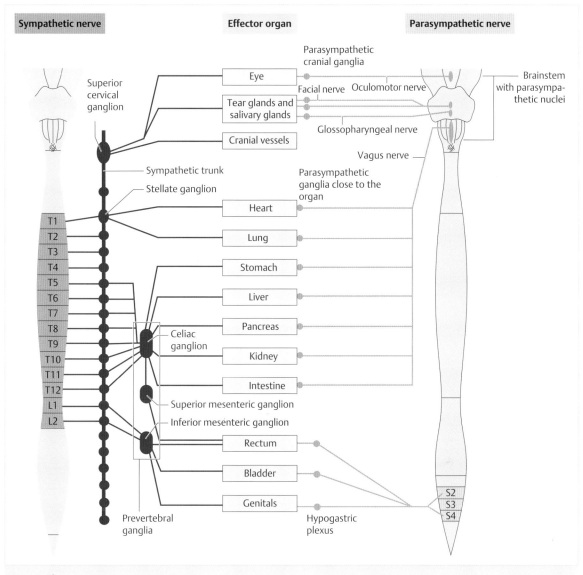

Sympathetic nerve	Effector organ	Parasympathetic nerve

Fig. 1.5 The autonomic nervous system.

same territory as the sensory nerve that accompanies them. There they innervate the blood vessels (constrictive effect), the sweat glands (secretion), and the erector muscles of the hair (creation of goose bumps). The sympathetic trunk through which the fibers run is structured in such a way that the fibers are massively fragmented and then redistributed in order to additionally supply the zones above the eighth cervical segment and below the second lumbar segment. At the same time, this results in the overlapping of multiple segments of sympathetic innervation zones of the skin, so that segmental stimuli trigger a multisegmental effect over an extensive area. This is one reason for the so-called remote effects of connective tissue massage (▶ Fig. 1.7).

What is known as the intramural system is a complex network of cells and nerve fibers in the intestinal wall (from Latin *murus*, wall), the walls of the urinary bladder and of the urinary tracts, the genital organs, and also the heart and the vessels, the bronchi, and other structures in the internal organs. It acts largely independently of the rest of the nervous system, but is at the same time significantly modulated by higher-level sympathetic and parasympathetic influences.

As suggested above, global sympathetic stimulation needs to be distinguished from global parasympathetic stimulation, although the mental, motor, and autonomic components are each simultaneously regulated in the same manner. During global sympathetic stimulation, the

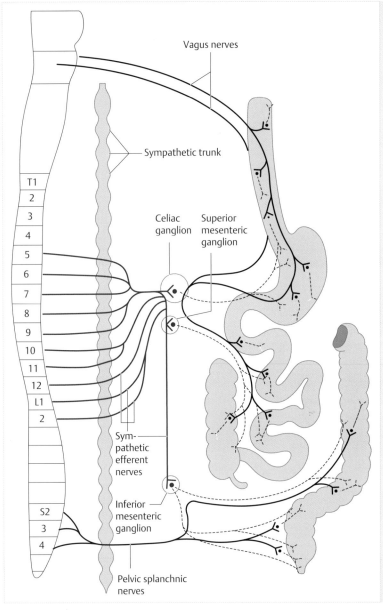

Fig. 1.6 Sympathetic and parasympathetic innervation of the gastrointestinal tract.

body is prepared for high performance, as well as acute pain or other threats or passionate excitation. For this reason, heart strength, heart rate, blood pressure, respiratory output, and muscle tone, as well as attention and alertness, are all increased. The pupils widen, the body hair is erect, sweating begins, the internal organs are inhibited, and defecation and urination, as well as sexual function, are not possible in this situation.

Global parasympathetic stimulation causes a lower heart rate and cardiac output, lower blood pressure, low respiratory activity, vascular dilation, narrowed pupils, and increased gastrointestinal activity, including glandular secretion and tendency to defecation and urination, as well as filling of the erectile tissue in the genital organs.

The muscles and mood relax. Of course, dealing with life's challenges requires various combinations of these global settings, as well as rapid switching from one mode to another.

By administering certain sensory skin stimuli, connective tissue massage can have a regulating and healing effect on these processes, usually by triggering reflexive motor and autonomic mechanisms via the segmental reflexes mentioned, and also by influencing the mental and psychosomatic state. The patient relaxes, lets the healing hands do their work, passively allows reflexes to happen, and becomes calm and relaxed. Connective tissue massage thus appears primarily to be a reflex therapy, although some psychotherapy is certainly also involved.

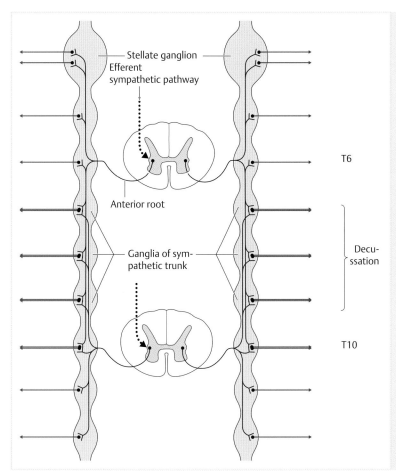

Stellate ganglion
Efferent
sympathetic pathway

Anterior root

Ganglia of sym-
pathetic trunk

T6

Decu-
ssation

T10

Fig. 1.7 Diagram showing distributor function in the sympathetic trunk.

1.2.3 Segmental Structure of the Body and Physiological Reflex Mechanisms

The sensory, motor, and autonomic systems are specially connected to each other at the level of body segments. Complex reflex mechanisms are made possible and can also be used for therapeutic purposes through connective tissue massage. Dicke pointed this out in her first monograph, *Massage of Reflex Zones and Connective Tissue,* published in 1942.

The segmental structure of the body is an ancient, time-honored anatomical principle that was so successful that it has been preserved virtually throughout the whole evolution of the animal kingdom, from the ringworm to reptiles and finally to humans (▶ Fig. 1.8).

It was used in particular for the "serpentine" locomotion and mobility of worms, fish, and snakes, but also appears to be an advantageous structural principle for higher vertebrates. The development of body segments can be well observed in embryonic development, whereas the formation of somites is an important intermediate stage. At the end, a complicated but uniform disk develops through differentiation of embryonic connective tissue and its "germinal sheets," consisting of different types of tissue and one paired nerve that innervates them all—namely, the segment. The paired nerve is in a sense "taken along" when the somite grows out. The segment is defined as the whole area influenced by a paired spinal nerve, the fibers of which course through the intervertebral foramina and innervate the corresponding organs and tissue parts (▶ Fig. 1.9).

The corresponding sections or tissue parts of the segment are called:
- Dermatome: related to the skin and subcutaneous tissue
- Myotome: related to the skeletal muscles
- Enterotome: related to the visceral organs
- Sclerotome: related to the bones and periosteum

Sensory fibers, including pain receptors, are detectable in all four compartments of this segmented structure, as are motor fibers to the parts of the musculoskeletal system and autonomic fibers to the visceral organs and vascular muscles, glands etc. Growth of the extremities causes a shift in these tissue layers relative to each other, and one needs to be aware of this (▶ Fig. 1.10).

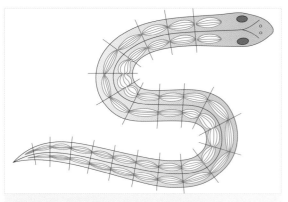

Fig. 1.8 The muscular system in a snake (diagram). A stretched body can only make serpentine movements with the help of segmented trunk muscles.

The **movement segment** of the spinal column refers to the functional unit of the intervertebral disk and adjacent vertebrae, with the corresponding spinous processes, joints, and intervertebral foramina, with the paired spinal nerve with the sensory posterior nerve root and the motor anterior nerve root. The sympathetic fibers leave the spinal cord together with the motor anterior nerve root fibers; the parasympathetic fibers connect to cranial nerves or vascular structures.

Overviews of innervation conditions are shown in ▶ Fig. 1.11 and ▶ Fig. 1.12 (dermatome scheme); ▶ Fig. 1.13 schematically illustrates mainly the reflex relationships between the skin (dermatome), muscles (myotome), visceral organs (enterotome), and spinal cord.

Sensory stimuli, including painful stimuli, can originate from the skin, muscles, visceral organs, and bones not included in the diagram (sclerotome). They are all

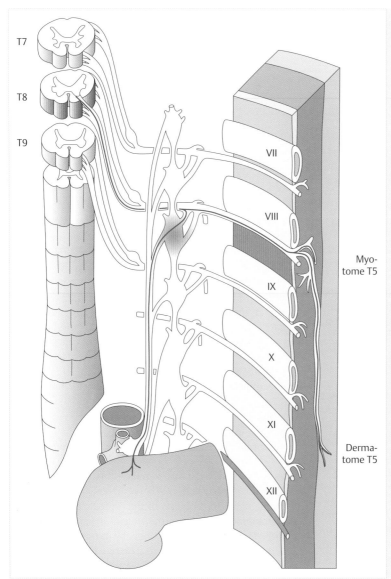

Fig. 1.9 Schematic illustrating a segment, with an enterotome (pancreas), myotome, dermatome, and neuromere (T8) and their most important neural connections. (Hansen K, Schliack H. Segmentale Innervation [Segmental Innervation]. Stuttgart: Thieme; 1962.)

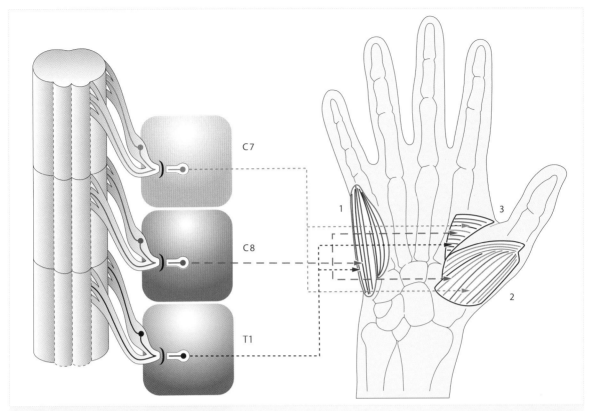

Fig. 1.10 Growth of somites, which carry the spinal nerves along with them.
1, Hypothenar (abductor, flexor digiti minimi brevis muscle); 2, thenar (abductor, flexor pollicis brevis and opponens pollicis muscles); 3, adductor pollicis muscle.

channeled into the spinal cord through sensory nerves, spinal ganglia, and posterior nerve roots. In the entry zone of the posterior nerve roots, the pain stimuli can be partly eliminated, as mentioned above, by the simultaneous arrival of additional stimuli such as connective tissue massage, acupuncture, etc. This is an approach to pain therapy. Every influence on this system, no matter from what side, can trigger reflex effects in all other compartments. According to Head, pain stimuli and other irritations from internal organs such as the heart, gallbladder, or stomach can cause paresthesia and hyperesthesia in the segment-associated skin zones, known as the **Head zones**. According to McKenzie, the same causes can trigger painful local segmental muscle cramps, known as the **McKenzie maximal points** or pressure points. They are also always found in the muscles of the corresponding segment—that is, in the corresponding myotome. Both mechanisms provide evidence of the effectiveness of segment reflexes and can be used as diagnostic signs and used for therapeutic intervention in the affected segments using connective tissue massage. For more information about the allocation of internal organs to their segments, see ▶ Table 1.1.

Segmental reflex mechanisms are probably also the essential mechanism of action of all other forms of massage therapy and most likely also of any nonmedicinal therapies that are applied to the skin, such as local heat applications, quaddle and stimulation therapies, including acupuncture and various types of balneotherapy. When warm mudpacks are applied to the skin, for example, with painful muscle tension, there have been various speculations that the underlying muscles are heated, causing the muscles to relax, vessels to dilate, the blood supply to improve and metabolic products to be removed more quickly, etc. This is certainly not correct. Heat applied to the skin is immediately "transported away" through convection and never reaches the muscles, for instance, through the hypodermis, which is rich in adipose tissue and vessels. In any case, the temperature of the muscles is optimally 37°C and raising it would not be desirable at all and might even be harmful. Vascular dilation and muscle relaxation occur anyway, however—not due to the local heat itself, but through a reflexive pathway triggered by the heat stimulus on the dermatome of the segment. The Schliack connection diagram can be consulted here to clarify these mechanisms (▶ Fig. 1.13).

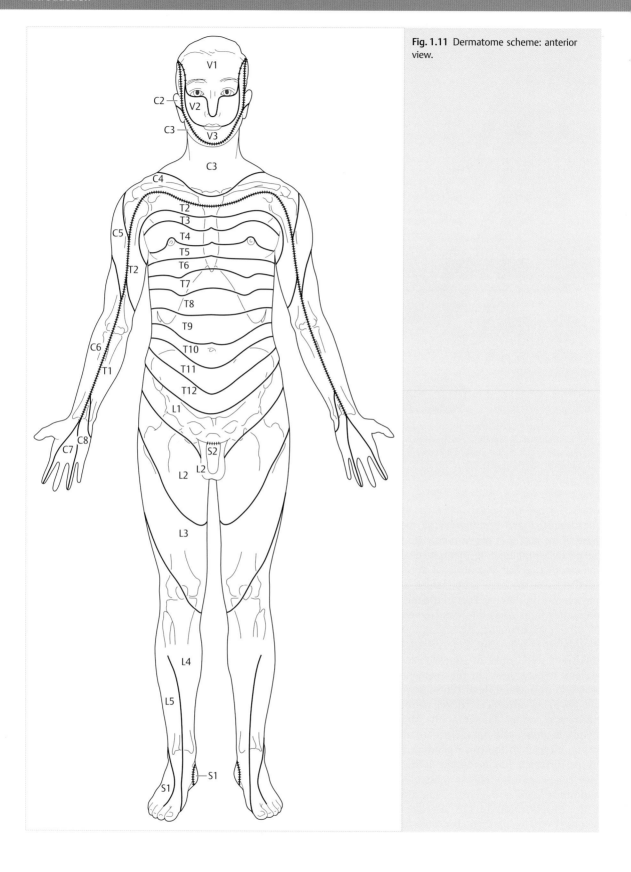

Fig. 1.11 Dermatome scheme: anterior view.

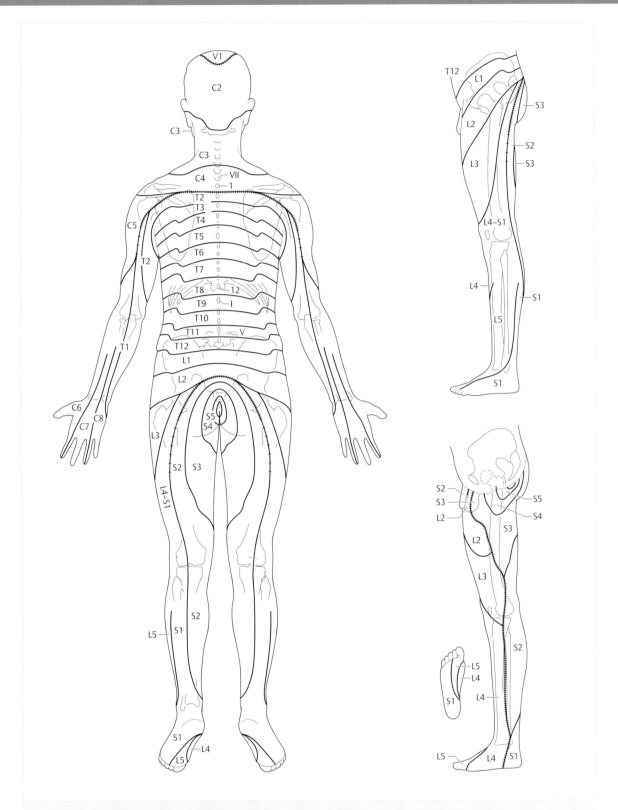

Fig. 1.12 Dermatome scheme: posterior view and lateral views of the lower extremities.

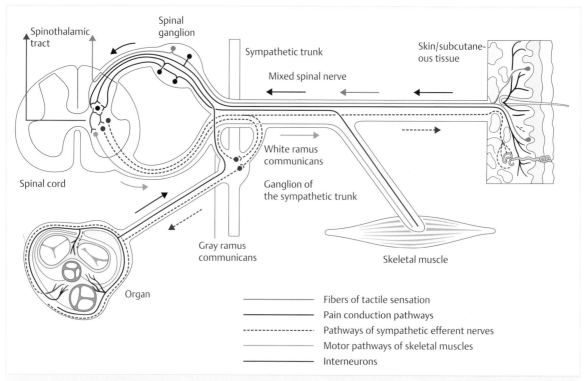

Fig. 1.13 Diagram illustrating neural connections between the internal organs, muscles, and skin–subcutaneous tissue: the viscerogenic and cutivisceral spinal reflexes.

Table 1.1 Segmental relations of the most important organs

Organ	Segmental relations / reflex zones
Segmental relations of paired organs	
Pleura, lung	T3–T10
Kidney, ureter	T9–T12, L1–L2
Gonads	T10–L1
Reflex zones on the right side of unpaired organs	
Duodenum	T6–T10
Ileum	T8/9–T11
Liver, gallbladder	C3/4, T6–T10
Appendix, ascending colon	T9–T12
Reflex zones on the left side of unpaired organs	
Heart	T1–T8
Stomach	T5–T9
Jejunum	T8–T11
Pancreas	T7–T9
Spleen	T7–T10
Descending colon, sigmoid colon	T9–L1

Intensive sensory skin stimulation—for example, using connective tissue massage—causes stimulation of the sensory afferent nerves, which block the efferent sympathetic flow of impulses, for instance, to the vessels, as a reflex at the level of the spinal cord segment, thus causing vascular dilation. At the same time, the stimuli reduce the corresponding tonic efferent impulses to the striated muscles, so that these relax and no longer cause pain. It is essential for the stimulated tissue—the skin zone and targeted tissue (vessels, muscles)—to belong to the same segment. One needs to be extremely familiar with the allocation of the tissue to dermatomes, myotomes, and enterotomes in order to be able to apply the therapy at the right location. Of course, connective tissue massage stimulates not only the skin, but also the underlying muscles themselves and can also cause a local reflex effect resulting in relaxation.

It should be repeated here that sensory stimuli such as those produced in connective tissue massage are able to eliminate simultaneously arriving pain stimuli at the entry zone of the posterior nerve roots. The complex processes involved have not yet been fully clarified. What was known as the "gate control theory" was thought for a time to be correct, but it is no longer accepted today. One mechanism that is based on the theory, however, must apply in the process. Segmental reflexes relax tensions in striated muscles or vascular spasms and relax or stimulate the intestinal muscles, as well as the ureter and urinary bladder, so that they are also effective in cases of colic and tenesmus. This is discussed in more detail below in the relevant sections.

1.2.4 Global Effects of Connective Tissue Massage

The "holistic effects" of connective tissue massage, which include even soothing effects on psychological wellbeing, can also be explained to a certain extent using a neurophysiological approach. As explained above in connection with sensory systems, connective tissue massage applies targeted sensory stimuli, the reflex effects of which are transmitted via the spinal cord pathway to the brain, where they can trigger global autonomic and motor responses as well as the psychological effects mentioned. They can have antihypertensive effects, reducing the heart rate, and can also have soothing and relaxing effects. Pulling fingers, balancing techniques (such as "branching" and balancing strokes), as well as flat strokes, can trigger general calmness, relaxation, and wellbeing in patients who respond positively to the therapy with projection of the stimuli into the limbic system of the brain, which is generally accompanied by muscle relaxation and a comfortable parasympathetic tone with the correspondingly calm basic mood. Connective tissue massage thus represents a holistic therapy and in the broadest sense also psychotherapy for stressed-out, rushed, or depressive individuals suffering from the pressures of everyday life, who may not necessarily be ill.

Creating a friendly—as it were "parasympathetic"—relaxed environment and thus a "therapeutic environment" while performing connective tissue massage is an important aspect of the therapist's task. Connective tissue massage is a holistic therapy for the whole body and more than just reflex therapy.

Chapter 2

Technique

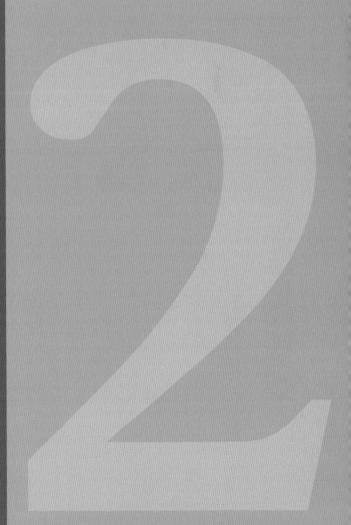

2 Technique

Elke Harms

2.1 Introduction

▶ Fig. 2.1 illustrates the medioclavicular and anterior axillary lines.

2.1.1 Anatomical Principles of the Technique

▶ Fig. 2.2 shows the posterior axillary line and ▶ Fig. 2.3 shows the tension lines on the skin (Langer lines, cleavage lines).

Manual Application

To create the "traction in connective tissue" characteristic of this method, pressure is applied with the fingertips (▶ Fig. 2.4). The third and fourth fingers, first applied in a flat, then in a raised fashion ("cutting"), usually pull the tissue toward the respective target. The tissue should not be "dropped," meaning that the traction on the tissue should stay the same at any point while following through on the stroke.

The fingertips are not removed immediately, but rather rest on the skin until the tissue has returned to its original position. The extent to which this happens depends on the degree of attachment of the tissue, which improves with each additional connective tissue massage (CTM).

Finger Technique

For flat strokes (▶ Fig. 2.5), the fingertips are positioned side by side or behind each other at a flat angle (position: finger, wrist and elbow joint) and pulled along the skin and subcutaneous tissue while using the skin's elasticity.

Traction from the fingers should be applied in the direction of the joints in the hand, so that pressure is applied to the finger joints in the axial direction. For counteracting or deflecting strokes, the fingers or the whole palm are used.

For cutting strokes (▶ Fig. 2.6), the fingers are applied at an oblique angle, which intensifies the traction and reaches the depth of the subcutaneous tissue and muscular fascia.

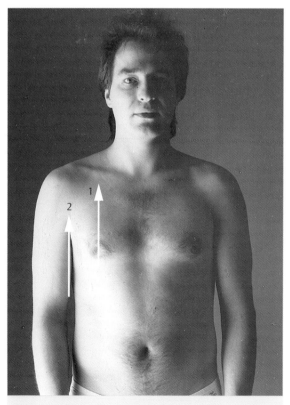

Fig. 2.1 Medioclavicular line (1) and anterior axillary line (2).

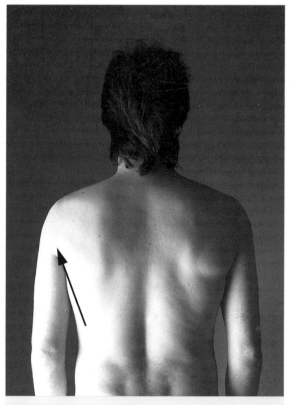

Fig. 2.2 Posterior axillary line.

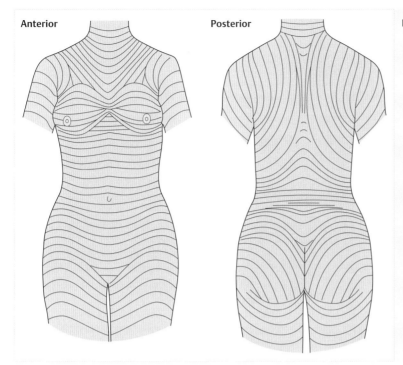

Anterior   **Posterior**

Fig. 2.3 Tension lines in the skin.

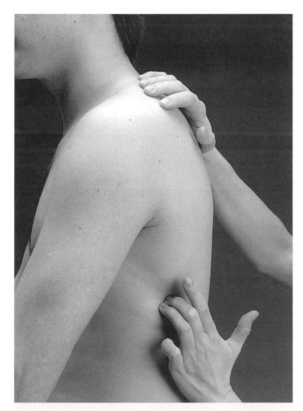

Fig. 2.4 Example of the characteristic traction in connective tissue.

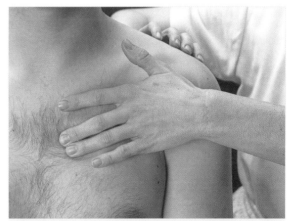

Fig. 2.5 Example of flat strokes with adjacent fingertips.

When both techniques are being applied, the joints have to remain fixed in their position by the muscles to prevent overstraining.

The following tips need to be followed in order to avoid ineffective treatment or possible injury:

- Do not slide over the tissue.
- Do not apply only pressure.
- Perform the strokes in a continuous and rhythmic fashion.
- Attach well and do not go deeper into the tissue layers too soon.
- Avoid traction in the opposite direction.

21

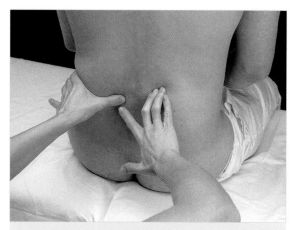

Fig. 2.6 Example of cutting strokes.

Traction Stimulus

Traction stimulus refers to the stimulus that results from different positions of the fingers on the dermis, subcutaneous tissue, and muscular fascia. According to Teirich-Leube, this is also referred to as "therapeutic stimulus."

The strokes should be transferred over loose shoulders, arms and hands to the fingertips, so that the stimuli are adequately applied. This in turn triggers the appropriate neural reflexes locally as well as throughout the entire organism (e.g., strokes are applied along the pelvis at first with the hands placed flat and elbows adducted, then the elbow is moved away from the body, ending in a "wide arm" position).

Depending on the tension in the tissue and the intensity of the traction (the connective tissue is pushed against a muscular, tendinous, and osseous sublayer), the patient will have the following sensations:
- Pulling with the fingers
- Scratching in the deeper layers (as if with the tip of a knife or a fingernail, for example)
- A sensation of being cut, although this is not experienced as discomfort

Dosage

The following factors need to be taken into account during *application* in order to achieve effective therapy and adapt to each patient's individual needs:
- Clinical picture
- Stage and severity of illness
- Stage of treatment (first day to last day of treatment)
- Patient's constitution, fitness, and age

To begin with, the upper tissue layers are loosened gently. As a reflex, the tension is also reduced in the deeper tissue layers.

The intensity of attachment to the skin, the type of application (flat or cutting strokes), and the speed of traction allow appropriate dosage.

> The greater the intensity and the traction speed, the more intense the traction stimulus.

Prescription

The physician determines when treatment should begin.

The **number** of CTM sessions in a treatment series depends on the type, stage, and severity of the illness. As can be seen from most treatment plans, long-term therapy can be expected—that is, more than six to 12 sessions of CTM in a series will be needed.

If possible, CTM should be administered every day to start with, and then three to four times a week. Later, if the patient's clinical condition improves, the sessions can be reduced to twice a week.

Interval treatment with pauses in between has proved to be effective for repeated series of treatment. The pauses can be used to administer other types of physical therapy.

CTM can be performed alternately with heat and ice applications, as well as with electrotherapy.

Heat and ice applications must be applied after CTM, as otherwise the findings in the tissue will be falsified.

The **duration** of the treatment depends on the patient's fitness, age, the clinical picture, and the stage of treatment. As a general rule, treatment can be expected to last 20 to 30 minutes.

The first session will take the most time, since determining the findings is very time-consuming and close attention needs to be given to the way in which the patient's autonomic nervous system reacts to the treatment. During the subsequent sessions, the autonomic nervous system response and the different levels of tension in the tissue will determine the further course.

Positioning and Posture

Patient

The small basic sequence, first to third sequences, treatment of the head, and treatment of the upper extremities are preferably performed with the patient sitting down. In this starting position, the tissue has postural tone and changes can be found easily.

If the patient has a low level of fitness, a lateral, prone, and/or supine position may be chosen instead.

The following points need to be observed when preparing the patient for CTM:
- Any tight clothing should be removed to ensure an unobstructed blood flow.
- Areas of the body that are not being treated should be carefully covered.
- Supports should be used to balance the patient's posture.

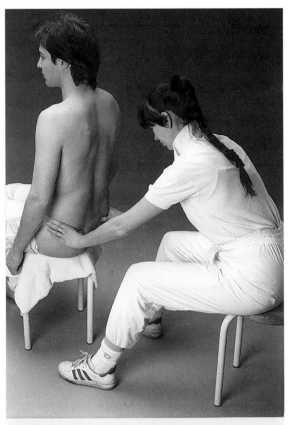

Fig. 2.7 Starting position: posture of therapist and patient.

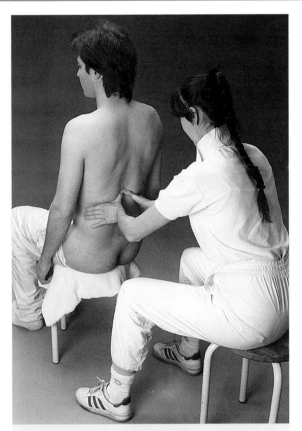

Fig. 2.8 Working position when the patient is seated.

- The room temperature should optimally be set to 22 to 24°C (72 to 75°F).
- One should always work in the same lighting conditions.
- The therapist's watch and any jewelry should be removed
- (▶ Fig. 2.7, ▶ Fig. 2.8, ▶ Fig. 2.9, ▶ Fig. 2.10)

Therapist

A rhythmic and fluent workflow promotes effectiveness and efficiency, stimulates the patient, and provides continuity to the technique, which is essential for working with the patient. A few points that should be observed are:

- One should always work with approximations of joints and muscle fixations.
- One should work with one leg advanced and shift one's balance.
- Leverage needs to be maintained.
- An active posture should be maintained—abnormal postures such a hunched or hollow back and unbalanced loads should be avoided.
- The origins and insertions of the muscles should be approximated.

Patient Reactions to CTM

CTM can have many effects on the patient, and the therapist should therefore be aware of all possible reactions:

- Local effects:
  - Hyperemization
  - Accelerated metabolism
  - Structural improvement in pathological tissue
- General effects:
  Improved venous backflow and arterial inflow, resulting in altered chemical reactions and a tendency to bind with water
- Local reflexive effects:
  Targeted, positive influence on motor functions, secretion, and hyperemization of one or more organs
- General reflexive effects—for example:
  - Warm/cold hands and/or feet
  - Sensation of hunger or even nausea
  - Effects on the cardiac, circulatory, and respiratory systems
  - Increased urge to urinate or defecate
  - Fatigue

When there are increased reactions or over-reactions that may also be caused by treatment being applied too fast or too intensively, the therapist needs to re-evaluate the technique used and reconsider the approach.

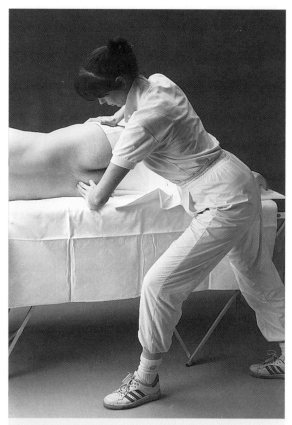

Fig. 2.9 Working position with one leg advanced to shift the balance.

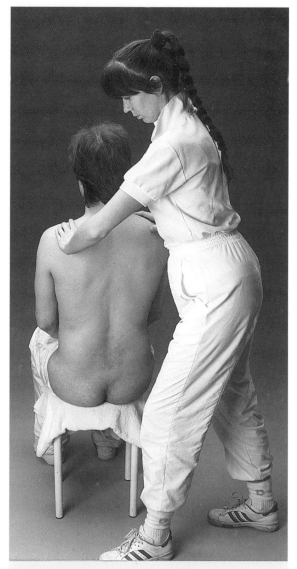

Fig. 2.10 Working position while standing.

Skin Reactions

In various descriptions of the treatment, Dicke mentions skin reactions that may be triggered by CTM. This phenomenon is known as dermographism and is a normal response of the sensory and sympathetic skin nerves, of the "axon reflex" type, which can lead to reddening (vasodilation) or paleness (vasoconstriction) in the stimulated skin. However, the empirical observations by Dicke and Teirich-Leube represent important tips for the therapist when administering CTM.

▶ **Red dermographism.** Thin, red, even streaks that remain only for a short time or immediately fade away indicate a normal process. A flaming red and flowing streak that remains for a longer period of time indicates a massive reaction by the autonomic nervous system. The therapist needs to pull the strokes gently along the tissue.

▶ **Examples**
• In polyarthritis in the back region
• Ventricular ulcer: upper rhomboid strokes on the left side, left edge of the rib cage

• In bronchial asthma, along the pectoral muscles and in the region of the sternal angle

▶ **Elevated dermographism.** The formation of welts is characteristic here. This is basically an acute irritable edema of the capillaries caused by increased histamine release. The therapist needs to check the condition of the tissue and carefully dose the strokes administered.

▶ **Example.** Muscular rheumatism in the area being treated.

▶ **White dermographism.** A white streak caused by a brief vascular spasm. This reaction may indicate a vascular disease or reduced blood flow in the tissue. The therapist needs to carefully dose the strokes until slight reddening shows better circulatory conditions.

▶ **Example.** White streaks can be seen in the region of the pelvis in patients with vascular diseases.

Distinct to severe skin reactions frequently occur in restless patients who are not used to the treatment. However, this cannot be regarded as a rule of thumb.

In fact, no rules can or should be applied with regard to the duration of skin reactions, since each patient responds differently.

Physical Responses

Cutivisceral reflexes and autonomic reactions are triggered by the sensory stimulus of the massage, which also includes transpiration of a thin, odorless sweat that is prominent during the first treatments and becomes less noticeable in the course of additional sessions. Patients are often astonished, as the sweating can already start during the first strokes and can extend over the whole back as well as the axilla and/or facial area.

Irritations such as goose bumps and changes in the pupils may also be observed after a short term and explained by physiological conditions (p. 11).

For cardiovascular reactions, refer to the general reflex mechanism of action (p. 17).

Also: sensations, such as a "light heart," hot or cold hands and feet, a general feeling of warmth, sometimes in conjunction with a "hot," often also red face, and hunger to the extent of feeling "emptiness in the stomach" may also be experienced. After the first treatments, "frequent urination" is reported also at night (▶ Table 2.1).

Reactions of the respiratory system include improved respiratory function and respiratory movements, which are caused by reflexes triggered by therapeutic applications in segments T3–T10. Deeper respiration is observed during and after the application of certain connective tissue strokes:
- When lifting and grasping tissue on the anterior superior iliac spine
- When crossing the transverse abdominal muscle
- When applying a large balancing stroke
- When stretching the latissimus dorsi muscle upward
- When applying grasping techniques—for example, on the anterior superior iliac spine
- When pulling out the lower edge of the rib cage
- When applying fanlike strokes, in the angle between the iliac crest and spinal column
- When strokes are applied along the respiratory angle
- When applying the liver stroke

The quadratus lumborum muscle, which often has increased tone, responds to the treatment with a reduction in tension and thus facilitates the respiratory movements, due to its complex relation to the diaphragm and the serratus posterior inferior muscle.

Reactions such as:
- Heart palpitations, tachycardia, and tightness in the chest
- Breathing difficulties, shortness of breath, and dyspnea
- Nausea and vomiting
- Dizziness or even fainting

are clear adverse reactions and alarm signals that should compel the therapist to reconsider the approach being used.

Remedies for Adverse Reactions and Abnormal Sensations

General Remedies

- Work primarily in the caudal area and, if necessary, in a lower section.
- Apply balancing strokes, branching out in large and small circles several times.
- Reassure the patient.
- Choose a relaxed position, cover the patient, and make sure he or she has enough fresh air.
- Check the working method again and adapt it to the new findings.

Specific Remedies

- For tightness in the chest or gastric pain, apply strokes along the left lower edge of the rib cage and the large balancing stroke.
- In the event of liver and gallbladder pain, the upper first pelvic strokes provide relief when applied several times.
- For pain in the kidneys, apply the upper pelvic strokes—if necessary, all three pelvic strokes—several times.
- If incorrect application of stimuli causes a spasm in the uterus muscles, apply the upper pelvic strokes several times.
- In the event of nausea or dizziness, the therapist should apply balancing strokes several times, calm the patient down, apply dispersion strokes, make sure there is enough fresh air, and have the patient lie supine.
- If the patient experiences sudden headaches, the following connective tissue strokes provide relief and have a balancing effect:
  - Pulling out the lower sacral bone and edge of the rib cage several times
  - Soft and flat balancing strokes on the pectoral muscles
  - Balancing strokes above the clavicle.

Table 2.1 Sensations experienced by the patient and information for the therapist

Sensation	Cause	Correction
Pulling finger	Correct technique/stimulus: turgor in the treated area or in partial sections is within normal limits	To convince unsure patients that one is working with the fingertips and not with the fingernails, one should perform the following test: applying traction (in front of the patient's eyes) on relaxed muscles illustrates the sensation of pulling fingers. Traction on tense muscles creates the sensation of scratching, the tip of a knife, or a fingernail (!) and/or a sensation resembling being cut
Sensation of being cut, which is not experienced as discomfort. The patient does not have an urge to "avoid" the application. The sensation of being cut is rarely recognized as such, and instead is felt like "deep scratching," the "tip of a knife," or a "fingernail underneath the skin"	Correctly applied therapeutic stimulus with increase in intensity where necessary: triggering of proper nervous reflex processes. The turgor in the treated area or in partial sections is increased or strongly increased	
Sensation resembling being cut that is perceived as uncomfortable, burning, and very painful, described as being razor-sharp to unbearable. The patient avoids the strokes	The technique (check finger/hand position, speed, and traction) is too intense. The area being worked on has been included too early. The tension level in the area being treated or in parts of it is too great	Reduce the intensity: Return to deeper structures (working caudally) Condition of the tissue should be checked Balancing strokes should be applied
A sensation described as stroking that is perceived as caressing, possibly even described as sliding over the skin	Usually the wrong technique	Check technique for: • Correct attachment • Finger/hand position • Speed
A sensation of pressure (according to Teirich-Leube) that is painful to unbearable, diffuse and cannot be exactly localized. The patient avoids the strokes	Wrong technique, and the area of increased turgor and tone has been included too soon: nerve reflex processes occur in the wrong sequence	Check technique (see above): Check condition of tissue Return to deeper structures, working caudally Apply balancing strokes
The patient experiences a mixture of sensations (according to Teirich-Leube) and is unable to stick to one description of what the sensation is. The patient responds hesitantly	Wrong technique, and the area of increased turgor and tone has been included too soon: nerve reflex processes occur in the wrong sequence	Check technique (see above): Check condition of tissue Return to deeper structures, working caudally. Apply balancing strokes

According to Dicke, the cutting sensation is not necessarily provoked, but may be generated by applying the correct technique—that is, depending on the findings present, the therapist should work with flat or cutting strokes.

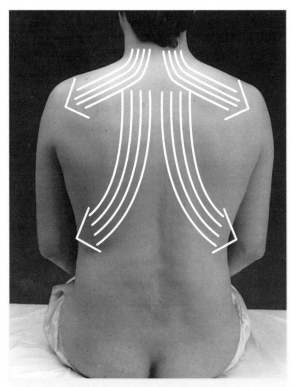

Fig. 2.11 Strokes for dyspnea during treatment.

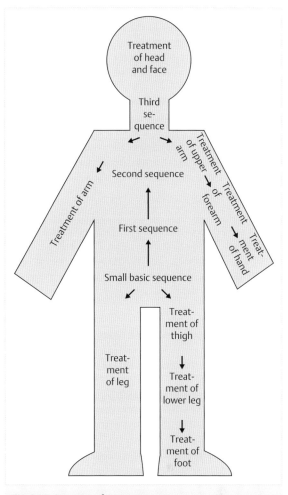

Fig. 2.12 Structure of treatment.

- Repeat strokes on the edge of the rib cage and lower rhomboid strokes
- Pull the fingers as if they were a "rake" several times from the neck, between the shoulder blades to the lower edge of the rib cage (▶ Fig. 2.11)
- Large, flat dispersion strokes
- If the patient is having difficulty in breathing and dyspnea, the following measures are recommended:
  - Apply balancing and dispersion strokes several times
  - Open the window and, if possible, place the patient in a favorable position
  - Pull the fingers like a "rake" several times (▶ Fig. 2.11).

It is important to apply the usual dispersion strokes after relieving measures and to give the patient enough time to rest after each measure.

2.2 Principles of CTM

2.2.1 Structure and Treatment

General Information

Connective tissue massage is performed in accordance with a systematic treatment plan; Dicke called this the "treatment build-up." It starts in the caudal area with the small basic sequence, which Dicke called the "basic build-up."

In the event of disorders of the lower extremity and/or of organs that lie in the pelvic space (such as the kidney or bladder), the legs are then treated after several CTMs with the small basic sequence. Depending on the condition, this includes either only the small basic sequence and treatment of the thighs, or the small basic sequence and treatment of the legs.

The first sequence follows in the cranial direction after sufficient treatment with the small basic sequence in the event of disturbances of the upper extremity and/or of organs that lie in the thorax (like the lungs, heart, liver, gallbladder, and stomach). Dicke called the small basic sequence and first sequence the "large build-up."

Depending on the response to the treatment and the positive influence and changes in the skin, muscle, and connective tissue zones, the second sequence and, if needed, later also the third sequence can be applied. All sequences together are called the "big basic build-up." Depending on the indication, treatment of the upper extremity follows the second or third sequences (▶ Fig. 2.12).

If it is not possible to start the treatment with the small basic sequence (e.g., due to the development of welts or mild swelling), treatment should be provided that includes the segments of the lower extremities until the acute event has improved or is no longer visible and/or palpable.

Experience shows that a connective tissue massage applied to the back with increasing intensity, from the caudal to cranial region, is tolerated better when ventral balancing strokes are applied at the end between the individual phases of treatment. The dispersion strokes in the dorsal region are also indispensable at the end of treatment.

> The more extensive and severe the findings and the clinical picture, the longer the individual treatment sequences have to be applied. Contralateral treatment—that is, using the consensual reaction—should be administered in the event of unilateral diseases (e.g., a heart illness).

The following points should also be considered:
- Patients should never be treated immediately after they have eaten, but they should also not be treated on an empty stomach.
- Any drug treatment the patient is receiving should be noted, as well as other physical therapy measures, and these should be discussed with the physician, if necessary.
- In all cases, resting phases after treatment must be observed and the treatment must be harmonized with other therapies.

Additional Information on the Hendrikx/Klein Small Basic Sequence

When one is triggering stimuli, the patient has to be observed closely so that their individual reaction can be assessed, as this often varies widely between patients. A slow, careful approach to the patient should be used, applying subtle stimuli during CTM to avoid over-reactions in the skin.

Safe work without risks is only possible below T12, where only effects on less sensitive organs can be triggered. This is the main idea behind the small basic sequence, and this kind of approach also has additional advantages. The sympathetic and parasympathetic nervous system can be influenced well from this area. The parasympathetic nervous system is known to cause reactions such as general relaxation, sleepiness, polyuria, and an urge to defecate, whereas the orthosympathetic nervous system triggers mydriasis, secretion of sweat, and piloerection, as well as muscle tension.

Three **principles** should guide the therapist's hand:
- At the beginning, the stimulus must be placed outside the affected body regions.
- All tissue layers should be treated one after the other.
- The dosage must be individually probed and should correspond to the responses of the patient's autonomic nervous system.

Rule of thumb:
- One should not apply stimuli that are too intense.
- One should not work immediately in the affected segment.

Later on, depending on the relaxation, the affected regions in the body and maximum points can be progressively integrated, if they have not already been normalized by the effects of previous treatment in the area.

The small basic sequence makes it possible to approach the individual reflex situation carefully and approximate the threshold, which is the only way to avoid undesired after effects.

It is also possible to balance sympathetic and parasympathetic stimuli, as neurons in both systems can be influenced here. Light massage in particular affects the parasympathetic nerve, while deeper massage particularly affects the sympathetic nerve, transmitting the triggered reflex to the surface and thus allowing remote effects from the lower area, outside the hazard zone.

2.2.2 Determination of Findings

During the first treatment session, the patient's medical history, visual findings (▶ Table 2.2), and palpable findings are noted first. Current findings are then briefly noted again during all follow-up appointments.

Inspection, palpation, and a conversation with the patient allow the therapist to establish an individual and meaningful treatment plan, always reacting to current situations with changes in the response and in the perception of pain by modifying the treatment.

The therapist should explain the treatment to the patient and inform him or her about the duration of the treatment, the objective, and also about the way in which connective tissue massage is applied and what reactions may occur during and after connective tissue massage.

The results are entered into the patient's record.

Medical History

The patient's medical history provides important information about the etiology and development of the disorder and needs to be noted in a sensitive fashion in order to create a harmonious, trusting atmosphere for treatment. The therapist is bound under oath to secrecy.

The following list of questions should be regarded as an example and can be adapted and expanded individually:
- General questions regarding:
  - Occupation

Table 2.2 Visual findings

Points to note	Points to evaluate
Habitual posture when standing and sitting	Relief postures and poor postures
	Postural damage in comparison
Gait:	Coordinated and rhythmic movements
Mobility of the joints	Relief posture and/or movements through:
Pelvis position (stabilization)	Contractures
Torso movements	Malposition of joints
Arm swing	Malformations
Head posture	
Dorsal:	
Calcaneus/Achilles tendon	Position of Achilles tendon
Popliteal cavities	Hyperextension or flexion
	Same level
Gluteal clefts	Same level
Leg	Knock-knee, bow leg
	Muscle contractures
	Bony structure
Pelvic crest	Symmetry
Waist triangle	
Sacral bone	
Spinal column	Scoliosis
	Muscle relief
Shoulder blades	Position and distance to each other
Shoulder girdle	Level
	Plane
	Width
Position of neck and head	Relief postures, poor postures
Lateral:	
Arch of foot	Position of the planes and axes to each other and possible deviations to neutral position—e.g., lordosis, kyphosis
Knee	
Pelvis position	
Spinal column	
Shoulder girdle	
Head position	
Abdominal wall	Tone
Ventral:	
Feet	Position (inward or outward), main point of stress
Knee	Patella position
Pelvis	Symmetry

Table 2.2 continued

Points to note	Points to evaluate
Costal arch	Epigastric angle
	Symmetry
Abdominal wall	Tone
Shoulder	Position of clavicle
Head	Position of planes and axes—e.g., wry neck
Face	Symmetry

- ○ Recreation
- ○ Hobbies
- ○ Sports
- ○ Stress situations, situation at home
- Questions regarding treatment:
  - ○ Has the patient ever received a prescription for CTM before; if yes, how was it tolerated?
  - ○ Has the patient already had other therapies or is the patient currently having other therapies?
  - ○ What medication is the patient taking?

Make sure to rule out contraindications.

- Questions about the illness:
  - ○ When did the disorder start and what triggered it?
  - ○ Is the condition associated with any other disorders, or is the patient aware of any other disorders?
  - ○ Is there a family disposition toward a certain disorder?
- Questions regarding pain:
  - ○ When, where, and how does the pain occur?
  - ○ In what conditions is the pain intensified?
  - ○ Is there a difference between day and night, between rest and activity?
  - ○ Does the pain radiate to other areas?
  - ○ Pressure pain?
  - ○ Stinging pain?
  - ○ Burning pain?
  - ○ Sensations of tension?
  - ○ Sensory disturbances?
- Questions regarding concomitant symptoms:
  - ○ Is breathing affected?
  - ○ Is there a different sensation of heat and cold between body regions?
  - ○ Does the patient know his or her blood pressure values?
  - ○ During or after eating, is there sensation of fullness or pressure in the gastric region?
  - ○ Is the patient quickly tired or listless during exertion?
  - ○ How does the patient sleep?

Visual Findings

If possible, lighting conditions and the general setting have to always be kept the same in order to allow an objective evaluation of the examination.

To begin with, the therapist has to determine the patient's physical build, weight, height, and habitual posture in order to evaluate any deviations from a correct axial posture.

The visual findings are noted while the patient is sitting or standing, from dorsal via lateral to ventral, and from caudal to cranial.

The two sides always have to be compared with each other. ▶ Table 2.2 summarizes the general visual findings.

In addition to static conditions and muscle structure, the therapist also needs to note the following points.

Skin

Skin diseases, hematomas, wounds, scars, and birthmarks should be recorded, in addition to complexion, blood supply, and dermographism.

Birthmarks should be very closely watched for any changes, in order to avoid overlooking a possible risk of melanoma for the patient.

Connective Tissue and Muscles

Not only disorders of the internal organs, but also static changes and deviations in the skeleton can alter tissue tone and the turgor of the skin.

Changes in the tone of the patient's connective tissue and muscles are signs of the patient's mental and physical condition.

Palpable Findings

Assessment of palpable findings is performed as described in the section "Palpation" (p. 31). In general, the therapist should always work from caudal to cranial and should always compare the two sides with each other.

Palpation is carried out with the patient in the sitting position, if possible.

Skin

- Temperature
- Skin texture
- Dermographism
- Tone level
- Skin changes
- Skin diseases
- Head's skin areas

Connective Tissue

- Disorders of connective tissue (e.g., benign tumors, malignant tumors or geloses)
- Adhesions of collagenous connective tissue
- Tone level
- Dicke and Teirich-Leube connective tissue zones

Muscles

- Tone changes (e.g., myogelosis and stiffness)
- Muscular disorders (e.g., sprained muscles, ruptured muscles, and myalgia)
- McKenzie muscle zones

Skin, Connective Tissue and Muscle Zones

Dicke did not use the term "zone," but it is the technical term currently in use today and is therefore also used in this presentation of Dicke connective tissue massage.

The skin and muscle zones have already been described in detail (Chapter 1).

The connective tissue zones can be discussed again here. To evaluate a connective tissue zone (CTZ), it is important to determine the basic tone of the connective tissue. People who are considered to be healthy by current medical standards present different basic tones. These can change due to age, sex, constitution, lifestyle, and stress components. A firm or flaccid basic tone in the connective tissue primarily says nothing about the patient's health status or disorders. It should also be noted that a different consistency in the connective tissue is found on the torso than, for example, in the region of the buttocks or the extremities.

Connective tissue zones are circumscribed areas of tissue that respond by reflex to functional disorders and/or disorders of the internal organs, static misloading, and trauma.

Tenseness: This is also sometimes referred to as adhesions. Between the dermis and subcutaneous tissue (Teirich-Leube's "upper mobile layer") and between the subcutaneous tissue and the superficial fascia (Teirich-Leube's "deep mobile layer"), adhesions and reduced mobility develop between the tissue layers due to reversible changes in tone and metabolism.

Retractions: The sliding capacity between the mobile layers is no longer present here. Lifting is not possible. This palpable sensation is also called adhesion.

Distension: The connective tissue may suffer infiltrations (Hanssen's "distension processes") due to changes in the physical and chemical state. Depending on the duration and progress of the disorder, the distension is described as follows:

- Soft, easily impressible distension (▶ Table 2.3)
- Firm distension: Feels firm and compact and is only impressible with difficulty, or not at all (▶ Table 2.3)

Silent zone: Connective tissue zones can also be described as "clinically silent" (Teirich-Leube) when the associated organs, nerves, vessels, and musculoskeletal system do not show, or no longer show, disorders and symptoms.

Zones of this type can indicate past disorders and/or a disposition.

Zones can only be described as silent if the corresponding organ functions also remain stable under stress, for example.

2.2.3 Palpation

The manual examination is used to examine skin texture and generally comprises the following components:

Sensitivity test: sharp/blunt contact (e.g., with the fingernail or fingertip), application of heat or cold, or when cooling fanning is used to test whether sensitivity is increased or decreased or is within normal limits.

Muscle test: muscle tone is checked through passive full motion and through pressure in the region of the junction between tendon and muscle and in the region of the abdominal muscles.

Paravertebral stroke (▶ Fig. 2.13): this diagnostic stroke is applied to the paravertebral region close to the spinal column, from L5 to C7. The speed at which the stroke is applied is determined by the mobility of the dermis.

Moving the tissue layers with the fingertips (displacement test) (▶ Fig. 2.14, ▶ Fig. 2.15): the therapist systematically works through the whole region of the buttocks and back on both sides, making use of dermal elasticity. Slipping must be avoided.

Lifting of tissue layers (▶ Fig. 2.16, ▶ Fig. 2.17): the tissue is lifted in the entire region of the back by trying to form a skin fold with the tip of the fingers and the thumb. The distance between thumb, index finger, and middle finger should not exceed 5 cm. Slipping must be avoided here, too. The tissue should not be dropped.

2.2.4 Balancing Strokes and Dispersion Strokes

Balancing strokes on the pectoral muscles (▶ Fig. 2.18): the flat strokes on the pectoral muscles are applied on the right and left sides of the body.

Table 2.3 Reaction zones and therapeutic consequences

Reaction zones	Examination method	Symptoms/reactions	Therapeutic consequences
Skin zones Head's zones Head's dermatomes	Sensitivity test: • Sharp/blunt • Stroking of the skin with an object or fingertip / fingernail • Warm/cold • Air movements Formation of skin folds (▶ Fig. 2.16)	Organs and organ systems (nerves and vessels), which are disturbed in their function, can trigger the following reactions/symptoms in the segment-dependent areas: • Reddening • Welts • Hyperalgesia • Hyperesthesia • Paresthesia (e.g., feelings of soreness, burning and pinching)	Remain below the affected dermatome or in the contralateral region until the acute condition is hardly noticeable any more
Dicke and Teirich-Leube connective tissue zones (CTZ)	Inspection palpation techniques (▶ Fig. 2.16)	Disturbances in organs and in different tissues trigger changes in the connective tissue by reflex: tone changes • Distensions:	
		• Soft, easily impressible distension indicates a pathological process	Initially, body regions that present distensions are omitted and the therapist works in lower segment sections (p. 27). Later, the therapist works around these until improvement is noticed (e.g., firm distension). The therapist first works with flat strokes.
		• Firm, barely impressible or unimpressible distensions show the therapist that this may mean one of the following: ○ Improved condition ○ Chronic course	Application of therapy in the area can be started here. The therapist needs to respond to the patient sympathetically and sensitively when working with any tension that may be present and the resulting pain
		• Tension/adhesions • Retractions • Silent zone (may be a retraction, adhesion, distension)	The therapist first applies flat and then cutting strokes, the dosage depending on the findings in the tissue. The strokes can be worked into the area here. Since there are no disturbances or irritation and the tissue can be distinguished from healthy tissue only through palpation, CTM can be applied in this area without restrictions
Muscles • McKenzie zones, myotome fields	Muscle test (p. 31)	Segment-related reaction of the muscles to functional disturbances or disorder of organs and organ systems: • Changes in tone • Pain on palpation and movement	Work in the affected area can be started now. The dosage must be adapted to the presented tone and the resulting pain
• Mackenzie maximum points		Maximum points Accumulation of pain stimuli and reflex muscle cramps.	The therapist applies the strokes in the contralateral area or below the painful muscle areas. The pain condition is an important indicator for further treatment

Note:
During all treatments, it should be taken into consideration that disturbances of sensitivity and perception (e.g., a mixed sensation of cutting and pressure) make it difficult for the patient to assess the traction stimulus that is so important for the therapy. For body regions that are not to be worked on directly, the therapist can use the consensual effect and segment-related work

Contraindications to the administration of connective tissue massage:
• Febrile and massively inflammatory disorders
• Infections
• Skin allergies

When the patient has an overly sensitive heart, only infra-clavicular and supraclavicular strokes are applied on the left half of the torso.

Dispersion strokes (▶ Fig. 2.19):
- Small dispersion strokes: when the treatment is concluded with the small basic sequence, the edges of the lower sacral bones are pulled out several times bimanually from the starting points at the rhomboid strokes to the intergluteal cleft as small dispersion strokes.
- Large flat dispersion strokes: after the small dispersion strokes, flat dispersion strokes are applied bimanually. They start in the neck, are pulled over the lateral part of the back downward, and end with strokes on the edges of the lower sacral bone. Paravertebral guidance of the hands is also possible.

Each treatment is concluded with balancing strokes on the pectoral muscles and dispersion strokes.

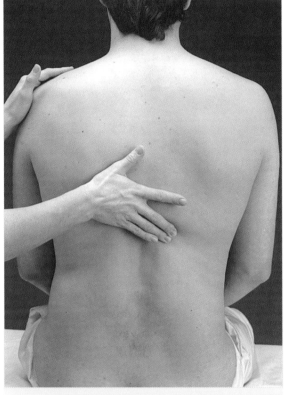

Fig. 2.13 Diagnostic stroke: paravertebral stroke.

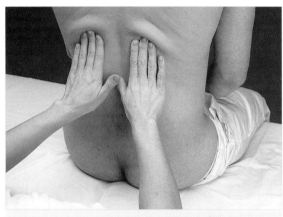

Fig. 2.15 Moving tissue layers with the distal phalanges of the fingers.

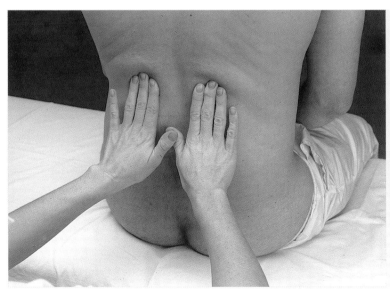

Fig. 2.14 Moving tissue layers with the fingertips.

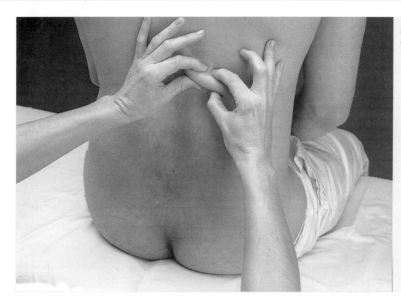

Fig. 2.16 Lifting tissue layers with the thumb and index finger.

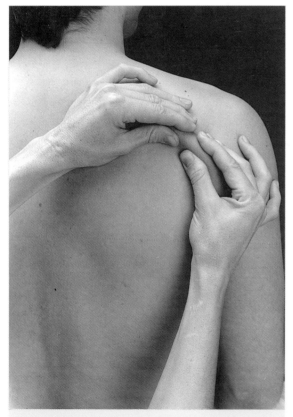

Fig. 2.17 Lifting tissue layers with the thumb, index finger, and middle finger.

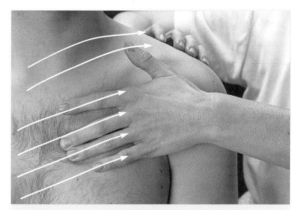

Fig. 2.18 Balancing strokes on the pectoral muscles.

2.2.5 Small Basic Sequence

Small Basic Sequence in Sitting Position

Overview

▶ Fig. 2.20 shows the strokes used in the small basic sequence.

Strokes

Rhomboid strokes (▶ Fig. 2.21) (synonym: sacral bone edge):
• Lower rhomboid strokes from the rhomboid end point to the intergluteal cleft

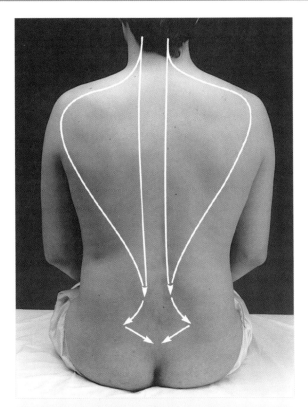

Fig. 2.19 Small and large extensive dispersion strokes.

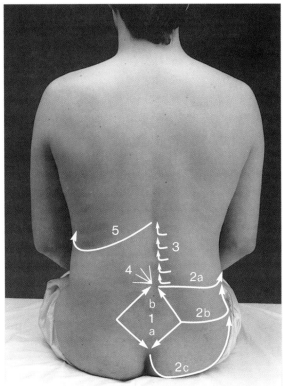

Fig. 2.20 Strokes in the small basic sequence with the patient in the sitting position.
1 Rhomboid strokes (**a, b**)
2 Pelvic strokes (**a, b, c**)
3 Hooks along the spinal column
4 Fan
5 Pulling out the rib cage edges

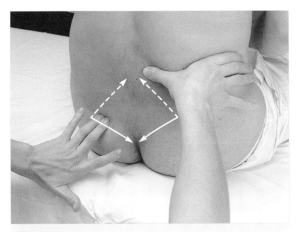

Fig. 2.21 Lower rhomboid strokes (——) and upper rhomboid strokes (- - - - - -).

- Upper rhomboid strokes from the rhomboid end point to L5

Three pelvic strokes (▶ Fig. 2.22) (synonym: strokes on the hip bones):
- **First pelvic strokes** from L5, extending along the iliac crest to the anterior superior iliac spine
- **Second pelvic strokes** from the rhomboid strokes point to the **anterior superior iliac spine**

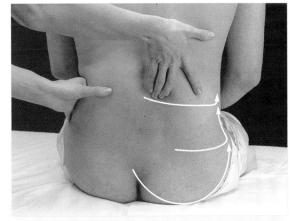

Fig. 2.22 Pelvic strokes 1 to 3.

- **Third pelvic strokes** starting at the intergluteal cleft, extending below the ischial tuberosity and the greater trochanter, also ending at the anterior superior iliac spine

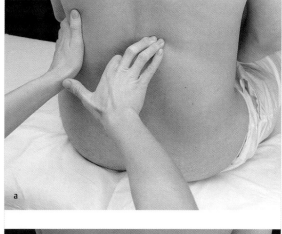

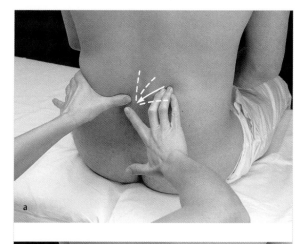

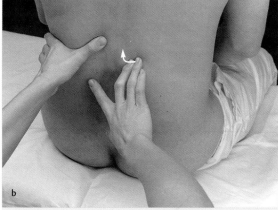

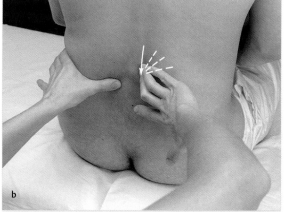

Fig. 2.23 Hook along the spinal column.
a Stroke.
b The thumb of the free hand fixates the next spinous process.

Fig. 2.24 The fan.
a Stroke and stroke length.
b L5 is fixated with the thumb of the free hand.

The pelvic strokes can also be applied in reverse order in accordance with the segmental structure.

- In all three strokes, the arm has to be extended widely to achieve continuous traction and to avoid slipping.
- The strokes always end with soft grasping of the anterior superior iliac spine.

Five hooks along the spinal column (▶ Fig. 2.23). These start at L5 and are pulled within the long erector muscle of the trunk toward the spinal column. The last hook ends at T12.

The fan (▶ Fig. 2.24). This is pulled in the angle between the iliac crest and the spinal column. A start is made at the iliac crest. The stroke length is approximately 5 cm.

Pulling out the rib cage edges (▶ Fig. 2.25). This stroke is started at the level of T12 and ends under mild traction at the medioclavicular line.

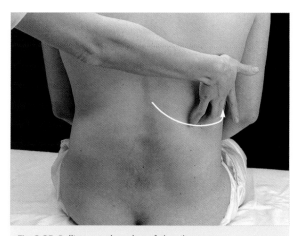

Fig. 2.25 Pulling out the edge of the rib cage.

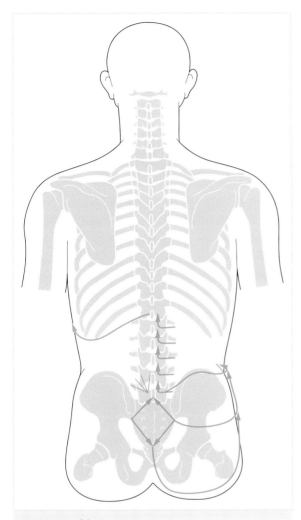

Fig. 2.26 Small basic sequence.

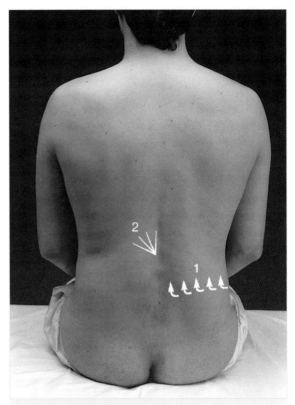

Fig. 2.27 Hooks along the first pelvic strokes (1) and upper fan-shaped stroke (2).

▶ Fig. 2.26 provides an anatomical overview of the strokes in the small basic sequence.

Additional Strokes

- **Hooks** to the sacral bone edges from caudal to cranial are performed after the rhomboid strokes.
- **Flat transverse strokes**. After the rhomboid strokes, flat transverse strokes can be applied from caudal upward to cranial over the sacral bone.
- **Hooks**, in the course of the first pelvic strokes (1) (▶ Fig. 2.27) applied after the rhomboid strokes; afterward, the upper and further pelvic strokes are applied.
- **Small, flat transverse strokes** are applied along the spinal column, within the area of the long extensor spinae muscles from L5 to T12, after the hooks in the direction of the spinal column.
- **Hook and stretching stroke** at the ischial tuberosity (▶ Fig. 2.28). The therapist stands and applies the stretching stroke with arm extended.

- **Stretching stroke** in the region of the lumbar triangle (▶ Fig. 2.29). These stimulating strokes are applied after the lower edges of the rib cage have been pulled out. The therapist sits behind the patient and gently stretches the tissue at the edge of the latissimus dorsi muscle toward the pelvic crest.
- The "upper fan," in the "respiratory angle" (2) (▶ Fig. 2.27). Flat fan-shaped strokes are applied along the angle between the lowest rib and the spinal column, starting at the lower edge of the rib cage and ending with the last stroke along the spinal column (L3 to T12).

Small Basic Sequence in the Lateral Position

Overview

▶ Fig. 2.30 shows the strokes of the small basic sequence in the lateral position.

Strokes

- If the patient is unable to sit, treatment can be performed in the lateral or prone position.

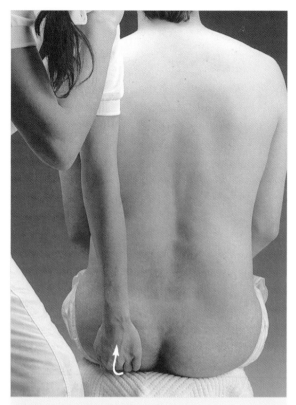

Fig. 2.28 Hook and stretching stroke on the ischial tuberosity. The therapist holds his or her own shoulder with the opposite hand to prevent it from pulling up.

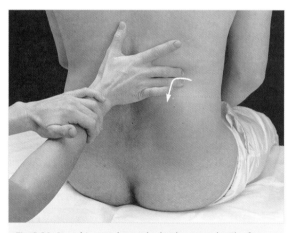

Fig. 2.29 Stretching stroke on the lumbar triangle. The free hand can be additionally used to support the traction.

- The small basic sequence (▶ Fig. 2.26) can also be applied in the sitting position. The sequences for the lateral position (and for the prone position as well) are thus alternatives.

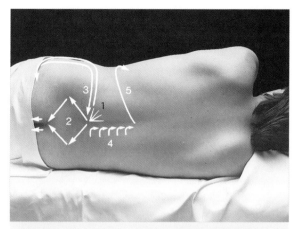

Fig. 2.30 Strokes in the small basic sequence in the lateral position.
1 Fan
2 Rhomboid strokes
3 Large pelvic strokes
4 Hooks along the spinal column
5 Pulling out the edge of the rib cage

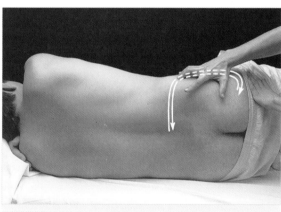

Fig. 2.31 Large pelvic strokes.

Fan: this stroke is pulled at an angle between the iliac crest and the spinal column. The therapist starts at the iliac crest, and the length of the strokes is approximately 5 cm (▶ Fig. 2.24).

Rhomboid strokes: short strokes are applied from L5 to the end point of the rhomboid strokes, from the end point of the rhomboid strokes to the gluteal cleft, and from there along the gluteal cleft (including the sacral segments) (▶ Fig. 2.30).

Large pelvic strokes: extending from L5, the therapist works his or her way along the iliac crest to the greater trochanter and from there back to L5 (▶ Fig. 2.31).

Five hooks along the spinal column: the strokes are pulled out in the paravertebral region toward L5–T12 (▶ Fig. 2.30).

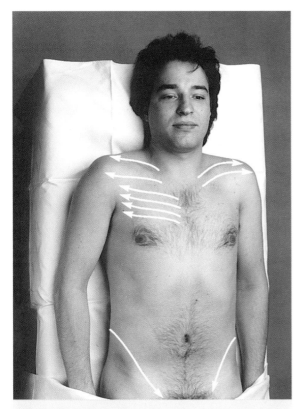

Fig. 2.32 Ventral balancing strokes.

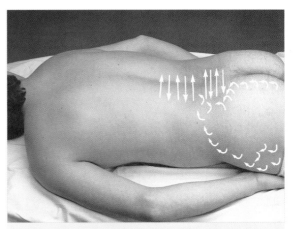

Fig. 2.33 Additional strokes from dorsal in the small basic sequence (possible in the lateral and prone positions).

Pulling out the edge of the rib cage: this stroke starts at the spinal column (T12) and ends at the ribs, in the region of the medioclavicular line (▶ Fig. 2.30).

The patient turns over to the other side and the treatment is repeated.

Balancing strokes on the pectoral muscles: with the patient in the **supine position** (▶ Fig. 2.32), flat balancing strokes are applied to the pectoral muscles, taking the patient's potential heart problems into consideration.

Ventral pelvis and abdominal strokes: balancing pelvis and abdominal strokes are applied to conclude the "small basic sequence in the supine position" (recumbent position). The pelvic strokes start at the level of the dorsal pelvic crest and work their way up to its upper edge. The fingertips are kept in close contact with the upper edge and move past the anterior superior iliac spine to the anterior inferior iliac spine and then flatly fan out toward the symphysis. These strokes are performed bimanually, first on one side then on the other. Flat transverse strokes are then applied between the anterior superior iliac spine, beginning at the hairline and moving toward the anterior iliac spines.

Additional Strokes

▶ **From dorsal** (▶ Fig. 2.33)
- **Hooks** toward the edges of the sacral bone, from cranial to caudal, starting at the level of L5, first along the sacroiliac joint, then downward along the edge of the sacral bone
- **Short transverse strokes** along the sternum
- **Small hooks** along the course of the large pelvic strokes, in both directions
- **Small hooks** around the greater trochanter
- **Flat balancing stroke,** starting above the greater trochanter toward the ischial tuberosity
- **Small, flat transverse strokes** along the spinal column, within the area of the long extensor spinae muscles, from L5 to T12

Small Basic Sequence in Prone Position

Overview

▶ Fig. 2.34 shows the strokes of the small basic sequence with the patient in the prone position.
- After the first three strokes, the therapist changes sides and performs the strokes on the other side in the same order.
- The remaining strokes are then performed. The flat balancing strokes on the pectoral muscles and in the pelvic area are performed with the patient in the supine or lateral position.
- The strokes are performed in the same way and in the same order as in the small basic sequence in the lateral position, except for the alterations mentioned above.

Additional Strokes

▶ **From dorsal** (▶ Fig. 2.33)
- **Short hooks** toward the edges of the sacral bone are applied in the same manner as in the small basic sequence in the lateral position.

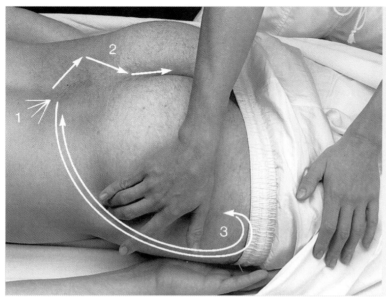

Fig. 2.34 Strokes in the small basic sequence with the patient in the prone position.
1 Fan
2 Rhomboid strokes
3 Large pelvic strokes
4 Hooks along the spinal column
5 Pulling out the rib cage edge

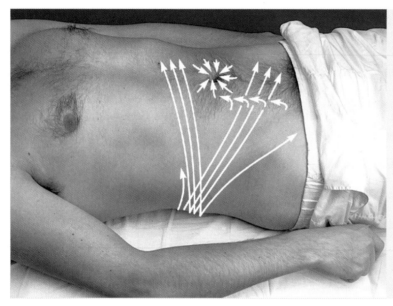

Fig. 2.35 Additional strokes from the ventral side in the small basic sequence, with the patient in the lateral and supine positions.

- **Short hooks** along the intergluteal cleft, pulling up from the side, are performed after the rhomboid strokes and a short stroke along the intergluteal cleft, followed by the long pelvic strokes.
- **Flat transverse strokes** are applied over the sacral bone, as described in the small basic sequence in the sitting position.
- **Hooks** during the large pelvic strokes and around the greater trochanter, as described for the small basic sequence in the lateral position.
- **Small, flat transverse strokes** within the area of the long extensor spinae muscles, from L5 to T12, after the hooks to the spinal column.

▶ **From ventral** (▶ Fig. 2.35)
- **Bimanual strokes**, starting from the dorsal side, pulling at the same time from the lower edge of the rib cage to the medioclavicular line and from the pelvic edge to the anterior superior iliac spine. These strokes are performed bimanually, first on one side then on the other.
- **Short hooks** along the rectus sheath from the symphysis to the level of the navel.
- **Short strokes**, like rays, pulling toward the navel.
- **Bimanual strokes crossing over** the abdominal walls, starting in the dorsal region and ending at the opposite edge of the rectus abdominis muscle.

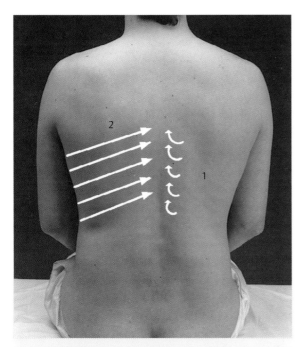

Fig. 2.36 Strokes for treating the intercostal area.
1 Hooks along the spinal column
2 Intercostal strokes

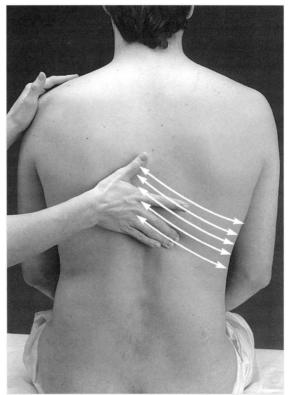

Fig. 2.37 Intercostal strokes.

• **Liver stroke**. This stroke starts on the ventral side at the medioclavicular line and is pulled along the right edge of the rib cage toward the dorsal side just before the spinal column. The strokes are applied with a flat hand. The intensity is slowly increased.

The patient should be in a lateral position.

Flat strokes are absolutely necessary in order to avoid irritation of the intercostal nerves.

For tips, see Remedies for Adverse Reactions and Abnormal Sensations (p. 25).

2.2.6 First Sequence

Treatment of the Intercostal Area (Lower Thoracic Sequence)

Overview

▶ Fig. 2.36 shows the strokes for treating the intercostal area.

Strokes

Five hooks along the spinal column: these are applied in the paravertebral region from T12 to T7.

Five to seven intercostal strokes: these are performed with flat strokes from the ventral axillary line along the intercostal spaces (rising cranially) toward the spinal column. After these five strokes, two additional strokes may be performed after the last stroke (▶ Fig. 2.37).

Balancing strokes on the pectoral muscles. *Special attention* is required for patients with heart problems (▶ Fig. 2.18).

Additional Strokes

▶ **From dorsal**
• **Change in direction.** The intercostal strokes are also performed in the opposite direction, from the spinal column along the lateral thoracic wall to the ventral axillary line, in order to gently grasp the tissue there (▶ Fig. 2.37).
• **The large balancing stroke** starts in the ventral axillary line at the level of the sixth/seventh intercostal space and is broadly pulled around the lower angle of the shoulder blade toward C7 (▶ Fig. 2.38).

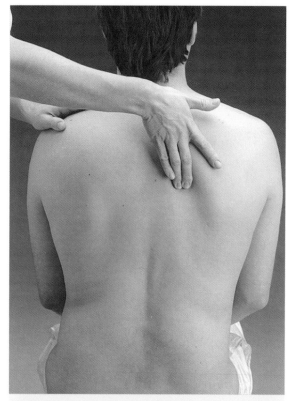

Fig. 2.38 Large balancing stroke. (The milk stroke is performed the same way, but applied at a more oblique angle.)

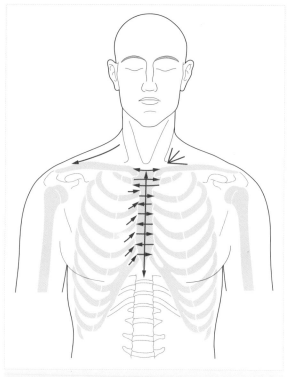

Fig. 2.39 Flat strokes in the ventral intercostal area.

When this stroke is pulled flatly but rapidly, with a stimulating function, it is called a "milk stroke." This stroke is performed after the intercostal strokes.

- The intercostal strokes are followed by a **stroke** from the lower angle of the shoulder blade to the spinal column at the level of T4.
- **Flat transverse strokes** over the spinal column, beginning at the level of T6 below the angle of the left shoulder joint and ending below the angle of the right shoulder blade, then pulled back to the starting point. This stroke is also performed after the intercostal strokes.
- **Small, flat transverse strokes** along the spinal column, within the area of the long extensor spinae muscles, from T12 to T7.

▶ **From ventral**
- **In the ventral intercostal area,** a set of flat strokes are pulled, starting at the lowest ribs, from the dorsal axillary line through the intercostal spaces (▶ Fig. 2.39).

▶ Fig. 2.40 shows the large basic sequence.

2.2.7 Second Sequence

Shoulder and Axilla Treatment

Overview

▶ Fig. 2.41 shows the strokes for treating the shoulder and axilla.

Strokes: Shoulder

Seven hooks are applied along the spinal column in the paravertebral region, from T7 to C7.

Short cutting strokes: from the spinal column (T9) to the medial border of the shoulder blade.

Border of the scapula: the strokes follow the border of the scapula:
- Medial border of the scapula
- Lateral border of the scapula
- Superior border of the scapula and spine of the scapula

When working on the shoulder blade, the therapist stands on the side that is to be treated. The starting position for the required traction stimulus is achieved by treating the right shoulder blade with the left hand, and vice versa. The strokes along the lateral border of the scapula are applied flatly and only up to approx. 1 cm

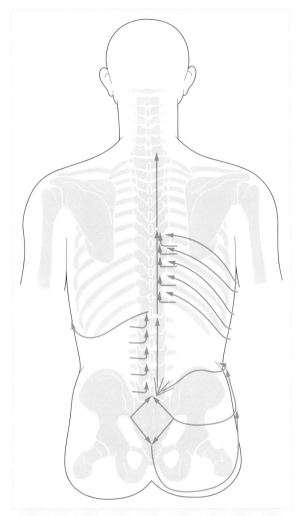

Fig. 2.40 Large basic sequence (small basic sequence and first sequence).

above the axillary gap, to avoid irritating what is known as the ulnar nerve spot.

The third stroke around the border of the scapula starts obliquely and ends at the acromion as a flat stroke.

Balancing strokes on the pectoral muscles.

When axillary treatment follows the treatment of the scapula, all balancing strokes on the pectoral muscles are omitted for the time being.

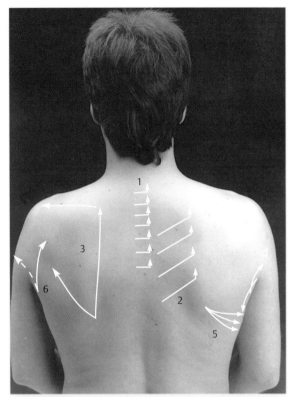

Fig. 2.41 Strokes for treating the shoulder and axilla.
1 Hooks
2 Short cutting strokes
3 Outlining the scapula with cutting strokes
4 Short upward and downward stretching
5 Garland
6 Bimanual stretching

Strokes: Axilla

Short downward stretching (▶ Fig. 2.42): The fingers are applied at the edge of the latissimus dorsi muscle, while the patient has the arm in abduction. Stretching is then performed with the arm in an adducted position in the dorsal direction, and then in the caudal direction toward the origin of the latissimus dorsi muscle.

Short upward stretching (▶ Fig. 2.43): strokes with marked traction are applied here in the dorsocranial direction toward the insertion tendon of the latissimus dorsi muscle.

Garland (▶ Fig. 2.44): Three flatly pulled strokes start from the inferior angle of the shoulder blade with an upward motion to the insertion tendon of the pectoralis major muscle.

Breast tissue and axilla need to be avoided here. The therapist stands in front of the patient.

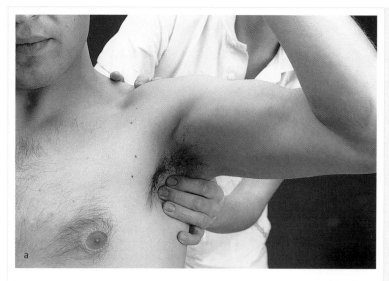

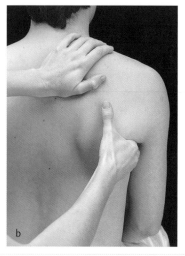

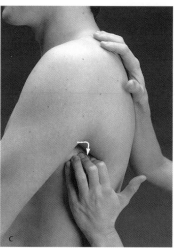

Fig. 2.42 Short downward stretching.
a The patient's arm is abducted in the starting position.
b With the arm adducted, traction is now applied in the dorsal direction.
c Traction in the dorsocaudal direction.

Bimanual axillary stretching (▶ Fig. 2.45): The stretching of the latissimus dorsi muscle and of the pectoralis major muscle starts with the patient's arm in abduction. The fingertips of both hands are placed below the axilla. Stretching is then performed in the cranial and lateral direction with the arm adducted. At the same time, the balls of the thumbs apply gentle pressure in the opposite direction.

- If both muscles are very tense, the individual muscles may be pre-stretched.
- The axilla is omitted.

Balancing strokes on the pectoral muscles. *Special attention* needs to be given in patients with heart problems.

Additional Strokes

Stretching strokes:
- **"Long downward stretching"** along the edge of the latissimus dorsi muscle toward its origin, which is performed after "short downward stretching" (▶ Fig. 2.46).
- **"Prolonged upward stretching"** on the edge of the latissimus dorsi muscle. This starts at the level of the sixth/seventh intercostal space.
- **Axillary stretching with elevated arm:** The patient places his/her arm on the therapist's shoulder, if the arm can be lifted to shoulder level. Connecting transverse strokes are applied again in the region of the serratus muscle in order to thoroughly loosen the dorsal and ventral axillary fold.

▶ **From dorsal**
- **A flat fan-shaped stroke** is pulled transversely over the scapula toward the shoulder joint, starting at the outer

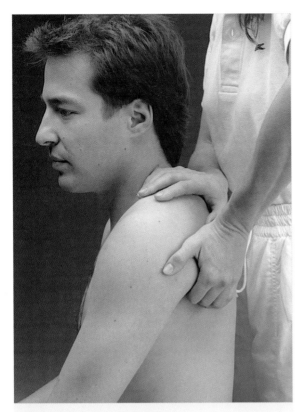

Fig. 2.43 Short upward stretching.

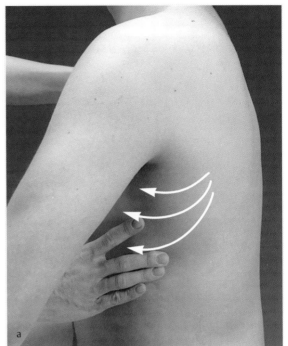

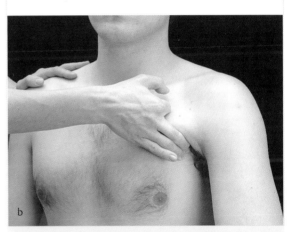

Fig. 2.44 Garland from dorsal to ventral.
a Strokes for the garland.
b End point of the third stroke.

edge of the scapula and ending at the lower edge of the spine of the scapula (▶ Fig. 2.47).

- **Small, flat transverse strokes** along the spinal column, within the area of the long extensor spinae muscles, from T12 to T7, to T3 or to C7. Short transverse strokes are applied after the hooks to the spinal column (1) (▶ Fig. 2.48).
- **Flat transverse strokes** from the inner side to the other inner side of the shoulder blades, starting at the level of T7 and ending at the spine of the scapula (2) (▶ Fig. 2.48).
- **Short hooks** around the angle of the scapula, followed by strokes around the edge along the same course (3) (▶ Fig. 2.48).

▶ **From ventral** (▶ Fig. 2.49)
- **The ventral edge** of the trapezius muscle is pulled out to the level of the shoulder, while applying resistance with the other hand.

▶ Fig. 2.50 illustrates the strokes in the second sequence.
- **Strokes** along the sternum, starting at the xiphoid process and passing to the jugular notch.
- **Short hooks** at the connection points between the ribs and sternum, pulling from the caudal to the cranial side.

- **Short transverse strokes** along the sternum. These start at the junction between the xiphoid process and the body of the sternum, along the area of the sternal angle. At the base of the second rib at the sternum, the strokes should become wider to just under the sternoclavicular joints.
- **Short strokes**, fanlike strokes over the jugular notch. These start with the first stroke on the clavicle and end with the last one on the dorsal edge of the sternocleido-mastoid muscle.
- **Strokes** on the interclavicular ligament.

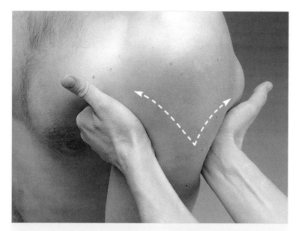

Fig. 2.45 Axillary stretching.

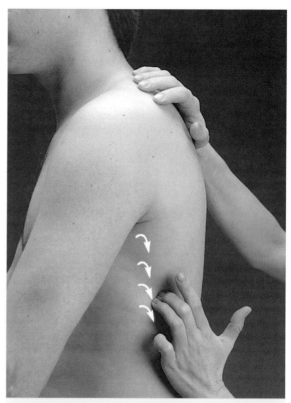

Fig. 2.46 Long downward stretching.

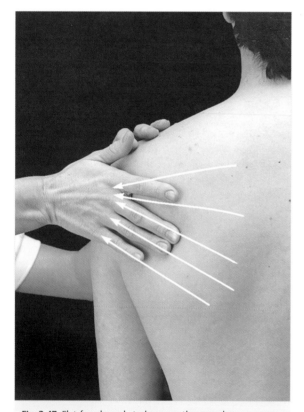

Fig. 2.47 Flat fan-shaped strokes over the scapula.

The types of ventral stroke used and when to apply them is indicated in the corresponding treatment plans and summaries. The strokes are administered with the patient in the supine position.

At the end of each treatment balancing strokes are applied to the pectoral muscles (▶ Fig. 2.18) and the strokes

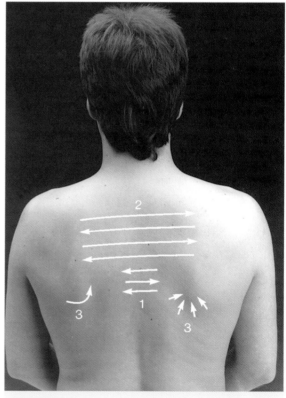

Fig. 2.48 Additional strokes, dorsal: flat transverse and small hooks.

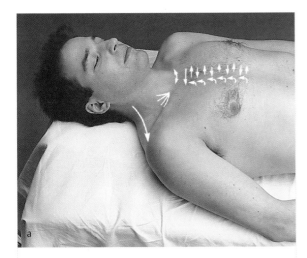

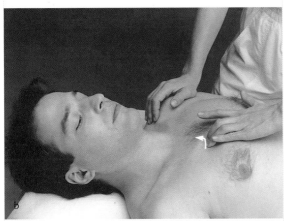

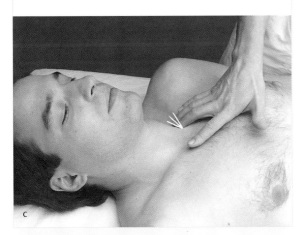

Fig. 2.49 Overview of additional ventral strokes, in vivo.
a Overview.
b Hooks toward the sternum.
c Fanlike short strokes toward the suprasternal notch.

above the clavicle, paying special attention to potential heart problems. The short and long flat strokes are applied in the dorsal direction (▶ Fig. 2.19).

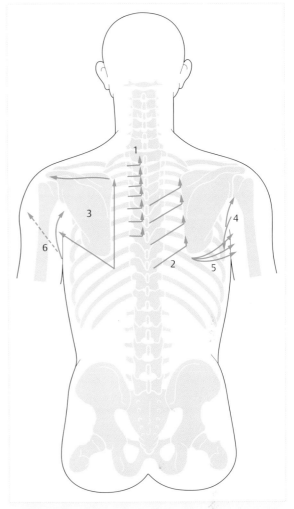

Fig. 2.50 Second sequence.

2.2.8 Third Sequence

Treatment of the Neck

Overview

▶ Fig. 2.51 shows the strokes for treating the neck area.

Strokes

Sun around the prominent vertebra: small strokes, only in the region of the trapezius muscle aponeurosis toward C7 (▶ Fig. 2.52).

Paravertebral stroke: from C7 to the occipital bone (▶ Fig. 2.51).

Seven hooks along the spinal column: from C7 to the occipital bone (1) (▶ Fig. 2.52).

Pulling out the nuchal ligament: traction starts at the spinal column and ends approximately 2 cm in front of the mastoid process.

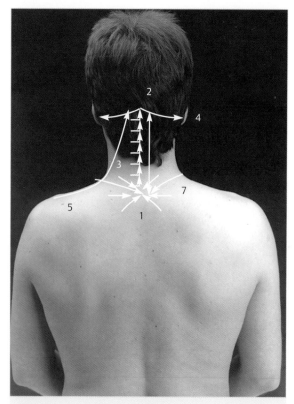

Fig. 2.51 Strokes for treating the neck area.
1 "Sun"
2 Paravertebral strokes
3 Hooks along the cervical spine
4 Pulling out the nuchal ligament
5 Strokes along the trapezius muscle (descending part)
6 Strokes along the dorsal edge of the sternocleidomastoid muscle (ventral strokes)
7 "Rabbit grip"

Strokes along the ventral edge of the trapezius muscle (descending part): the strokes start on the lateral third of the clavicle and end at the external occipital protuberance (2) (▶ Fig. 2.52).

Strokes along the dorsal edge of the sternocleidomastoid muscle: traction starts at the clavicle and ends at the mastoid process.

Stretching stroke (rabbit grip): the two hands are positioned with the fingertips on the trapezius muscle, are lightly attached, and the muscle is then stretched with force toward C7.

Balancing strokes on the pectoral muscles: *Special attention* needs to be given in patients with heart problems.

If this concludes the treatment, it ends with the usual dispersion strokes.

2.2.9 Treatment of the Upper Extremity

Upper Arm

Overview

▶ Fig. 2.53 shows the strokes on the upper arm.

Strokes

Capsule stroke (▶ Fig. 2.54): on each side, the strokes start in the region of the axillary space (ventral/dorsal) and end at the acromion.

Hooks (▶ Fig. 2.54): along the capsule stroke.

Biceps stroke (▶ Fig. 2.55): this is pulled along the long biceps tendon and ends at the acromion.

Pulling out the deltoid muscle (▶ Fig. 2.56): this stroke starts flatly and softly at the acromion and ends with marked traction at the deltoid tuberosity of the humerus. The other hand has to be placed firmly on the opposite side. *This can also be done bimanually.*

Two short transverse strokes (▶ Fig. 2.56): over the insertion tendon of the deltoid muscle.

Additional Strokes

• **Bimanual soft stretching** of the flexor and extensor on the upper arm in the lateral direction.
  These are pulled in the tissue between the biceps/triceps muscles of the upper arm up to near the elbow.

Forearm

Overview

▶ Fig. 2.57 shows the strokes on the forearm.

Strokes

Two short biceps strokes (▶ Fig. 2.58): The strokes are applied on both sides along the tendon and under traction, toward the crook of the elbow.

Two short strokes from distal to proximal to the crook of the elbow (▶ Fig. 2.58): on the medial edge of the brachioradialis muscle and along the medial edge of the palmaris longus muscle. The middle of the crook of the elbow has to be omitted with this stroke, due to the nerves and vessels located there.

Two strokes, along the muscle edges of the flexor carpi radialis muscle, starting in the lower third of the forearm.

Strokes, along the medial edge of the flexor carpi ulnaris muscle.

Strokes, along the extensor digitorum muscle (▶ Fig. 2.59), starting in the lower third of the forearm.

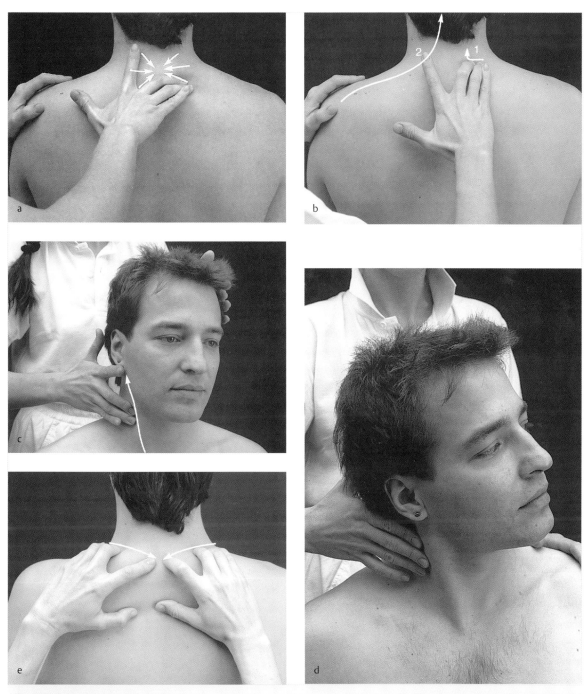

Fig. 2.52 Strokes in the third sequence.
a Sun around the prominent vertebra.
b Hooks along the spinal column (1) and strokes on the descending part of the trapezius muscle (2).
c Strokes along the sternocleidomastoid muscle toward the mastoid process.
d Presentation of the position of the sternocleidomastoid muscle.
e Stretching stroke from the trapezius muscle toward C7.

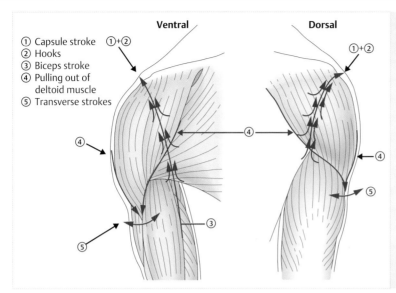

① Capsule stroke
② Hooks
③ Biceps stroke
④ Pulling out of deltoid muscle
⑤ Transverse strokes

Ventral ①+②

Dorsal ①+②

Fig. 2.53 Ventral and dorsal strokes on the upper arm.

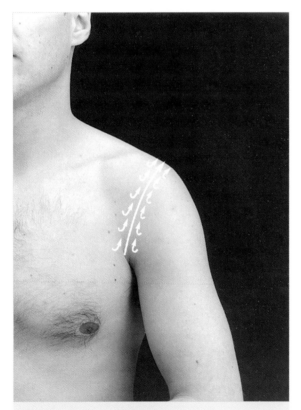

Fig. 2.54 Capsule stroke (ventral) (1) and hooks (2).

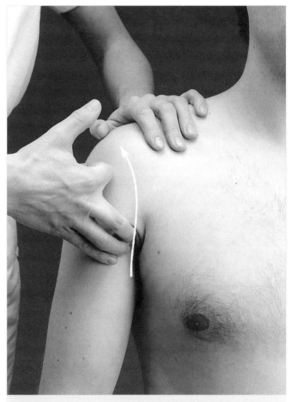

Fig. 2.55 Biceps stroke.

Soft bimanual stretching in the crook of the elbow (▶ Fig. 2.60): the stretching is performed bimanually in a soft fashion and directed toward the outside.

If the treatment is concluded, the usual balancing strokes and dispersion strokes are applied.

Hand

Overview

▶ Fig. 2.61 shows the strokes for treatment of the hand.
  Palmar start:
- Medial edges of the flexor carpi radialis/ulnaris muscles
- Space between these two flexors
- Flexor retinaculum

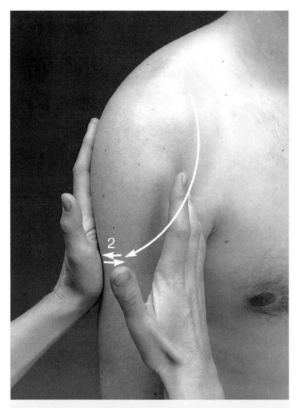

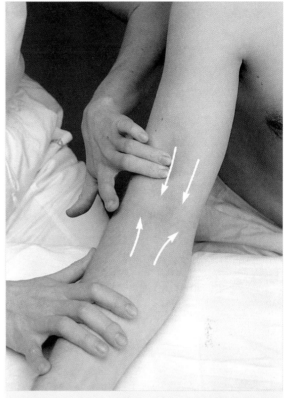

Fig. 2.56 Pulling out the deltoid muscle (1); transverse strokes (2).

Fig. 2.58 Strokes along the biceps tendon and along the medial edge of the palmaris longus and brachioradialis muscles.

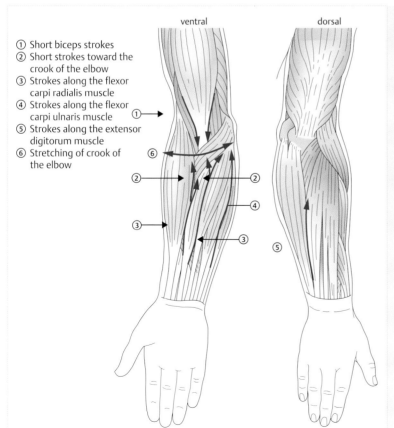

① Short biceps strokes
② Short strokes toward the crook of the elbow
③ Strokes along the flexor carpi radialis muscle
④ Strokes along the flexor carpi ulnaris muscle
⑤ Strokes along the extensor digitorum muscle
⑥ Stretching of crook of the elbow

ventral

dorsal

Fig. 2.57 Ventral and dorsal strokes on the forearm.

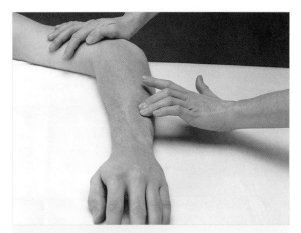

Fig. 2.59 From the extensor digitorum muscle to the elbow.

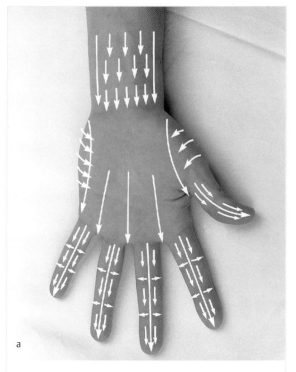

a

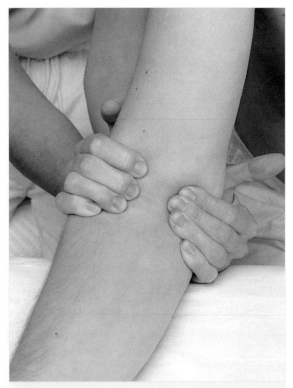

Fig. 2.60 Bimanual stretching in the crook of the elbow.

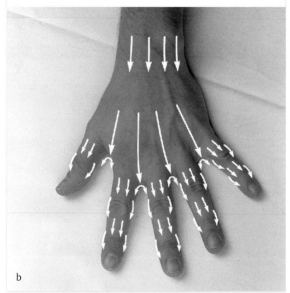

b

Fig. 2.61 Strokes for treatment of the hand.
a Palmar strokes.
b Dorsal strokes.

- Metacarpals
- Thenar
- Hypothenar
- Finger joints

Dorsal continuation:
- Extensor retinaculum
- Metacarpals

- Interdigital webs
- Metacarpophalangeal joint to fingertip
- Collateral ligaments
- Finger joints
- Hand

- One should always start in the palmar region when treating the hand. ▶ Fig. 2.61a, however, contains two strokes running from dorsal to palmar, which do not show up again in ▶ Fig. 2.61b.
- In contrast to the previous instructions, the sequence of anatomical structures is listed for the hand and their designation is omitted from the illustration.

Strokes

Palmar

Two strokes each are applied from proximal to distal along the medial edges of the flexor carpi radialis and flexor carpi ulnaris muscles toward the wrist.

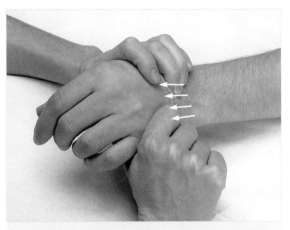

Fig. 2.62 Small strokes over the extensor retinaculum, applied with traction from the extension position to the flexion position.

Three short strokes between both **flexor tendons** of the flexor carpi radialis and flexor carpi ulnaris muscles.

Strokes in the region of the flexor retinaculum:
- Short strokes above the flexor retinaculum
- Short strokes on the flexor retinaculum

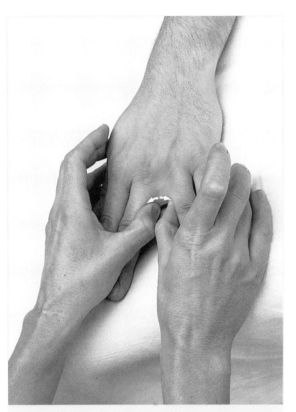

Fig. 2.63 Stretching of the interdigital webs.

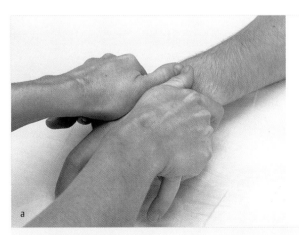

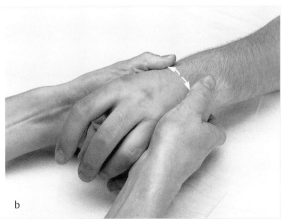

a

b

Fig. 2.64 Stretching of the hand.
a In the dorsal direction.
b In the palmar direction.

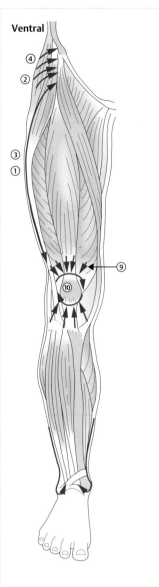

Ventral

④
②
③
①
⑨
⑩

Dorsal

⑥
⑤
⑧
⑦
⑪
⑫

Fig. 2.65 Ventral and dorsal strokes on the thigh and lower leg.

① Tract stroke from proximal to distal
② Strokes around the trochanter
③ Tract stroke from distal to proximal
④ Strokes between trochanter
  and iliac spine
⑤ Internal stroke
⑥ Bimanual stretching with flat pulling out

⑦ Traction on the gastrocnemius muscle
⑧ Bimanual stretching of popliteal cavity
⑨ Hooks toward the patella
⑩ Strokes around the patella
⑪ Pulling out of the Achilles tendon
⑫ Pulling strokes around the malleoli

Three interosseous strokes between:
- Metacarpals 5 and 4
- Metacarpals 4 and 3
- Metacarpals 3 and 2

Thenar strokes as vertical and transverse strokes.
  Hypothenar strokes as vertical and transverse strokes.
  Short strokes between the individual finger joints.

Dorsal

Small strokes over the extensor retinaculum (▶ Fig. 2.62).
  Four interosseous strokes between:
- Metacarpals 5 and 4
- Metacarpals 4 and 3
- Metacarpals 3 and 2
- Metacarpals 2 and 1

Careful stretching of the interdigital webs with the thumb toward both sides (▶ Fig. 2.63).

Pulling out the individual fingers from the metacarpophalangeal joint to the fingertip. This stroke is applied in the palmar direction, but fixated on the opposite dorsal side. The hand is in the palmar position.

Pulling out the collateral ligaments.

Bimanual stretching in the region of the finger joints from palmar to dorsal.

Small strokes between the individual finger joints ▶ Fig. 2.61b.

Stretching of the hand in the palmar and dorsal direction (▶ Fig. 2.64).

2.2.10 Treatment of the Lower Extremity

Overview

▶ Fig. 2.65 shows the strokes on the thigh and lower leg.

Thigh/Knee (Patella)

Strokes

Tract stroke from proximal to distal (▶ Fig. 2.66). Starting above the greater trochanter and flatly along the edge of the dorsal iliotibial tract, pulling to the insertion tendon of the biceps femoris muscle.

Pulling around the greater trochanter from dorsal to ventral (▶ Fig. 2.67).

Tract stroke from distal to proximal. This stroke starts in the distal third of the thigh and ends above the greater trochanter (▶ Fig. 2.68a).

Strokes between the greater trochanter and the anterior superior iliac spine (1) (▶ Fig. 2.67).

The internal stroke (▶ Fig. 2.68b, ▶ Fig. 2.69). Start in the distal third of the thigh and pull from proximal to distal between the semimembranosus and semitendinosus muscles.

Bimanual stretching. This starts on the dorsal, transverse vascular fold and is flatly pulled out toward the popliteal cavity (▶ Fig. 2.68b).

Bimanual traction in the fold of the gastrocnemius muscle. We start lightly and bimanually and pull in the proximal direction under traction toward the popliteal cavity and to the insertion spots of the gastrocnemius muscle (▶ Fig. 2.68, ▶ Fig. 2.70).

Bimanual flat stretching of the popliteal cavity (▶ Fig. 2.68b).

Hooks to the patella (▶ Fig. 2.68a).

Strokes around the patella (▶ Fig. 2.68a).

Additional Strokes

- Short strokes from the last third of the fascia lata, in the shape of a fan toward the patella.
- The thigh stroke starts in the upper third of the thigh, on the lateral edge of the sartorius muscle, and ends shortly before the groin.
- Short hooks, which must be pulled from the transverse intergluteal cleft to the popliteal cavity.

Lower Leg

Strokes

Bimanually pulling out of the Achilles tendon toward the calcaneus (▶ Fig. 2.68b).

Strokes around the lateral malleolus and medial malleolus, at first one by one, then bimanually. (▶ Fig. 2.68a).

Additional Strokes

- Strokes from the inner side of the thigh, starting below the patella and traveling around the medial malleolus.
- Bimanual stretching between the muscle bellies of the gastrocnemius muscle, from top to bottom, pulling in the direction of the Achilles tendon.

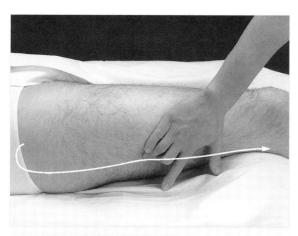

Fig. 2.66 Tract stroke in the distal direction.

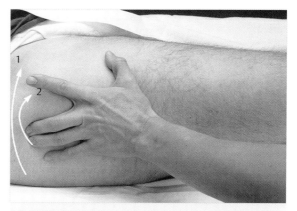

Fig. 2.67 One of four strokes between the greater trochanter (1) and anterior superior iliac spine, applied around the greater trochanter (2).

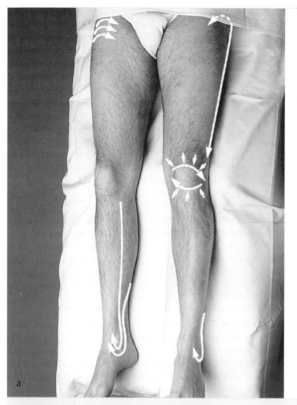

Fig. 2.68 Treatment of the thigh and lower leg.
a Ventral strokes.
b Dorsal strokes.

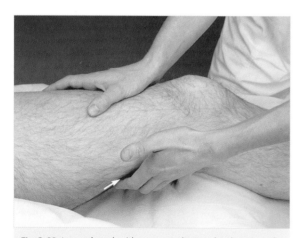

Fig. 2.69 Internal stroke (the arrow indicates the direction of the traction. Its course can be seen in ▶ Fig. 2.65.

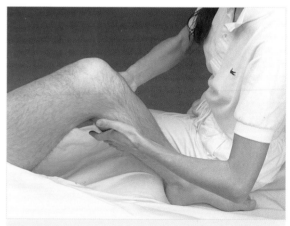

Fig. 2.70 Bimanual traction in the fold of the gastrocnemius muscle.

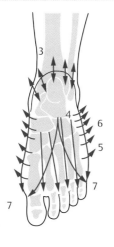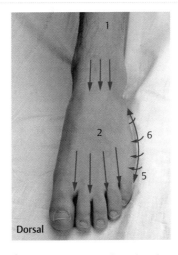

Fig. 2.71 Plantar and dorsal strokes in foot treatment.

Plantar

Dorsal

① Hooks over the upper ankle joint
② Strokes between the metatarsals
③ Strokes on the calcaneal tuberosity
④ Plantar strokes
⑤ Transverse strokes along the edge of the foot
⑥ Hooks on the edge of the foot
⑦ Stretching

Foot

Overview

▶ Fig. 2.71 shows the strokes for foot treatment.

Strokes

Hooks, over the upper ankle joint, in the distal direction.
   Four strokes, between metatarsals I–V.
   Small strokes on the calcaneal tuberosity:
• Between the lateral malleolus and the edge of the foot
• Between the medial malleolus and the edge of the foot (not illustrated)
• From plantar to dorsal along the edge of the calcaneal tuberosity (not illustrated)
• From dorsal to plantar along the edge of the calcaneal tuberosity

These last two strokes both start in the middle of the heel.
   Four plantar strokes, pulling from the calcaneal tuberosity in the direction of the interdigital spaces.
   Transverse strokes, along the lateral and medial edge of the foot.
   Hooks, along the lateral and medial edge of the foot.
   The strokes are pulled from plantar to dorsal.
   Bimanual stretching of the plantar aponeurosis.

Treatment of the toes, if necessary, can be performed in the same way as when treating the fingers.

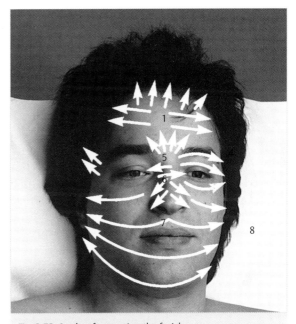

Fig. 2.72 Strokes for treating the facial area.
1 Initial flat strokes
2 Small hooks along the hairline
3 Pulling out the temporal area
4 Strokes around the eye sockets
5 Short, fan-shaped strokes
6 Short strokes from one corner of the eye to the other
7 Bimanual nasal strokes
8 Bimanual balancing strokes

2.2.11 Treatment of the Head

Face

Overview

▶ Fig. 2.72 shows the strokes for treating the facial area.

Strokes

Initial flat strokes, applied bimanually, moving from the center of the forehead with traction to the temple.

Small hooks along the hairline (▶ Fig. 2.73).

Pulling out from the temporal area to the hairline.

Strokes around the eye socket. With a well-supported hand, the eyebrow and the upper and lower parts of the eye socket are approached with three strokes, each time with traction applied toward the temple.

Short, fan-shaped strokes, applied from the root of the nose (nasal bone) to the forehead (glabella) (▶ Fig. 2.74).

Two short strokes, with firmly supported hand, pulling the thenar region from one corner of the eye toward the other over the nasal root.

Bimanual nasal strokes.

Make sure that the patient is breathing properly.

Bimanual balancing strokes:

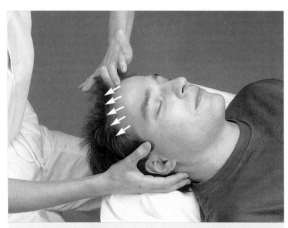

Fig. 2.73 Small hooks along the hairline.

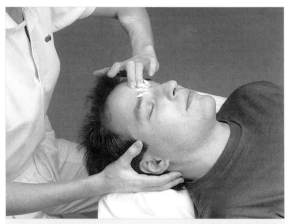

Fig. 2.74 Fan-shaped strokes to the glabella.

- Pull from the middle of the nose over the zygomatic bone
- Above the lip over the maxilla
- Below the lip over the mandible
- From the tip of the chin (mental protuberance) over the mandible

Head

Overview

▶ Fig. 2.75 shows the strokes of head treatment.

Strokes

Hooks:
- Along the ventral edge
- Along the lateral edge
- With hooks along the ventral and lateral edge omitting the area of the temples
- Along the dorsal edge
- Along the skull seams

Transverse strokes toward the mastoid process.
　Stroke around the ears from ventral to dorsal.
　Smaller strokes behind the ear.

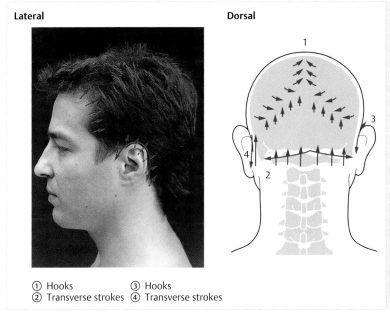

Lateral　　　　　　　　　　**Dorsal**

① Hooks　　　　　③ Hooks
② Transverse strokes　④ Transverse strokes

Fig. 2.75 Lateral and dorsal view of head treatment.

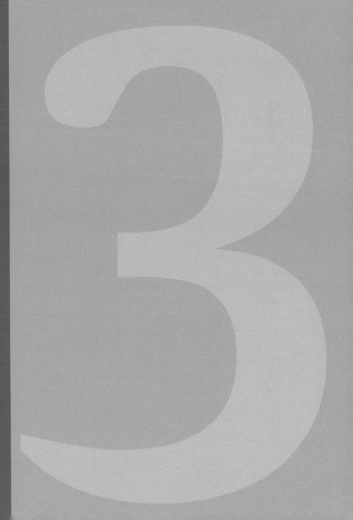

Chapter 3
Clinical Pictures

3 Clinical Pictures

3.1 Indications, Contraindications, Prescriptions

Roland Schiffter

Connective tissue massage (CTM) is a form of symptomatic therapy that is primarily helpful in the treatment of subacute and chronic functional disorders and complaints. This applies in particular to the sequelae of diverse disorders and injuries. "Functional" in this sense refers mainly to pain and local and global cramp, and also to pareses of the striated muscles and spasm or dysfunction in the smooth muscles—for example, circulatory disturbances; disorders of the stomach, intestines, and urination; and other regulatory disorders of the autonomic nervous system. Psychosomatic symptoms and disturbances of mental wellbeing also need to be taken into consideration.

Connective tissue massage is unsuitable or contraindicated for acute inflammation; infarctions of the heart, brain, or other organs; hypertensive crises; hemorrhage; new traumatic injuries; and certainly in the acute phase of slipped disks, fractures, and the like. However, once the acute or florid symptoms have subsided, CTM, if deemed necessary by a physician is even more effective on subsequent functional disorders and syndromes. CTM may also be beneficial to tumor patients undergoing surgical, radiological, or chemotherapeutic treatment, so long as no contraindications such as bone metastases—which pose a risk of pathological fractures—have been determined by the attending physician.

Connective tissue massage may be indicated for patients with psychological and psychosomatic disorders, but not for patients with acute psychosis, aroused states of confusion, or symptoms of intoxication.

Patients sensitive to mechanical skin irritation who develop reddening (red dermographism [p.24]) or even welts must be treated with the greatest care or by the use of a different form of therapy.

It is important to monitor the patient's cardiovascular functions carefully. CTM can trigger massive reflexes involving the circulatory system, such as hypertensive crises or orthostatic fainting, especially in patients predisposed to these types of reactions. If there is doubt, CTM should not be applied or should be applied only with extreme caution or at longer intervals.

Connective tissue massage can usually be combined with all other physical therapy treatment methods; but the attending physician must be consulted for the decision on the appropriate treatment plan.

Connective tissue massage is a therapy that involves the body as a whole and should follow a structured scheme. There is no such thing as application to just one part of the body, such as to the right arm only or to the left hip only.

3.2 Medical Guidelines

Each health insurance company has its own binding regulations concerning the coverage of medical treatment, including physical therapy. Physicians and physical therapists should know the health insurance regulations applicable for each form of treatment. Those bound by contractual agreement must ensure that their representatives and assistants follow these regulations.

Connective tissue massage may not be covered by health insurance, unless specific conditions are met. However, even if this form of treatment is not covered, out-of-pocket fees may represent a worthwhile investment for the patient in the long run, given that CTM may help to

- Cure a disorder, prevent its progress or alleviate complaints
- Improve the patient's health in such a way that he or she is less likely to become ill
- Promote a child's development that is at risk
- Avoid or reduce the need for medical care in the near future

Most insurances provide documentation with a list of treatments and remedies covered. The documentation regulates

- The indications for which the insurance will provide coverage
- The type of coverable remedies for these indications
- The amount of coverable remedies per diagnosis, and special conditions for follow-up prescriptions (follow-up and long-term prescriptions)

The prescription may only be issued by physicians who have a contract with the insurance company.

Connective tissue massage may be covered according to these regulations, but one must check with the health insurance company first. CTM is also often categorized as "reflex zone therapy," because its effects are primarily based on reflex mechanisms.

The following are possible indications for CTM that may be found in the insurer's regulations, among others:

- Muscle tension caused by the spine including disturbances of blood supply and metabolism in these affected muscles
- Radicular syndromes
- Causes of intervertebral disk surgery
- Complaints caused by scars and contractures

- Reflex neurovascular dystrophy (Sudeck atrophy)
- Causes of arthritis, osteoarthritis, and traumatic joint damage
- Periarthropathies, tendinopathies, central and peripheral pareses
- Bronchial disorders and the subsequent conditions of various lung diseases
- Arterial vascular disease
- Chronic intestinal disease (e.g., Crohn disease or irritable bowel syndrome)
- Chronic prostatitis or salpingitis
- Scleroderma

One must always refer to the information provided in the guidelines, and every physician bound by contractual agreement with a health insurance company should own a copy of these.

3.3 Orthopedic Disorders

Michael Weber, Rauthgundis Gleich von Muenster

Physical treatment methods such as physical therapy, massages, balneotherapy, electrotherapy, and the like were integrated early into the methods available to orthopedists.

Many orthopedic illnesses are expressions of a localized or extensive dystrophy. For example, contractures or some conditions caused by humeroscapular periarthritis or disorders of the spine with radicular or pseudoradicular symptoms are often caused by disturbances of the sensory motor system.

Connective tissue massage plays a special role here and, from the orthopedist's perspective, thorough diagnosis and correct application of the small basic sequence are decisively important. The small basic sequence is what Elisabeth Dicke called the "basic build-up."

The more severe the disorder and the condition, the longer must the therapist administer the small basic sequence, before slowly proceeding to the reflex zones of the affected area.

In the field of orthopedics especially, time-consuming therapeutic measures may be required for application of CTM in a proper and timely manner.

Connective tissue massage can also be applied together with other methods and, due to its universal and safe effects, it is often combined with tried and proven physical measures such as physical therapy, heat application, and electrotherapy. It should be noted that application of heat and/or mud packs can make the skin swell, which could interfere with correct diagnosis and make the correct administration of CTM more difficult. Thus, the application of heat and/or mud packs is advisable only on days when no CTM is to be applied.

If the prescription reads "connective tissue massage and physical therapy," then CTM should always be administered *after* physical therapy, because it is important that the patient rests after the connective tissue massage.

3.3.1 Disorders of the Spinal Column

The risk of developing back pain depends on many endogenous and exogenous factors. Endogenous factors include the physique, muscle composition, pathological changes of the spine (e.g., damaged intervertebral disks), and numerous very various disorders of the spine. Exogenous factors primarily describe mechanical influences on the spine, especially in the workplace, as well as psychosocial factors.

With age the frequency of pain increases and usually peaks when people reach their sixties. Because many different causes of pain often occur together, chronic neck or back pain is usually difficult to explain and to treat.

The concept of the movement segment makes it decidedly easier to understand the pathological mechanics behind degenerative disorders of the spine. The moving spaces between two vertebrae are called the "movement segment." These movable parts of the spine are not coextensive with the ontogenic segments. Since the supply of vessels and nerves follows the ontogenic segmentation, the movement segments are not supplied by only one vessel or nerve.

The afferent nerves, for instance, of a spinal nerve (segment nerve) stem from at least two movement segments. A vertebral joint is supplied by at least two branches of the spinal nerve. Different branches from multiple spinal nerves are involved in the innervation of a movement segment.

The anterior ligament, the intervertebral disk itself, and the vertebra are only scantly supplied by pain receptors with the exception of the posterior one-fourth. The internal parts of the intervertebral disk have no sensory innervation at all.

By comparison the vertebral joints are rather abundantly innervated. Accordingly pathological processes of the spine, in the region of the anterior ligament, vertebrae, and intervertebral disk can remain clinically silent for a long time, while disorders in the rest of the movement segment (posterior ligament, vertebral canal, vertebral joints, space between spinal processes, and autochthonous muscles) usually present at an early stage.

In general, so-called *receptor pain* can be distinguished from *neuralgic pain* (see also "Sensory System" [p. 6] and "Nerve Root Lesions" [p. 110]). Receptor pain is caused by activation of the nociceptors in the area of the pathological process. It is perceived as blunt and pulling. The patients describe it as "rheumatic."

Neuralgic pain has a drilling character and is perceived as being sharper. While receptor pain cannot always be exactly located, neuralgic pain is characterized by the consistency of its extent within certain boundaries of sensory territories. The neuralgia is caused by compression of peripheral nerves or nerve roots (radicular syndrome). Receptor pain, however, is not accompanied by sensory or motor deficits; some forms are also called "pseudoradicular."

Because of the connection of the individual parts of the movement segment through reflexes, syndromes of the spine with and without peripheral nerve deficits and disturbances of blood supply are accompanied by verifiable changes in the region of those muscles and bone and joint structures that belong to the affected segment.

Certain trigger points with particular tenderness can be determined for individual movement segments. Trigger points are spots of increased sensitivity due to a located pathological process or "zones" that are particularly excitable due to referred pain. There are cutaneous, fascial, and periosteal trigger points.

Most disorders of the spine have a degenerative etiology. Lumbar syndromes occur most often, with a rate of 62%.

Spine syndrome can be caused by a number of pathological changes in the movement segment. There are also often concomitant dysfunctions of the vertebral joints. In almost every case they originate from changes in the intervertebral disks.

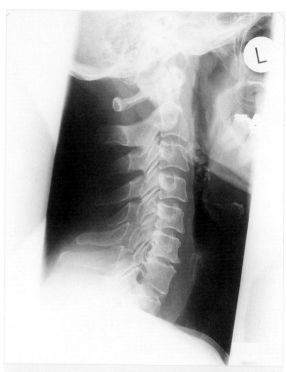

Fig. 3.1 Chondrosis and spondylosis of the cervical spine in segment C6/C7.

Acute and Chronic Cervical Syndrome

Definition

The pathogenesis and clinical picture mirror those of sciatica and the cause is degenerative changes in the region of the movement segment. There is an upper, a medial, and a lower cervical syndrome.

The upper cervical syndrome is characterized by pain in the neck and back of the head (cervical migraine).

The symptoms of the medial cervical syndrome are particularly manifold because, in addition to pain in the shoulder and neck, there can also develop disturbances of diaphragmatic innervation, heart sensations similar to angina pectoris, and dysfunctions of other organs. Additionally, dizziness, tinnitus, and impaired vision are reported, although the causal relationship is not discernible. These symptoms also develop with dysfunctions of the upper cervical spine—that is, of the so-called head joints (▸ Fig. 3.1). They are often combined with sometimes very severe paresthesia. The pathology, anatomy, and neurophysiology of these symptoms have not been fully elucidated, as opposed to those caused by the medial and lower cervical spine. There is a close relation to psychosomatic disorders.

Leading symptoms of the lower cervical syndrome are radicular pain and disturbed innervation of arms and hands. For all cervical syndromes it must be determined whether or not the vertebral artery is injured before applying a more intensive or even conservative therapy.

Findings

Increased turgor and muscle tone of the tissue can be found in the region of the cervical spine, shoulder, neck, and rib cage in segments C5–C8, T1–T6 and T12.

Tissue changes can be found in the following areas on the back of the body:
- Above the sacral bone, under the pelvic edges and on both sides along the lumbar spine
- On the edge of the latissimus dorsi muscle and of the teres major muscle
- Along the angle of the shoulder and neck along the trapezius muscle, descending part, the scalene muscles, the sternocleidomastoid and levator scapulae muscles, and the short extensors in the region of the head joints

The muscles of the neck and the anterior rib cage are permanently tense. The movements of the cervical spine are very limited and particular attention must be paid to the organ/segment relationship. For example, there may be heart disease, which triggers complaints in the neck/nape region.

Treatment Plan

Starting position: sitting, supine position, prone position.
- Small basic sequence, flat strokes over the back from caudal toward cranial.

- Small basic sequence, first sequence, flat strokes over the rib cage.
- Small basic sequence, first and second sequence, ventral side.
- Small basic sequence, first, second, and third sequence, ventral side.
- Small basic sequence, first, second, and third sequence, ventral side, treatment of face.

Balancing strokes over the pectoral muscles and dorsal dispersion strokes end each treatment session.

Additional Strokes

First Sequence (▶ Fig. 2.37, ▶ Fig. 2.38, ▶ Fig. 2.39)

▶ From dorsal
- When changing the direction, the intercostal strokes are also performed in the opposite direction, from the spine along the lateral thoracic wall to the ventral axillary line, in order to gently grasp the tissue there.
- The large balancing stroke starts in the ventral axillary line at the level of the sixth/seventh intercostal space and is broadly pulled around the lower angle of the scapula toward C7.
- Short strokes from the lower angle of the scapula to the spine at the level of segment T4.
- Flat transverse strokes over the spine, beginning at the level of T6 under the angle of the left scapula and ending under the angle of the right scapula and then back again.
- Small, flat transverse strokes along the spine, within the area of the long extensor spinae muscles, from T12 to T7.

▶ From ventral
- In the ventral intercostal area a set of flat strokes are pulled beginning at the dorsal axillary line through the intercostal spaces. These should start at the lowest ribs.

Second Sequence (▶ Fig. 2.46, ▶ Fig. 2.47, ▶ Fig. 2.48, ▶ Fig. 2.49)

▶ From dorsal
- Long downward stretching, along the edge of the latissimus dorsi muscle in the direction of the iliac crest.
- Prolonged upward stretching, beginning at the level of the sixth/seventh intercostal space, along the edge of the latissimus dorsi muscle in the direction of the axilla.
- Axillary stretching with elevated arm: the patient puts his or her arm on the therapist's shoulder. Connecting transverse strokes are applied through the axilla to thoroughly loosen the axillary fold.
- A flat fan-shaped stroke is pulled transversely over the scapula toward the shoulder joint, starting at the outer edge of the scapula and ending at the lower edge of the spine of the scapula.
- Small, flat transverse strokes over the spine, within the area of the long extensor spinae muscles, from T7 to T3 or C7.
- Flat transverse strokes from the inner side to the lateral edge of the scapulae, starting at the level of T7, ending at the spine of the scapula.
- Small hooks around the upper angle of the scapula followed by outlining the edge of the scapula with cutting strokes.

▶ From ventral
- The ventral edge of the trapezius muscle is pulled out starting from the cervical base, while pressing against it with the free hand.
- Strokes over the sternum, beginning at the xiphoid process, pulling toward the jugular notch.
- Short hooks on the connection points between the ribs and sternum, pulling from caudal to cranial.
- Short transverse strokes along the sternum. These start at the junction between the xiphoid process and the body of the sternum, along the area of the sternal angle. At the base of the second rib at the sternum, the strokes should become wider to just under the sternoclavicular joints.
- Short fanlike strokes on the suprasternal notch, beginning on the clavicle and ending on the dorsal edge of the sternocleidomastoid muscle.
- Short strokes on the interclavicular ligament.

Comments
- The treatment structure depends on the tension in the tissues.
- The small basic sequence should be performed two or three times and only then do the additional sequences follow.
- In the first sequence the intercostal strokes are applied in both directions to improve the mobility of the ribs to lift the rib cage and the posture of the head.
- In the second sequence the therapist should intensively work through the area of the scapula.
- In the third sequence when the complaints are only on one side, the neck stroke is to be applied on the unaffected side first. When the tension in the tissue loosens, treatment is administered to the affected side.
- The patient's posture at work should be analyzed.

Thoracic Syndrome

Definition

Thoracic syndrome with dysfunction of the costovertebral joints is more frequently found in younger people in comparison with the number of cervical and lumbar syndromes because damage of the intervertebral disk mostly develops in the thoracic spine before developing in the cervical and lumbar spine. Thoracic syndromes are typical after surgery involving extensive stretching of the rib cage.

Root irritations in the chest area manifest themselves as intercostal neuralgia. The spreading of the pain to the torso cannot always be distinctively attributed to a dermatome as with the extremities. This may easily lead to confusion due to the projection of pain into the Head's zones in disorders of intestinal organs. Slipped disks must also be taken into consideration if the thoracic spine is involved. They are rare but they are dangerous, since they can lead to paraplegia.

In the differential diagnosis, the sternal syndrome that originates in the sternocostal joints must be distinguished.

Findings

The patients complain about pain radiating into the intercostal spaces, which is mostly present on only one side. There is increased tone in the lateral part of the erector spinae muscle.

Treatment Plan

Starting position: sitting, supine position.
- Small basic sequence, flat strokes over the back from caudal to cranial.
- Small basic sequence, first sequence, flat strokes over the rib cage.
- Small basic sequence, first and second sequence.

Balancing strokes over the pectoral muscles and dorsal dispersion strokes end each treatment session.

Additional Strokes

First Sequence

(See ► Fig. 2.37, ► Fig. 2.38, ► Fig. 2.39.)

► From dorsal
- When changing the direction, the intercostal strokes are also performed in the opposite direction from the spine along the lateral thoracic wall to the axillary line in order to gently grasp the tissue there.
- The large balancing stroke begins in the ventral axillary line at the level of the sixth/seventh intercostal space and is broadly pulled around the lower angle of the scapula toward C7.
- Short strokes from the lower angle of the scapula to the spine at the level of segment T4.
- Flat transverse strokes are made over the spine, beginning at the level of T6 under the angle of the left scapula and ending under the angle of the right scapula and then back again.

- Small, flat transverse strokes along the spine, within the area of the long extensor spinae muscles, from T12 to T7.

► From ventral
- In the ventral intercostal area a set of flat strokes are pulled beginning at the dorsal axillary line through the intercostal spaces. These should start at the lowest ribs.

Second Sequence (► Fig. 2.46, ► Fig. 2.47, ► Fig. 2.48, ► Fig. 2.49)

► From dorsal
- Long downward stretching, along the edge of the latissimus dorsi muscle in the direction of the iliac crest.
- Prolonged upward stretching, beginning at the level of the sixth/seventh intercostal space, along the edge of the latissimus dorsi muscle in the direction of the axilla.
- Axillary stretching with elevated arm: the patient puts his or her arm on the therapist's shoulder. Connecting transverse strokes are applied through the axilla to thoroughly loosen the axillary fold.
- A flat fan-shaped stroke is pulled transversely over the scapula toward the shoulder joint, starting at the outer edge of the scapula and ending at the lower edge of the spine of the scapula.
- Small, flat transverse strokes over the spine, within the area of the long extensor spinae muscles, from T7 to T3 or C7.
- Flat transverse strokes from the inner side to the lateral edge of the scapulae, starting at the level of T7, ending at the spine of the scapula.
- Small hooks around the upper angle of the scapula followed by outlining the edge of the scapula with cutting strokes.

► From ventral
- The ventral edge of the trapezius muscle is pulled out starting from the cervical base, while pressing against it with the free hand.
- Strokes over the sternum, beginning at the xiphoid process and pulling toward the jugular notch.
- Short hooks on the connection points between the ribs and sternum, pulling from caudal to cranial.
- Short transverse strokes along the sternum. These start at the junction between the xiphoid process and the body of the sternum, along the area of the sternal angle. At the base of the second rib at the sternum, the strokes should become wider to just under the sternoclavicular joints.
- Short fanlike strokes on the suprasternal notch, beginning on the clavicle and ending on the dorsal edge of the sternocleidomastoid muscle.
- Short strokes on the interclavicular ligament.

Comments

- If a block of the costovertebral joints is diagnosed, it should be treated with manual therapy. Mobilization of the joints may itself alleviate the pain.
- The patient's posture at the workplace should be analyzed.

Sciatica and Chronic Lumbar Syndrome

Definition

Sciatica is the acute onset of back pain that subsides after a few days with fast developing reflex tension of the all of the back muscles that fixates the lumbar spine in malposition. The extremely hard back muscles extend and intensify the pain. All abdominal muscles are also involved.

The goal of treatment with CTM, physical therapy, and other physical measures is to interrupt the pain reflex and to loosen the muscles. In administering CTM, the therapist carefully approaches the center from the marginal areas.

The muscles do not always show the characteristic increase of tone with chronic lumbar syndrome. Remarkable, however, is the persistent spasm of the quadratus lumborum muscle. Chronic pain requires exact diagnosis—for example, in respect to neurological disorders, gynecological conditions, osteoporosis, vertebral metastases, or onset of ankylosing spondylitis.

The orthopedist must clarify whether damage to the intervertebral disk (chondrosis) has caused a slipped disk, narrowing of the spinal canal (spinal canal stenosis), or instability (abnormal mobility of two vertebrae with respect to each other) (▸ Fig. 3.2).

Findings

Increased turgor and muscle tone of the tissue can be found in the region of the lumbar spine, pelvis, and leg, in segments T12, L1–L5, and S1–S3. The abdominal wall is particularly tense. The external and internal oblique muscles of the abdomen, the transverse muscle of the abdomen, and the iliopsoas muscle are affected by this. Pain foci are found on the edges of the sacral bone and in the erector spinae muscle along the course of the spine.

Special tissue changes can be found under the pelvic edges, in the lesser gluteal muscles, and around the trochanters. Also in the region of the attachment of pelvitrochanteric muscles, in the course of the iliotibial tract, on

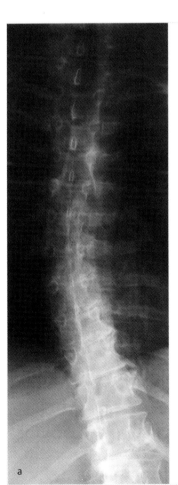
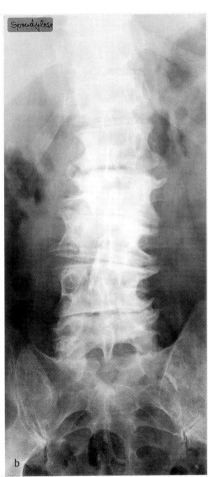

Fig. 3.2 Spondylosis of the thoracic spine with degenerative changes on the costovertebral joints.
a With severe chondrosis and spondylosis of the lumbar spine.
b With osseous protuberances on the vertebral edges and reduced height of the intervertebral spaces.

the muscular edges of the adductor muscles, and in the region of the pubic bone tissue there are palpable changes that extend to the abdominal wall.

Treatment Plan

Starting position: lateral position, lying on the affected side.
- Small basic sequence, flat strokes over the back from caudal toward cranial.
- Small basic sequence, first sequence, ventral side of the body, flat strokes over the rib cage.
- Small basic sequence, first sequence, ventral side of the body, treatment of the thighs, flat strokes over lower leg and foot.

Balancing strokes over the pectoral muscles, dorsal dispersion strokes, and flat strokes of the legs are applied at the end of each treatment session to support the venous back flow.

Additional Strokes

Basic Sequence (▶ Fig. 2.27, ▶ Fig. 2.28, ▶ Fig. 2.29)

▶ **From dorsal**
- Hooks to the sacral bone edges from caudal to cranial.
- Flat transverse strokes over the sacral bone, from caudal to cranial.
- Hooks, in the course of the first pelvic stroke.
- Small, flat transverse strokes along the spine, within the area of the long extensor spinae muscles, from L5 to T12.
- Grasping and stretching stroke at the ischial tuberosity.
- Stretching stroke in the region of the lumbar triangle.

First Sequence (▶ Fig. 2.37, ▶ Fig. 2.38, ▶ Fig. 2.39)

▶ **From dorsal**
- When changing the direction, the intercostal strokes are also performed in the opposite direction from the spine along the lateral thoracic wall to the ventral axillary line in order to gently grasp the tissue there.
- The large balancing stroke starts in the ventral axillary line at the level of the sixth/seventh intercostal space and is broadly pulled around the lower angle of the scapula toward C7.
- Short strokes from the lower angle of the scapula to the spine at the level of segment T4.
- Flat transverse strokes over the spine, beginning at the level of T6 under the angle of the left scapula and ending under the angle of the right scapula and then back again.
- Small, flat transverse strokes along the spine, within the area of the long extensor spinae muscles, from T12 to T7.

▶ **From ventral**
- In the ventral intercostal area a set of flat strokes are pulled beginning at the dorsal axillary line through the intercostal spaces. These should start at the lowest ribs.
- Bimanual strokes, from dorsal at the lower edge of the rib cage to the medioclavicular line and from the pelvic edge to the anterior superior iliac spine. These strokes are performed bimanually, first on one side then on the other side of the body.
- Short hooks along the rectus sheath from the symphysis to the level of the navel.
- Short strokes, like rays, pulling toward the navel.
- Bimanual strokes crossing over the abdominal walls, starting in the dorsal region and ending at the opposite edge of the rectus abdominis muscle.

▶ **On the leg** (▶ Fig. 2.70)
- Short hooks from the last third of the fascia lata, in the shape of a fan toward the patella.
- The thigh stroke starts in the upper third of the thigh, on the lateral edge of the sartorius muscle, and ends shortly before the groin.
- Flat strokes, which are pulled from the transverse intergluteal cleft to the popliteal cavity.
- Flat strokes from the inner side of the thigh, starting below the patella and traveling around the medial malleolus.
- Bimanual stretching between the muscle bellies of the gastrocnemius muscle, from cranial to caudal, pulling in the direction of the Achilles tendon.

Comments

- Due to the extensive tension the pull can be perceived as very painful in the skin tissue. If this is the case, the therapist should not continue to treat with CTM. When the tension decreases, the strokes of the small basic sequence are performed.
- After CTM, a rolled-up hot pack is moved over the upper abdomen, over the lower edges of the ribs, over the quadratus lumborum muscle, and along the pelvic edges to the area of the trochanter.
- The therapist should pay particular attention to the patient's constitution and physical reaction. Sitting incorrectly at work or in furniture that is too low, and faulty posture involving the head, rib cage, and pelvis of the patient frequently triggers these recurrent complaints.

Ankylosing Spondylitis (Bekhterev Disease)

Definition

This is a chronic form of rheumatic systemic disease, occurring in bouts, that especially affects the spine. The inflammatory changes start on both sacroiliac joints and on the thoracolumbar junction. From there they can spread to other parts of the spine. The inflammatory changes affect not only the ligaments and intervertebral disks but also the vertebral joints.

The ossification of the ligaments that is so typical of this disease is an independent, inflammation-independent process, which can cause eventual fusion of the spine (bamboo pole). Women and men are equally affected, but disease usually takes a less severe course in women.

In its initial stage, the inflammatory lower back pain is the leading diagnostic finding. In contrast to the back pain caused by degeneration, this type of back pain mostly develops before the age of 45 years. It responds immediately to the administration of nonsteroidal antirheumatics.

If left untreated, the disease lasts longer than 3 months and usually progresses. Nocturnal pain, morning stiffness, and pseudoradicular pain radiation are characteristic. The soft tissue symptoms at the torso are the same as those of lumbar syndrome.

Almost no therapeutic success can be expected once the patient reaches the end stage with complete fusion and malformation of the spine. The most important treatment goals in the early stages of the disease are to maintain the mobility of the costovertebral joints, vertebral joints, and respiratory movements of the rib cage and to avoid malformation of the spine (round back). This helps to prevent the frequently developing disturbances of lung function and cardiopulmonary insufficiency.

In addition to the physical therapy and CTM, complex treatment measures must be employed as with all other rheumatic diseases.

Findings

Increased turgor and muscle tone affect the torso and the area of the shoulder and hip joints close to the torso. They are located in the segments C3–C8, T1–T12, L1–L4.

▶ **On the posterior side of the body**
- On the sacral bone and on the edges of the sacral bone
- Along the erector spinae muscle and on the lower edges of the ribs
- Around the scapula and in the region of the neck and shoulder

▶ **On the anterior side of the body**
- On the edges of the sternocleidomastoid, levator scapulae, and scalene muscles
- On and under the clavicle
- On the muscle edges of the latissimus dorsi muscle, on the anterior delta portion, and on the pectoralis major muscle
- On the origin of the rectus abdominis muscle in the epigastric angle, extending in the caudal direction to both sides of the rectus sheath
- On the far bottom edge of the ribs
- In the intercostal spaces

- On the leg: on the adductors, around the greater trochanter and the iliotibial tract

Treatment Plan

Starting position: sitting, lateral position, supine position.
- Small basic sequence, flat strokes over the back from caudal toward cranial.
- Small basic sequence, first sequence, flat strokes over the rib cage.
- Small basic sequence, first and second sequence, ventral side.
- Small basic sequence, first, second, and third sequence, ventral side.

Balancing strokes over the pectoral muscles and dorsal dispersion strokes end each treatment session.

Additional Strokes
Small Basic Sequence (▶ Fig. 2.27, ▶ Fig. 2.28, ▶ Fig. 2.29)

▶ **From dorsal**
- Hooks to the sacral bone edges from caudal to cranial.
- Flat transverse strokes over the sacral bone, from caudal to cranial.
- Hooks, in the course of the first pelvic stroke.
- Small, flat transverse strokes along the spine, within the area of the long extensor spinae muscles, from L5 to T12.
- Hooks and stretching strokes at the ischial tuberosity.
- Stretching strokes in the region of the lumbar triangle.
- Fanlike strokes in the upper respiratory angle: Fanlike strokes are applied to the angle between the lowest rib and the spine in flat strokes. These should start at the lower edge of the rib cage and end with the last strokes along the spine (L3 to T12).

Small Basic Sequence in Lateral Position (▶ Fig. 2.33)

▶ **From dorsal**
- Small hooks around the greater trochanter.
- Flat balancing stroke, starting above the greater trochanter toward the ischial tuberosity.

Small Basic Sequence in Prone Position (▶ Fig. 2.33)

▶ **From dorsal**
- Short hooks along the intergluteal cleft pulling up from the lateral side.

First Sequence (▶ Fig. 2.37, ▶ Fig. 2.38, ▶ Fig. 2.39)

▶ **From dorsal**
- When changing the direction, the intercostal strokes are also performed in the opposite direction from the

spine along the lateral thoracic wall to the ventral axillary line in order to gently grasp the tissue there.

- The large balancing stroke starts in the ventral axillary line at the level of the sixth/seventh intercostal space and is broadly pulled around the lower angle of the scapula toward C7.
- Short strokes from the lower angle of the scapula to the spine at the level of segment T4.
- Flat transverse strokes over the spine, beginning at the level of T6 under the angle of the left scapula and ending under the angle of the right scapula and then back again.
- Small, flat transverse strokes along the spine, within the area of the long extensor spinae muscles, from T12 to T7.

▶ **From ventral**
- In the ventral intercostal area a set of flat strokes are pulled beginning at the dorsal axillary line through the intercostal spaces. These should start at the lowest ribs.
- Bimanual strokes, from dorsal on the lower edge of the rib cage to the medioclavicular line and from the pelvic edge to the anterior superior iliac spine. These strokes are performed bimanually, first on one side then on the other side of the body.
- Short hooks along the rectus sheath from the symphysis to the level of the navel.
- Short strokes, like rays, pulling toward the navel.
- Bimanual strokes crossing over the abdominal walls, starting in the dorsal region and ending at the opposite edge of the rectus abdominis muscle.

Second Sequence (▶ Fig. 2.46, ▶ Fig. 2.47, ▶ Fig. 2.48, ▶ Fig. 2.49)

▶ **From dorsal**
- Long downward stretching, along the edge of the latissimus dorsi muscle in the direction of the iliac crest.
- Prolonged upward stretching, beginning at the level of the sixth/seventh intercostal space, along the edge of the latissimus dorsi muscle in the direction of the axilla.
- Axillary stretching with elevated arm: the patient puts his or her arm on the therapist's shoulder. Connecting transverse strokes are applied through the axilla to thoroughly loosen the axillary fold.
- A flat fan-shaped stroke is pulled transversely over the scapula toward the shoulder joint, starting at the outer edge of the scapula and ending at the lower edge of the spine of the scapula.
- Small, flat transverse strokes over the spine, within the area of the long extensor spinae muscles, from T7 to T3 or C7.
- Flat transverse strokes from the inner side to the lateral edge of the scapulae, starting at the level of T7, ending at the spine of the scapula.
- Small hooks around the upper angle of the scapula followed by outlining the edge of the scapula with cutting strokes.

▶ **From ventral**
- The ventral edge of the trapezius muscle is pulled out starting from the cervical base, while pressing against it with the free hand.
- Strokes over the sternum, beginning at the xiphoid process, pulling toward the jugular notch.
- Short hooks on the connection points between the ribs and sternum, pulling from caudal to cranial.
- Short transverse strokes along the sternum. These start at the junction between the xiphoid process and the body of the sternum, along the area of the sternal angle. At the base of the second rib at the sternum, the strokes should become wider to just under the sternoclavicular joints.
- Short fanlike strokes on the suprasternal notch, beginning on the clavicle and ending on the dorsal edge of the sternocleidomastoid muscle.
- Short strokes on the right interclavicular ligament.

▶ **On the leg** (▶ **Fig. 2.70**)
- Short hooks from the last third of the fascia lata, in the shape of a fan toward the patella.
- The thigh stroke starts in the upper third of the thigh, on the lateral edge of the sartorius muscle, and ends shortly before the groin.
- Flat strokes, which are pulled from the transverse intergluteal cleft to the popliteal cavity.
- Flat strokes from the inner side of the thigh, starting below the patella and running around the medial malleolus.
- Bimanual stretching between the muscle bellies of the gastrocnemius muscle, from cranial to caudal, pulling in the direction of the Achilles tendon.

Comments

- The small basic sequence must be applied intensively. In the additional sequences special emphasis is placed on working the tissue next to the spine. The region of the neck and anterior rib cage must be carefully integrated into the treatment process.
- The best way to relax the tissue in the region of the rib cage is to first apply just the right amount of CTM and then slowly advance to the technique with cutting strokes depending on the condition of the tissue. This enables deeper respiration, which subsequently significantly improves wellbeing.
- The application of CTM must be planned as long-term therapy with pauses in treatment.

Scoliosis

Definition

Scoliosis is a lateral, fixed curvature of the spine with rotation of the vertebrae against each other. Idiopathic scoliosis is the most frequent form and is determined

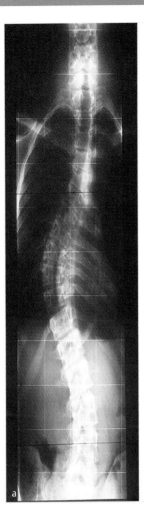
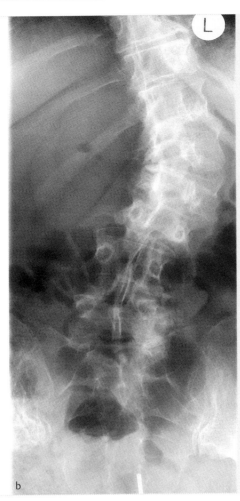

Fig. 3.3 S-shaped scolioses.
a S-shaped scoliosis.
b Severe secondary degenerations with gliding vertebrae can be seen.

genetically. Unlike in the congenital form, no changes of the spine are present at birth. Secondary scoliosis develops after inflammations or injuries of the spine. Various other pathological conditions can also lead to the development of scoliosis: for example, neuromuscular diseases or Scheuermann disease.

Scoliosis as a malformation of the spine must be distinguished from the scoliotic malposition, which is caused, for example, when the legs differ in length or in the event of a slipped disk (sciatic scoliosis).

Scoliosis results in a deformation of the thorax, because the ribs follow the rotation of the spine toward convexity and are pushed into each other on the concave side of the curvature (▸ Fig. 3.3).

The severity of the scoliosis is determined by measuring the angle of the curvature. Severe scoliosis leads to respiratory disturbances, which may subsequently lead to cardiac insufficiency. Due to the special significance of the complications affecting the intrathoracic organs, these thoracic deformations are discussed in the section Disorders in Internal Medicine (p. 124) later in this chapter.

The administration of CTM and physical therapy treatment primarily reduces muscular dysfunctions and thereby has a positive effect on the malposition of the spine that is present in scoliosis. For the same reason, CTM and physical therapy can be employed effectively with other deformities of the spine and thorax (roundback, hollow back, flat back, funnel chest, pigeon chest).

Findings

Increased turgor and muscle tone are located over the back and abdominal area. They are most distinctively palpable on the vertex of the scoliosis. The tissue of the dermis and hypodermis is in an elevated state of tension due to the changed turgor and tone. This may be intensified by uneven traction on the muscles.

The torso must be palpated very thoroughly with scoliosis that has persisted for some time, because tissue changes may obscure organic findings. Checking with the patient can help to ascertain the findings.

Treatment Plan

Starting position: sitting, supine position.
- Small basic sequence, flat strokes over the back from caudal toward cranial.
- Small basic sequence, first sequence, flat strokes over the rib cage.
- Small basic sequence, first and second sequence, ventral side.

Balancing strokes over the pectoral muscles and dorsal dispersion strokes end each treatment session.

Additional Strokes

Small Basic Sequence (▶ Fig. 2.27, ▶ Fig. 2.28, ▶ Fig. 2.29)

▶ **From dorsal**
- Hooks to the sacral bone edges from caudal to cranial.
- Flat transverse strokes over the sacral bone, from caudal to cranial.
- Hooks, in the course of the first pelvic stroke.
- Small, flat transverse strokes along the spine, within the area of the long extensor spinae muscles, from L5 to T12.
- Grasping and stretching stroke at the ischial tuberosity.
- Stretching stroke in the region of the lumbar triangle.
- Fanlike strokes in the upper respiratory angle: Fanlike strokes are broadly applied to the angle between the lowest rib and the spine. These should start on the lower edge of the rib cage and end with the last strokes along the spine (L3 to T12).

First Sequence (▶ Fig. 2.37, ▶ Fig. 2.38, ▶ Fig. 2.39)

▶ **From dorsal**
- When changing the direction, the intercostal strokes are also performed in the opposite direction, from the spine along the lateral thoracic wall to the ventral axillary line, in order to gently grasp the tissue there.
- The large balancing stroke starts in the ventral axillary line at the level of the sixth/seventh intercostal space and is broadly pulled around the lower angle of the scapula toward C7.
- Short strokes from the lower angle of the scapula to the spine at the level of segment T4.
- Flat transverse strokes over the spine, beginning at the level of T6 under the angle of the left scapula and ending under the angle of the right scapula and then back again.
- Small, flat transverse strokes along the spine, within the area of the long extensor spinae muscles, from T12 to T7.

▶ **From ventral**
- In the ventral intercostal area a set of flat strokes are pulled beginning at the dorsal axillary line through the intercostal spaces. These should start at the lowest ribs.

- Bimanual strokes, from dorsal on the lower edge of the rib cage to the medioclavicular line and from the pelvic edge to the anterior superior iliac spine. These strokes are performed bimanually, first on one side then on the other.
- Short hooks along the rectus sheath from the symphysis to the level of the navel.
- Short strokes, like rays, pulling toward the navel.
- Bimanual strokes crossing over the abdominal walls, starting in the dorsal region and ending at the opposite edge of the rectus abdominis muscle.

Second Sequence (▶ Fig. 2.46, ▶ Fig. 2.47, ▶ Fig. 2.48, ▶ Fig. 2.49)

▶ **From dorsal**
- Long downward stretching, along the edge of the latissimus dorsi muscle in the direction of the iliac crest.
- Prolonged upward stretching, beginning at the level of the sixth/seventh intercostal space, along the edge of the latissimus dorsi muscle in the direction of the axilla.
- Axillary stretching with elevated arm: the patient puts his or her arm on the therapist's shoulder. Connecting transverse strokes are applied through the axilla to thoroughly loosen the axillary fold.
- A flat fan-shaped stroke is pulled transversely over the scapula toward the shoulder joint, starting at the outer edge of the scapula and ending at the lower edge of the spine of the scapula.
- Small, flat transverse strokes over the spine, within the area of the long extensor spinae muscles, from T7 to T3 or C7.
- Flat transverse strokes from the inner side to the lateral edge of the scapulae, starting at the level of T7, ending at the spine of the scapula.
- Small hooks around the upper angle of the scapula followed by outlining the edge of the scapula with cutting strokes.

▶ **From ventral**
- The ventral edge of the trapezius muscle is pulled out starting from the cervical base, while pressing against it with the free hand.
- Strokes over the sternum, beginning at the xiphoid process pulling toward the jugular notch.
- Short hooks on the connection points between the ribs and sternum, pulling from caudal to cranial.
- Short transverse strokes along the sternum. These start at the junction between the xiphoid process and the body of the sternum, along the area of the sternal angle. At the base of the second rib at the sternum, the strokes should become wider to just under the sternoclavicular joints.

Comments

- The effects produced by CTM offer an excellent starting point for the success of subsequent physical therapy.

- CTM improves the blood supply of the muscles in poor postures, round back, flat back, and funnel chest and makes them more stretchable for physical therapy treatment. Lifting the sternum and thorax has a particularly beneficial effect on posture. The patient should be advised to use backstroke when swimming.

Congenital Torticollis

Definition

During breech delivery there may be pulling of the sternocleidomastoid muscle, with bleeding into the muscles. These hematomas lead to a reconfiguration of the affected muscle fiber parts at the level of the connective tissue, with shortening and loss of their elasticity as well as tilting of the head to one side. The child's head is tilted to the affected side and the face is turned to the opposite side. Such a wry neck can also be caused by a forced posture of the fetus while in the uterus. Osseous malformations may also be a cause of torticollis.

Physical therapy with redressing of the cervical spine, and long-term regular CTM (if necessary with fixation of the head in overcorrection) are implemented. Surgical correction of the shortened muscle can also be considered.

Findings

Increased turgor and muscle tone of the tissue are found in the area of the neck and shoulder girdle and even in the rib cage. These findings are located in the segments C2–C8, T1–T6. Tissue changes can be palpated on the attachment and origin of the sternocleidomastoid, levator scapulae, and scalene muscles. The latissimus dorsi and teres major muscles, the trapezius muscle, descending, transverse and ascending part, and the pectoralis major muscle show reduced mobility on the muscle edges.

Treatment Plan

Starting position: lateral position, lying on the unaffected side, prone position.
- Small basic sequence, flat strokes over the rib cage from caudal toward cranial.
- Small basic sequence, first sequence, flat strokes over the rib cage.
- Small basic sequence, first and second sequence, ventral side.
- Small basic sequence, first and second sequence, treatment of upper arm, ventral side.
- Small basic sequence, first, second, and third sequence, treatment of upper arm, ventral side.
- Small basic sequence, first, second, and third sequence, treatment of upper arm, ventral side, treatment of face.

Balancing strokes over the pectoral muscles and dorsal dispersion strokes end each treatment session.

Additional Strokes

First Sequence (▶ Fig. 2.37, ▶ Fig. 2.38, ▶ Fig. 2.39)

▶ **From dorsal**
- When changing the direction, the intercostal strokes are also performed in the opposite direction from the spine along the lateral thoracic wall to the ventral axillary line in order to gently grasp the tissue there.
- The large balancing stroke starts in the ventral axillary line at the level of the sixth/seventh intercostal space and is broadly pulled around the lower angle of the scapula toward C7.
- Short strokes from the lower angle of the scapula to the spine at the level of segment T4.
- Flat transverse strokes over the spinal column, beginning at the level of T6 under the angle of the left scapula and ending under the angle of the right scapula and then back again.
- Small, flat transverse strokes along the spine, within the area of the long extensor spinae muscles, from T12 to T7.

▶ **From ventral**
- In the ventral intercostal area a set of flat strokes are pulled, beginning at the dorsal axillary line through the intercostal spaces. These should start at the lowest ribs.

Second Sequence (▶ Fig. 2.46, ▶ Fig. 2.47, ▶ Fig. 2.48, ▶ Fig. 2.49)

▶ **From dorsal**
- Long downward stretching strokes, along the edge of the latissimus dorsi muscle in the direction of the iliac crest.
- Prolonged upward stretching strokes, beginning at the level of the sixth/seventh intercostal space, along the edge of the latissimus dorsi muscle in the direction of the axilla.
- Axillary stretching with elevated arm: the patient puts his or her arm on the therapist's shoulder. Connecting transverse strokes are applied through the axilla to thoroughly loosen the axillary fold.
- A flat fan-shaped stroke is pulled transversely over the scapula toward the shoulder joint, starting at the outer edge of the scapula and ending at the lower edge of the spine of the scapula.
- Small, flat transverse strokes over the spine, within the area of the long extensor spinae muscles, from T7 to T3 or C7.
- Flat transverse strokes from the inner side to the lateral edge of the scapulae, starting at the level of T7, ending at the spine of the scapula.
- Small hooks around the upper angle of the scapula followed by outlining the edge of the scapula with cutting strokes.

▶ **From ventral**
- The ventral edge of the trapezius muscle is pulled out starting from the cervical base, while pressing against it with the free hand.
- Strokes over the sternum, beginning at the xiphoid process pulling toward the jugular notch.
- Short hooks on the connection points between the ribs and sternum, pulling from caudal to cranial.
- Short transverse strokes along the sternum. These start at the junction between the xiphoid process and the body of the sternum, along the area of the sternal angle. At the base of the second rib at the sternum, the strokes should become wider to just under the sternoclavicular joints.
- Short fanlike strokes on the suprasternal notch, beginning on the clavicle and ending on the dorsal edge of the sternocleidomastoid muscle.
- Short strokes on the interclavicular ligament.

Comments

- The strokes on the shoulder girdle and neck are first applied to the unaffected side. When the tension in the tissue of the affected side subsides, the strokes are moved to that side.
- Physical therapy treatment should always be administered before CTM, since after CTM the patient requires sufficient rest with good positioning of the head.

3.3.2 Fractures and Contractures of the Upper Extremity

Connective tissue massage is not indicated in fractures that have healed without complications. Treatment by physical therapy plays the major role here.

CTM can be applied when immobilization or concomitant injuries of soft tissue cause hardening of muscles, adhesions in the connective tissue of the muscular septa obstructing gliding systems, or even stiffening of the joints. Post-traumatic circulatory disturbances, edemas, and the effects of compartment syndrome can be successfully treated with CTM. Treatment should be administered as early as possible.

The diagnostics provide information for selecting the technique and the intensity of its application. When the tissue's response demands it, additional strokes are applied for relaxation or stimulation.

As a rule of thumb, CTM should be applied after physical therapy, since the patient must rest after the treatment.

The treatment goals are the same for the upper and for the lower extremities. These are to
- Loosen the hardening and adhesions in the periarticular and subcutaneous connective tissue
- Restore the obstructed gliding function of muscles and tendons
- Loosen muscle attachments and origins
- Support circulation from the segments C5–T1 and L2.

Fractures and Contractures of the Shoulders

Findings

Increased turgor and muscle tone are located in the region of the shoulder and arm in segments C5–C8, T1–T6, T12, and L2.

▶ **Tense tissue on the posterior side of the body**
- Extending below the spine of the scapula into the posterior axillary wall
- On the lower angle of the scapula, along the latissimus dorsi muscle toward the pelvic edge and along the axillary line extending under the axilla

▶ **On the anterior side of the body**
- Extending over the clavicle toward the shoulder joint
- Below the clavicle, on the sternoclavicular joint, along the subclavius muscle
- On the anterior part of the deltoid muscle extending to the upper arm
- Along the lower edge of the ribs, extending toward the rectus abdominis muscle

▶ **On the arm**
- Extending from the origin of the triceps muscle of the upper arm to the insertion of the elbow
- In the region of the flexor of the elbow and hand, on the medial epicondyle of the upper arm, extending into the wrist

Treatment Plan

Starting position: sitting, supine position.
- Small basic sequence, flat strokes over back and arms.
- Small basic sequence, first sequence, flat strokes over rib cage and arms.
- Small basic sequence, first and second sequence, ventral side, flat strokes on the arms.
- Small basic sequence, first and second sequence, ventral side of the body, treatment of the upper arm, flat strokes of forearm and hand.
- Small basic sequence, first, second, and third sequence, ventral side, treatment of arm.

Balancing strokes over the pectoral muscles and dorsal dispersion strokes and strokes on the arms to support the venous backflow end each treatment session.

Additional Strokes

First Sequence (▶ Fig. 2.37, ▶ Fig. 2.38, ▶ Fig. 2.39)

▶ **From dorsal**
- When changing the direction, the intercostal strokes are also performed in the opposite direction from the

spine along the lateral thoracic wall to the ventral axillary line in order to gently grasp the tissue there.
- The large balancing stroke starts in the ventral axillary line at the level of the sixth/seventh intercostal space and is broadly pulled around the lower angle of the scapula toward C7.
- Short strokes from the lower angle of the scapula to the spine at the level of segment T4.
- Flat transverse strokes over the spine, beginning at the level of T6 under the angle of the left scapula and ending under the angle of the right scapula and then back again.
- Small, flat transverse strokes along the spine, within the area of the long extensor spinae muscles, from T12 to T7.

▶ **From ventral**
- In the ventral intercostal area a set of flat strokes are pulled, beginning at the dorsal axillary line through the intercostal spaces. These should start at the lowest ribs.
- Bimanual strokes, from dorsal on the lower edge of the rib cage to the medioclavicular line and from the pelvic edge to the anterior superior iliac spine. These strokes are performed bimanually, first on one side of the body, then on the other side.
- Short hooks along the rectus sheath from the symphysis up to the navel.
- Short strokes, like rays, pulling toward the navel.
- Bimanual strokes crossing over the abdominal walls, starting in the dorsal region and ending at the opposite edge of the rectus abdominis muscle.

Second Sequence (▶ Fig. 2.46, ▶ Fig. 2.47, ▶ Fig. 2.48, ▶ Fig. 2.49)

▶ **From dorsal**
- Long downward stretching, along the edge of the latissimus dorsi muscle in the direction of the iliac crest.
- Prolonged upward stretching, beginning at the level of the sixth/seventh intercostal space, along the edge of the latissimus dorsi muscle in the direction of the axilla.
- Axillary stretching with elevated arm: the patient puts his or her arm on the therapist's shoulder. Connecting transverse strokes are applied through the axilla to thoroughly loosen the axillary fold.
- A flat fan-shaped stroke is pulled transversely over the scapula toward the shoulder joint, starting at the outer edge of the scapula and ending at the lower edge of the spine of the scapula.
- Small, flat transverse strokes over the spine, within the area of the long extensor spinae muscles, from T7 to T3 or C7.
- Flat transverse strokes from the inner side to the lateral edge of the scapulae, starting at the level of T7, ending at the spine of the scapula.

- Small hooks around the upper angle of the scapula followed by outlining the edge of the scapula with cutting strokes.

▶ **From ventral**
- The ventral edge of the trapezius muscle is pulled out starting from the cervical base, while pressing against it with the free hand.
- Strokes over the sternum, beginning at the xiphoid process pulling toward the jugular notch.
- Short hooks on the connection points between the ribs and sternum, pulling from caudal to cranial.
- Short transverse strokes along the sternum. These start at the junction between the xiphoid process and the body of the sternum, along the area of the sternal angle. At the base of the second rib at the sternum, the strokes should become wider to just under the sternoclavicular joints.
- Short fanlike strokes on the suprasternal notch, beginning on the clavicle and ending on the dorsal edge of the sternocleidomastoid muscle.
- Short strokes on the interclavicular ligament.

▶ **On the arm**
- Bimanual soft stretching of flexor and extensor of the upper arm.

Comments

- The first sequence immediately follows the small basic sequence in one session depending on the condition of the tissue.
- If the tension in the tissue has not yet sufficiently loosened, the second sequence can be applied first to the unaffected side.
- Experience shows that applying the third sequence has proven effective in extremely stubborn cases.
- The same treatment plan is employed for the treatment of contracture in the shoulder joint. Special emphasis should be placed then on the additional strokes. Application of a rolled-up hot pack in the region of neck, shoulder, and arm after CTM supports the effects of CTM and improves the gliding between the muscular septa.

Fractures and Contractures of the Elbow

Findings

Increased turgor and muscle tone are located in segments C3–C8, especially segment C6. Almost all segments are affected in the thoracic area, probably caused by the cervical innervation of the latissimus dorsi muscle.

▶ **On the posterior side of the body**
- Increased tension is located in the area of the entire back, the shoulder girdle, along the spinous processes

of the thoracic vertebrae, and on the edge of the latissimus dorsi muscle up to the axilla.
- There is an especially tender spot on the scapula, just under the spine of the scapula in T2, which must be considered and treated as the maximal point.
- Distensions can often be observed between the spinal column and on the scapula of the affected side.

▶ **Arm**
- The tissue of the deltoid muscle and triceps muscle of the upper arm is in a higher state of tension.
- Also the tissue in the crook of the elbow and the forearm down to the wrist has altered stretchability.
- Atrophy of the muscles develops when the illness lasts for extended periods.

Treatment Plan

Starting position: sitting, supine position
- Small basic sequence, flat strokes over back and arm.
- Small basic sequence, first sequence, flat strokes over back and arm.
- Small basic sequence, first and second sequence, ventral side, flat strokes over back and arm.
- Small basic sequence, first and second sequence, ventral side, treatment of upper arm, flat strokes on the arm.
- Small basic sequence, first and second sequence, ventral side, treatment of arm.
- Small basic sequence, first, second, and third sequence, treatment of the arm, ventral side, flat strokes on the arm.

Balancing strokes over the pectoral muscles, dorsal dispersion strokes, and strokes on the arms to support the venous backflow end each treatment session.

Additional Strokes

First Sequence (▶ Fig. 2.37, ▶ Fig. 2.38, ▶ Fig. 2.39)

▶ **From dorsal**
- When changing the direction, the intercostal strokes are also performed in the opposite direction from the spine along the lateral thoracic wall to the ventral axillary line in order to gently grasp the tissue there.
- The large balancing stroke starts in the ventral axillary line at the level of the sixth/seventh intercostal space and is broadly pulled around the lower angle of the scapula toward C7.
- Short strokes from the lower angle of the scapula to the spine at the level of segment T4.
- Flat transverse strokes over the spine, beginning at the level of T6 under the angle of the left scapula and ending under the angle of the right scapula and then back again.
- Small, flat transverse strokes along the spine, within the area of the long extensor spinae muscles, from T12 to T7.

▶ **From ventral**
- In the ventral intercostal area a set of flat strokes are pulled beginning at the dorsal axillary line through the intercostal spaces. These should start at the lowest ribs.

Second Sequence (▶ Fig. 2.46, ▶ Fig. 2.47, ▶ Fig. 2.48, ▶ Fig. 2.49)

▶ **From dorsal**
- Long downward stretching, along the edge of the latissimus dorsi muscle in the direction of the iliac crest.
- Prolonged upward stretching, beginning at the level of the sixth/seventh intercostal space, along the edge of the latissimus dorsi muscle in the direction of the axilla.
- Axillary stretching with elevated arm: the patient puts his or her arm on the therapist's shoulder. Connecting transverse strokes are applied through the axilla to thoroughly loosen the axillary fold.
- A flat fan-shaped stroke is pulled transversely over the scapula toward the shoulder joint, starting at the outer edge of the scapula and ending at the lower edge of the spine of the scapula.
- Small, flat transverse strokes over the spine, within the area of the long extensor spinae muscles, from T7 to T3 or C7.
- Flat transverse strokes from the inner side to the lateral edge of the scapulae, starting at the level of T7, ending at the spine of the scapula.
- Small hooks around the upper angle of the scapula followed by outlining the edge of the scapula with cutting strokes.

▶ **From ventral**
- The ventral edge of the trapezius muscle is pulled out starting from the cervical base, while pressing against it with the free hand.
- Strokes over the sternum, beginning at the xiphoid process pulling toward the jugular notch.
- Short hooks on the connection points between the ribs and sternum, pulling from caudal to cranial.
- Short transverse strokes along the sternum. These start at the junction between the xiphoid process and the body of the sternum, along the area of the sternal angle. At the base of the second rib at the sternum, the strokes should become wider to just under the sternoclavicular joints.
- Short fanlike strokes on the suprasternal notch, beginning on the clavicle and ending on the dorsal edge of the sternocleidomastoid muscle.
- Short strokes on the interclavicular ligament.

▶ **On the arm**
- Bimanual soft stretching of flexor and extensor of the upper arm.

Comments

- Depending on the condition of the tissue, the first sequence can immediately follow the small basic sequence in the same session.
- Only light traction is applied during the strokes on the elbow, since this area is at risk of developing myositis ossificans. The risk of developing stiffness of the elbow caused by inappropriate treatment with CTM must be considered here.
- The same treatment plan is used to treat contracture in the elbow. After treatment having started in the lumbodorsal area, the strokes of first and second sequences are applied together with work in the region of the upper arm. Again the effects of segmental reflex responses are employed here, while the connective tissue of the upper arm and elbow can be treated locally with strokes adapted to the particular condition.
- The work on the contracture itself starts after the second sequence. Particular care is required in the treatment of the capsule.
- If the traction applied can be seen as a white streak in the tissue, this means that the circulation is disturbed here. More second sequences must be applied in segments T5–T7, since the autonomic nervous system of the arms are located in these segments of the spinal cord.

3.3.3 Fractures and Contractures of the Lower Extremity

Fractures of the Thigh and Femoral Neck

Findings

Increased muscle tone and turgor are located in the segments L1–L5 and S1–S3.

On the posterior side of the body
- On the edges of the sacral bone (origin of the gluteus maximus muscle) pulling down to the ischiorectal fossa
- Under the edges of the pelvis in the region of the origin of the lesser gluteal muscles

▶ On the anterior side of the body
- On the anterior superior iliac spine extending to the groin
- Along the edges of the abdominal muscles

▶ On the leg
- Extending from the iliotibial tract to the popliteal cavity
- Along the course of the adductors and the fascial tube of the sartorius muscle
- Around the knee joint
- On the outside of the calf
- Between the heads of the gastrocnemius toward the heel
- Along the edge of the anterior tibial muscle

- On the sole of the foot and the inner edge of the foot, and over the metatarsophalangeal joints of the toes

Treatment Plan

Starting position: lateral position, lying on the unaffected side.
- Small basic sequence, flat strokes on the leg.
- Small basic sequence, treatment of the thigh, flat strokes on lower leg and foot.
- Small basic sequence, first sequence, ventral side of the body, treatment of thigh and knee, flat strokes over lower leg and foot.
- Small basic sequence, first sequence, ventral side of the body, treatment of thigh, knee, lower leg, and foot.

Balancing strokes over the pectoral muscles, dorsal dispersion strokes, and flat strokes of the legs are applied at the end of each treatment session to support the venous backflow.

Additional Strokes

Basic Sequence (▶ Fig. 2.27, ▶ Fig. 2.28, ▶ Fig. 2.29)

▶ From dorsal
- Hooks to the sacral bone edges from caudal to cranial.
- Flat transverse strokes over the sacral bone, from caudal to cranial.
- Hooks in the course of the first pelvic stroke.
- Small, flat transverse strokes along the spine, within the area of the long extensor spinae muscles, from L5 to T12.
- Grasping and stretching stroke at the ischial tuberosity.
- Stretching stroke in the region of the lumbar triangle.

Small Basic Sequence in Lateral Position (▶ Fig. 2.33)

▶ From dorsal
- Small hooks around the greater trochanter.
- Flat balancing stroke, starting above the greater trochanter toward the ischial tuberosity.

Small basic sequence in prone position (▶ Fig. 2.33).

▶ From dorsal
- Short hooks along the intergluteal cleft pulling up from the lateral side.

▶ On the leg (▶ Fig. 2.70)
- Short hooks from the last third of the fascia lata, in the shape of a fan toward the patella.
- The thigh stroke starts in the upper third of the thigh, on the lateral edge of the sartorius muscle, and ends shortly before the groin.

- Flat strokes pulled from the transverse intergluteal cleft to the popliteal cavity.
- Flat strokes from the inner side of the thigh, starting below the patella and running around the medial malleolus.
- Bimanual stretching between the muscle bellies of the gastrocnemius muscle, from cranial to caudal, pulling in the direction of the Achilles tendon.

Comments

- Frequent repetitions of the large pelvic stroke supports circulation.
- The focus of the treatment moves from the torso to the extremities after the fourth or fifth CTM session. The strokes of the small basic sequence are pulled through only once or twice.
- This concept can also be adapted for treatment after hip surgery.
- Vibration may be applied to the lower leg to loosen the adductors, which usually have a very high tone. Heat packs, placed on the adductors between the legs after treatment at night, also have a tone-relieving effect.

Fractures of the Lower Leg and Mortise, Sprained Ankle Joints

Findings

Increased muscle tone and turgor are located in the tissue around the pelvis within segments L1–L5 and S1–S3.

▶ **On the posterior side of the body**
- On the dorsal edges of the sacral bone (origin of the gluteus maximus muscle) pulling down to the ischiorectal fossa
- Under the edges of the pelvis in the region of the lesser gluteal muscles' origin

▶ **On the anterior side of the body**
- On the anterior superior iliac spine extending to the groin

▶ **On the leg**
- Extending from the iliotibial tract to the popliteal cavity
- Along the course of the adductors and the fascial tube of the sartorius muscle
- Around the knee joint
- On the outside of the calf
- Between the gastrocnemius traveling toward the heel
- Over the tibia to the ankle joint
- On the sole and the back of the foot over the metatarsophalangeal joints and the metatarsal bone, on the inner edge of the foot

Treatment Plan

Starting position: sitting, supine position.
- Small basic sequence, flat strokes on the leg.
- Small basic sequence, treatment of the thigh, flat strokes on the leg.
- Small basic sequence, treatment of the thigh and knee, flat strokes on the leg.
- Small basic sequence, treatment of the leg.

Balancing strokes over the pectoral muscles, dorsal dispersion strokes, and flat strokes of the legs are applied at the end of each treatment session to support the venous backflow.

Additional Strokes

Basic Sequence (▶ Fig. 2.27, ▶ Fig. 2.28, ▶ Fig. 2.29)

▶ **From dorsal**
- Hooks to the sacral bone edges from caudal to cranial.
- Flat transverse strokes over the sacral bone, from caudal to cranial.
- Hooks, in the course of the first pelvic stroke.
- Small, flat transverse strokes along the spine, within the area of the long extensor spinae muscles, from L5 to T12.
- Hooks and stretching strokes at the ischial tuberosity.
- Stretching strokes in the region of the lumbar triangle.

▶ **On the leg (▶ Fig. 2.70)**
- Short hooks from the last third of the fascia lata, in the shape of a fan toward the patella.
- The thigh stroke starts in the upper third of the thigh, on the lateral edge of the sartorius muscle, and ends shortly before the groin.
- Flat strokes, which are pulled from the transverse intergluteal cleft to the popliteal cavity.
- Flat strokes from the inner side of the thigh, starting below the patella and running around the medial malleolus.
- Bimanual stretching between the muscle bellies of the gastrocnemius muscle, from cranial to caudal, pulling in the direction of the Achilles tendon.

Comments

- In the treatment of *fractures of the lower leg*, especially with compartment syndromes, the adhesions in the muscular septa (extensor, peroneus, and superficial and deep calf muscle beds) with reduced gliding capacity and contractures of the muscles and their appendages must be accounted for.
- The same treatment plan can be adapted for the treatment after surgery of *internal knee joint injuries*. The following must be considered:

○ The strokes on the knee joint are in the foreground. Stretching of the dorsal thigh muscles and the gastrocnemius is performed from the middle of the calf several times.

○ In the region of the greater trochanter and iliotibial tract the therapist first works in the proximal, and then slowly in the distal direction. Should circulatory disturbances develop in the foot, the distal strokes in the region of the tract must be omitted.

• Treatment of the foot must be emphasized for *ankle fractures.*

○ Loosening of the capsule of the ankle joints and improvement of the circulation are key objectives of local strokes on the foot.

○ The four interosseous spaces are distinctly pulled out from dorsal and ventral and the forefoot is stretched with both hands in the dorsal and plantar direction.

○ In the event of insufficient blood supply, build-up of heat, and edema, the onset of dystrophy should be taken into consideration.

It is advisable to administer physical therapy after CTM because CTM loosens the deeper tissue structures, activates the capsule, and benefits the gliding capacity of the structures.

Contractures of the Hip and Knee Joint

Findings

Increased muscle tone and turgor are located in segments L1–L5 and S1–S3. Tissue changes are located on the **posterior side of the body**:

• Lateral side of the lumbar spine

▶ **On the anterior side of the body**
• On the edges of the abdominal muscles
• On the leg
• On the edges of the hip flexors and adductors
• In the region of the trochanter, on the origins of the pelvitrochanterian muscle and along the fascia of the iliotibial tract
• On the muscle edges of the flexors and extensors in the region of the knee joint
• Around the patella
• Along the edges of the peroneal and anterior tibial muscles
• In the region of the capsule around the mortise

Treatment Plan

Starting position: sitting, lateral position, supine position.
• Small basic sequence, flat strokes on the leg.
• Small basic sequence, first sequence, ventral side of the body, flat strokes over the leg.

• Small basic sequence, first sequence, ventral side of the body, treatment of the thigh, flat strokes over the leg.
• Small basic sequence, first sequence, ventral side of the body, treatment of thigh and lower leg.
• Small basic sequence, first sequence, ventral side of the body, treatment of thigh, lower leg and foot.

Balancing strokes over the pectoral muscles, dorsal dispersion strokes, and flat strokes of the legs are applied at the end of each treatment session to support the venous backflow.

Additional Strokes
Small Basic Sequence (▶ Fig. 2.27, ▶ Fig. 2.28, ▶ Fig. 2.29)

▶ **From dorsal**
• Hooks to the sacral bone edges from caudal to cranial.
• Flat transverse strokes over the sacral bone, from caudal to cranial.
• Hooks, in the course of the first pelvic stroke.
• Small, flat transverse strokes along the spine, within the area of the long extensor spinae muscles, from L5 to T12.
• Hook and stretching stroke at the ischial tuberosity.
• Stretching stroke in the region of the lumbar triangle.

Small Basic Sequence in Lateral Position (▶ Fig. 2.33)

▶ **From dorsal**
• Small hooks around the greater trochanter.
• Flat balancing stroke, starting above the greater trochanter toward the ischial tuberosity.

Small Basic Sequence in Prone Position (▶ Fig. 2.33)

▶ **From dorsal**
• Short hooks along the intergluteal cleft pulling up from the lateral side.

▶ **On the leg** (▶ Fig. 2.70)
• Short hooks from the last third of the fascia lata, in the shape of a fan toward the patella.
• The thigh stroke starts in the upper third of the thigh, on the lateral edge of the sartorius muscle, and ends shortly before the groin.
• Flat strokes, which are pulled from the transverse intergluteal cleft to the popliteal cavity.
• Flat strokes from the inner side of the thigh, starting below the patella and running around the medial malleolus.
• Bimanual stretching between the muscle bellies of the gastrocnemius muscle, from cranial to caudal, pulling in the direction of the Achilles tendon.

Comments

- Intensive strokes in small basic sequence.
- Treatment of the thigh should be started only after the fourth or fifth session.
- The treatment should not be diverted to the periphery too soon. First, the tension in the tissue around the trochanter and in the adductors must be reduced.
- The iliopsoas muscle attachment on the lesser trochanter and the attachment of the adductors on the inner side of the thigh should be treated with a rolled-up hot pack after CTM.
- The originating tendons of the rectus muscle of the femur as well as the sartorius and tensor fasciae latae muscles on the anterior spinae are palpated and integrated into the treatment if there is increased tension.
- With contracture of the knee, the structures of the knee joint are remotely influenced by the segmental treatment in the lumbodorsal area (small basic sequence). The success of the treatment is supported by strokes that are adapted to the respective findings around the greater trochanter and on the iliotibial tract. The following must especially be taken into consideration:
  - Stretching of the structures that surround the knee joint from the dorsal side (popliteal muscle).
  - Strokes around the patella, hooks, and movement are applied to support gliding.
  - Palpation of tissue mobility in the course of the pes anserinus: this can be improved through hooks, if necessary.

3.3.4 Amputations

Amputation of the Arm

Findings

Increased turgor and muscle tone are located in segments C5–C8, T1–T5. Tense tissue is especially found in the thoracic area and around the scapula of the affected arm:

▶ **On the posterior side of the body**
- On both sides along the spinal column, in the region of the erector spinae muscle, up to the neck to the insertion point of the trapezius muscle
- On the edge of the latissimus dorsi muscle extending into the upper arm
- On the lower angle of the scapula around the medial side of the scapula
- On the spine of the scapula toward the level of the shoulder, along the edge of the trapezius muscle and the descending part

▶ **On the anterior side of the body**
- Under the clavicle, affecting the subclavius muscle
- On the clavicle, in the surrounding area of the sternoclavicular joint, along the sternocleidomastoid muscle

- In the region of the pectoral muscles, extending into the axilla

▶ **On the arm**
- Along the muscle edges of the upper arm, primarily the flexors
- Along the muscle edges of the forearm, primarily the extensors

In all cases the unaffected side of the body should also be palpated and the findings integrated into the treatment plan.

Treatment Plan

Starting position: sitting, lateral position.
- Small basic sequence, flat strokes over back and arms.
- Small basic sequence, first sequence, flat strokes over rib cage and arms.
- Small basic sequence, first and second sequence, treatment of the upper arm on the unaffected side, flat strokes of the arms.
- Small basic sequence, first and second sequence, treatment of the upper arm on the affected side.
- Small basic sequence, first, second, and third sequence, treatment of the affected arm.

Balancing strokes over the pectoral muscles, dorsal dispersion strokes, and flat strokes of the arms are applied at the end of each treatment session to support the venous backflow.

Additional Strokes

First Sequence (▶ Fig. 2.37, ▶ Fig. 2.38, ▶ Fig. 2.39)

▶ **From dorsal**
- When changing the direction, the intercostal strokes are also performed in the opposite direction from the spine along the lateral thoracic wall to the ventral axillary line in order to gently grasp the tissue there.
- The large balancing stroke starts in the ventral axillary line at the level of the sixth/seventh intercostal space and is broadly pulled around the lower angle of the scapula toward C7.
- Short strokes from the lower angle of the scapula to the spine at the level of segment T4.
- Flat transverse strokes over the spinal column, beginning at the level of T6 under the angle of the left scapula and ending under the angle of the right scapula and then back again.
- Small, flat transverse strokes along the spine, within the area of the long extensor spinae muscles, from T12 to T7.

► **From ventral**
- In the ventral intercostal area a set of flat strokes are pulled beginning at the dorsal axillary line through the intercostal spaces. These should start at the lowest ribs.

Second Sequence (► Fig. 2.46, ► Fig. 2.47, ► Fig. 2.48, ► Fig. 2.49)

► **From dorsal**
- Long downward stretching, along the edge of the latissimus dorsi muscle in the direction of the iliac crest.
- Prolonged upward stretching, beginning at the level of the sixth/seventh intercostal space, along the edge of the latissimus dorsi muscle in the direction of the axilla.
- Axillary stretching with elevated arm: the patient puts his or her arm on the therapist's shoulder. Connecting transverse strokes are applied through the axilla to thoroughly loosen the axillary fold.
- A flat fan-shaped stroke is pulled transversely over the scapula toward the shoulder joint, starting at the outer edge of the scapula and ending at the lower edge of the spine of the scapula.
- Small, flat transverse strokes over the spine, within the area of the long extensor spinae muscles, from T7 to T3 or C7.
- Flat transverse strokes from the inner side to the lateral edge of the scapulae, starting at the level of T7, ending at the spine of the scapula.
- Small hooks around the upper angle of the scapula followed by outlining the scapula with cutting strokes.

► **From ventral**
- The ventral edge of the trapezius muscle is pulled out starting from the cervical base, while pressing against it with the free hand.
- Strokes over the sternum, beginning at the xiphoid process and pulling toward the jugular notch.
- Short hooks on the connection points between the ribs and sternum, pulling from caudal to cranial.
- Short transverse strokes along the sternum. These start at the junction between the xiphoid process and the body of the sternum, along the area of the sternal angle. At the base of the second rib at the sternum, the strokes should become wider to just under the sternoclavicular joints.
- Short fanlike strokes on the suprasternal notch, beginning on the clavicle and ending on the dorsal edge of the sternocleidomastoid muscle.
- Short strokes on the interclavicular ligament.
- On the arm: bimanual soft stretching of flexor and extensor of the upper arm.

Comments

- The therapists should work swiftly through the basic and first sequences.

- One should start with the strokes of second sequence first on the unaffected side to trigger the consensual reaction. The strokes of the second sequence are also applied on the affected side but only after satisfactory reaction of the tissue.
- After five or six sessions the amputation scar is treated (p. 98). The goal of the treatment is to toughen the tissue and to support the blood supply around the stump. This means that the traction can be applied using cutting and firm pulls through the tissue. The reactions of the tissue should be carefully noted. If there is an ischemic reaction, the strokes must be directed back into the segment and then again toward the periphery.
- The cutting sensation must be distinctively felt.
- For amputations of the hand or fingers, treatment is increasingly directed toward the periphery to improve the blood supply.

Amputation of the Leg

Findings

Increased turgor and muscle tone are located in segments C5–C8, T1–T12, L1–L5.

Tension on the posterior side of the body:
- On the edges of the sacral bone (origin of the gluteus maximus muscle) pulling down to the ischiorectal fossa
- Under the edges of the pelvis in the region of the origin of the lesser gluteal muscles

► **On the anterior side of the body**
- On the anterior superior iliac spine extending to the groin
- Along the edges of the abdominal muscles
- On the leg: along the course of the iliotibial tract to the popliteal cavity
- Along the adductors and the fascial tube of the sartorius muscle.
- Around the knee joint
- On the outside of the calf
- Between the heads of the gastrocnemius muscle toward the heel
- Along the edge of the anterior tibial muscle.

Treatment Plan

Starting position: lateral position, supine position.
- Small basic sequence, flat strokes on both legs.
- Small basic sequence, treatment of the thigh on the unaffected side, flat strokes on both legs.
- Small basic sequence, treatment of the thigh and lower leg on the unaffected side, flat strokes on both legs.
- Small basic sequence, treatment of the thigh on the amputated leg, flat strokes on both legs.
- Small basic sequence, treatment of the thigh and possibly lower leg on the amputated leg, flat strokes on both legs.

Balancing strokes over the pectoral muscles, dorsal dispersion strokes, and flat strokes of the legs are applied at the end of each treatment session to support the venous backflow.

Additional Strokes

Small Basic Sequence (▶ Fig. 2.27, ▶ Fig. 2.28, ▶ Fig. 2.29)

▶ **From dorsal**
- Hooks to the sacral bone edges from caudal to cranial.
- Flat transverse strokes over the sacral bone, from caudal to cranial.
- Hooks, in the course of the first pelvic stroke.
- Small, flat transverse strokes along the spine, within the area of the long extensor spinae muscles, from L5 to T12.
- Hook and stretching stroke at the ischial tuberosity.
- Stretching stroke in the region of the lumbar triangle.

Small Basic Sequence in Lateral Position (▶ Fig. 2.33)

▶ **From dorsal**
- Small hooks around the greater trochanter.
- Flat balancing stroke, starting above the greater trochanter toward the ischial tuberosity.

Small Basic Sequence in Prone Position (▶ Fig. 2.33)

▶ **From dorsal**
- Short hooks along the intergluteal cleft pulling up from the lateral side.

▶ **On the leg** (▶ Fig. 2.70)
- Short hooks from the last third of the fascia lata, in the shape of a fan toward the patella.
- The thigh stroke starts in the upper third of the thigh, on the lateral edge of the sartorius muscle, and ends shortly before the groin.
- Flat strokes, which are pulled from the transverse intergluteal cleft to the popliteal cavity.
- Flat strokes from the inner side of the thigh, starting below the patella and running around the medial malleolus.
- Bimanual stretching between the muscle bellies of the gastrocnemius muscle, from cranial to caudal, pulling in the direction of the Achilles tendon.
- In the region of the scar.

Comments

- Scars may maintain disruptive connections to segmentally associated organs.
- The treatment of the lower extremity in contractures is started on the healthy leg, since this triggers the consensual response.

- When applying short hooks to the scar tissue, the response of the tissue must be observed and the techniques adapted to the healing process:
  - Local treatment can be continued in the event of hyperemia.
  - If there is an ischemic reaction, there are still significant circulatory disturbances. The therapist must focus more on the tissue segments above the amputated spot or return to the strokes of the small basic sequence.
- When the patient reports the cutting sensation in the tissue, this is proof to the therapist that adequate traction has been applied to this scar area and the autonomic nervous system is responding.
- Treatment is focused more on the periphery for amputations of the foot or forefoot in order to improve the blood supply.

3.3.5 Osteoarthritis

Definition

Osteoarthritis, which is often a slow and progressive process, is the destruction of the joint with pathological changes in all joint structures caused by a primary cartilaginous lesion. The cartilaginous lesion can have very different causes, defined as *prodromes of arthritis*, which include axial deviations, joint instabilities, joint diseases, neurological and metabolic disorders, and rheumatic and infectious inflammations of joints. These must be distinguished from abacterial joint inflammations, which may occur in phases during osteoarthritis (activated arthritis).

Factors that cause arthritis must be distinguished from those that promote arthritis (e.g., obesity or overexertion). The aged joint is more liable to develop arthritis, so that arthritis becomes more frequent with age. Genetic factors must be assumed for systemic arthritis in particular. If the cause of arthritis cannot be determined, it is termed primary or idiopathic arthritis. There is no spontaneous remission of arthritis, nor is there a causal therapy.

Knee and shoulder joints are most often affected, followed by hip and finger joints. Clinical consequences include painful limitations of mobility, typically associated with exertion, and often malposition.

▶ **Treatment measures**
- Elimination of factors promoting arthritis
- Symptomatic physical and medicinal therapies (analgesic and anti-inflammatory drugs)
- Surgical procedures in the form of joint-preserving measures (joint replacement surgery, resection arthroplasty).

Treatment depends on the age, general health, and individual needs of the patient; on the number and location of affected joints; and on the stage of the arthritis.

The application of CTM can improve the nutrient supply of the tissue through reactions of the autonomic nervous system, but should primarily alleviate pain and muscle tension. Subsequent local treatment of tissue structures around the joint itself intensifies this reaction.

Acute, inflammatory pain with joint effusion is a contraindication for CTM.

Arthritis of the Upper Extremity

Connective tissue massage triggers the same response in arthritis of the upper as of the lower extremity. The general reactions of the autonomic nervous system that are induced by CTM can even be intensified by the local treatment of tissue.

The combination of physical therapy and CTM is successful with arthritis as it is with all joint diseases. CTM is always applied after physical therapy, since the patient must definitely rest after the treatment

Findings

Increased turgor and muscle tone are located in the region of the shoulder and arm in segments C5–C8, T12 and L2.

▶ **Tense tissue on the posterior side of the body**
- Extending below the spine of the scapula into the posterior axillary wall
- On the lower angle of the scapula, along the latissimus dorsi muscle toward the pelvic edge and along the axillary line extending under the axilla

▶ **On the anterior side of the body**
- Extending over the clavicle toward the shoulder joint
- Below the clavicle, on the sternoclavicular joint, along the subclavius muscle
- Along the lower edge of the ribs, extending toward the rectus abdominis muscle

▶ **On the arm**
- On the anterior part of the deltoid muscle extending to the upper arm
- From the origin of the triceps muscle of the upper arm to the attachment on the elbow
- In the region of the flexor of elbow and hand, on the medial epicondyle of the upper arm, extending into the wrist

Treatment Plan

Starting position: sitting, supine position.
- Small basic sequence, flat strokes over back and arm.
- Small basic sequence, first sequence, flat strokes over back and arm.
- Small basic sequence, first and second sequence, ventral side, flat strokes on the arm.

- Small basic sequence, first and second sequence, ventral side of the body, treatment of the upper arm, flat strokes of forearm and hand.
- Small basic sequence, first, second, and third sequence, ventral side of the body, treatment of the upper arm, flat strokes on forearm and hand.
- Small basic sequence, first, second, and third sequence, ventral side, treatment of arm.

Balancing strokes over the pectoral muscles, dorsal dispersion strokes, and flat strokes of the arms are applied at the end of each treatment session to support the venous backflow.

Additional Strokes

First Sequence (▶ Fig. 2.37, ▶ Fig. 2.38, ▶ Fig. 2.39)

▶ **From dorsal**
- When changing the direction, the intercostal strokes are also performed in the opposite direction from the spine along the lateral thoracic wall to the ventral axillary line in order to gently grasp the tissue there.
- The large balancing stroke starts in the ventral axillary line at the level of the sixth/seventh intercostal space and is broadly pulled around the lower angle of the scapula toward C7.
- Short strokes from the lower angle of the scapula to the spine at the level of segment T4.
- Flat transverse strokes over the spine, beginning at the level of T6 under the angle of the left scapula and ending under the angle of the right scapula and then back again.
- Small, flat transverse strokes along the spine, within the area of the long extensor spinae muscles, from T12 to T7.

▶ **From ventral**
- In the ventral intercostal area a set of flat strokes are pulled, beginning at the dorsal axillary line through the intercostal spaces. These should start at the lowest ribs.

Second Sequence (▶ Fig. 2.46, ▶ Fig. 2.47, ▶ Fig. 2.48, ▶ Fig. 2.49)

▶ **From dorsal**
- Long downward stretching, along the edge of the latissimus dorsi muscle in the direction of the iliac crest.
- Prolonged upward stretching, beginning at the level of the sixth/seventh intercostal space, along the edge of the latissimus dorsi muscle in the direction of the axilla.
- Axillary stretching with the arm elevated: the patient puts his or her arm on the therapist's shoulder. Connecting transverse strokes are applied through the axilla to thoroughly loosen the axillary fold.
- A flat fan-shaped stroke is pulled transversely over the scapula toward the shoulder joint, starting at the outer

edge of the scapula and ending at the lower edge of the spine of the scapula.

- Small, flat transverse strokes over the spine, within the area of the long extensor spinae muscles, from T7 to T3 or C7.
- Flat transverse strokes from the inner side to the lateral edge of the scapulae, starting at the level of T7, ending at the spine of the scapula.
- Small hooks around the upper angle of the scapula followed by outlining the scapula with cutting strokes.

▶ From ventral

- The ventral edge of the trapezius muscle is pulled out starting from the cervical base, while pressing against it with the free hand.
- Strokes over the sternum, beginning at the xiphoid process, pulling toward the jugular notch.
- Short hooks on the connection points between the ribs and the sternum, pulling from caudal to cranial.
- Short transverse strokes along the sternum. These start at the junction between the xiphoid process and the body of the sternum, along the area of the sternal angle. At the base of the second rib at the sternum, the strokes should become wider to just under the sternoclavicular joints.
- Short fanlike strokes on the suprasternal notch, beginning on the clavicle and ending on the dorsal edge of the sternocleidomastoid muscle.
- Short strokes on the interclavicular ligament.

▶ On the arm

- Bimanual soft stretching of flexor and extensor of the upper arm.

Comments

- Depending on the condition of the tissue, the first sequence can immediately follow the small basic sequence in the same session. Treatment is focused on the region of the affected joints.
- Since arthritis of the shoulder joint generally has a chronic course, cutting and strong strokes are applied to the tissue.
- The strokes along the joint capsule are the most important for all joints.
- Special attention must be paid to the carpometacarpal joint of the thumb. Short hooks are applied to the joint capsule, the thenar eminence (ball of the thumb), and on the dorsal side between D1 and D2 in the radial and ulnar direction.
- CTM of the affected region is not suitable for inflammatory processes (e.g., effusion) in the joints.

Hip Joint Arthritis and Surgery

The exclusively conservative therapy of hip joint arthritis partially corresponds to the measures after surgery (e.g.,

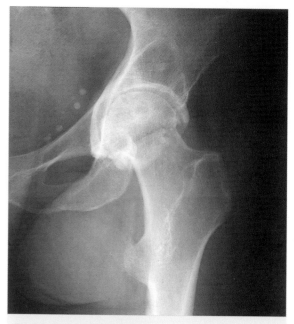

Fig. 3.4 Hip joint arthritis.

hip joint-preserving procedures [reconfiguration osteotomy] or artificial joint replacement [endoprosthetics]). The focus of the conservative therapy is to allow movement without exertion (▶ Fig. 3.4).

In the treatment of the so-called Girdlestone hip (removal of hip endoprosthesis without replacement), CTM may be applied in addition to physical therapy exercises. CTM may be started about 6 weeks after the surgical procedure.

Findings

Tissue imbalances are found in the affected areas of fractures in the thigh and the femoral neck.

The adhesions are located in the mobile layers of hypodermis and muscle fascia, when the pathology has persisted for longer periods.

▶ On the posterior side of the body

- In the lateral region on both sides of the lumbar spine as seen with hypertonia
- Hypotonic muscular changes can be found in the region of the lesser gluteus muscles

▶ On the anterior side of the body

- On the edges of the abdominal muscles, especially of the rectus abdominis muscle

▶ On the leg

- On the edges of the flexor muscles of the hip, here especially on the hypertonic sartorius and rectus femoris muscles
- On the origin of the short adductors at the pubic bone

Treatment Plan

Starting position: lateral position, lying on the unaffected side, supine position.
- Small basic sequence, flat strokes over back and legs.
- Small basic sequence, first sequence, ventral side of the body, flat strokes over the leg.
- Small basic sequence, first sequence, ventral side of the body, treatment of the thighs, flat strokes on lower leg and foot.

Balancing strokes over the pectoral muscles, dorsal dispersion strokes, and flat strokes on the legs are applied at the end of each treatment session to support the venous backflow.

Additional Strokes

Basic Sequence (▶ Fig. 2.27, ▶ Fig. 2.28, ▶ Fig. 2.29)

▶ **From dorsal**
- Hooks to the sacral bone edges from caudal to cranial.
- Flat transverse strokes over the sacral bone, from caudal to cranial.
- Hooks, in the course of the first pelvic stroke.
- Small, flat transverse strokes along the spine, within the area of the long extensor spinae muscles, from L5 to T12.
- Hook and stretching stroke at the ischial tuberosity.
- Stretching stroke in the region of the lumbar triangle.

Small Basic Sequence in Lateral Position (▶ Fig. 2.33)

▶ **From dorsal**
- Small hooks around the greater trochanter.
- Flat balancing stroke, starting above the greater trochanter toward the ischial tuberosity.

Small Basic Sequence in Prone Position (▶ Fig. 2.33)

▶ **From dorsal**
- Short hooks along the intergluteal cleft pulling up from the lateral side.

▶ **On the leg (▶ Fig. 2.70)**
- Short hooks from the last third of the fascia lata, in the shape of a fan toward the patella.
- The thigh stroke starts in the upper third of the thigh, on the lateral edge of the sartorius muscle, and ends shortly before the groin.
- Flat strokes, which are pulled from the transverse intergluteal cleft to the popliteal cavity.
- Flat strokes from the inner side of the thigh, starting below the patella and running around the medial malleolus.
- Bimanual stretching between the muscle bellies of the gastrocnemius muscle, from cranial to caudal, pulling in the direction of the Achilles tendon.

Comments

- Depending on the tension of the tissue, the small basic sequence may also be applied immediately to the area of the trochanter.
- Special attention is paid to relaxing the adductors. This can be achieved with vibration, shaking or also heat packs, which are placed between the legs while resting afterward.
- Depending on the condition of the tissue the fingers should be in a slightly more raised position to enable a good pull through the tissue.

Arthritis of the Knee and Ankle Joints

Findings

Increased muscle tone and turgor are located in the tissue around the pelvis within segments L1–L5 and S1–S3.

▶ **On the posterior side of the body**
- On the lateral edges of the sacral bone, the edges of the gluteus maximus muscle, down to the ischiorectal fossa
- Under the edges of the pelvis in the region of the lesser gluteal muscles' origin

▶ **On the anterior side of the body**
- On the anterior superior iliac spine extending to the groin

▶ **On the leg**
- Along the course of the iliotibial tract to the popliteal cavity
- Along the adductors and the fascial tube of the sartorius muscle
- Around the knee joint
- On the outside of the calf
- Between the gastrocnemius heads toward the heel
- Over the tibia to the ankle joint
- On the sole and the back of the foot over the metatarsophalangeal joints and the metatarsal bone
- On the inner edge of the foot

Treatment Plan

Starting position: sitting, supine position, lateral position.
- Small basic sequence, flat strokes on the leg.
- Small basic sequence, treatment of the thigh, flat strokes on lower leg and foot.
- Small basic sequence, treatment of the thigh and knee, flat strokes on the lower leg and foot.
- Small basic sequence, treatment of thigh, knee and lower leg.
- Small basic sequence, treatment of the leg.

Balancing strokes over the pectoral muscles, dorsal dispersion strokes, and flat strokes of the legs are applied at the end of each treatment session to support the venous backflow.

Additional Strokes

Basic Sequence (▶ Fig. 2.27, ▶ Fig. 2.28, ▶ Fig. 2.29)

▶ From dorsal
- Hooks to the sacral bone edges from caudal to cranial.
- Flat transverse strokes over the sacral bone, from caudal to cranial.
- Hooks, in the course of the first pelvic stroke.
- Small, flat transverse strokes along the spine, within the area of the long extensor spinae muscles, from L5 to T12.
- Hook and stretching stroke at the ischial tuberosity.
- Stretching stroke in the region of the lumbar triangle.

Small Basic Sequence in Lateral Position (▶ Fig. 2.33)

▶ From dorsal
- Small hooks around the greater trochanter.
- Flat balancing stroke, starting above the greater trochanter toward the ischial tuberosity.

Small Basic Sequence in Prone Position (▶ Fig. 2.33)

▶ From dorsal
- Short hooks along the intergluteal cleft pulling up from the lateral side.

▶ On the leg (▶ Fig. 2.70)
- Short hooks from the last third of the fascia lata, in the shape of a fan toward the patella.
- The thigh stroke starts in the upper third of the thigh, on the lateral edge of the sartorius muscle, and ends shortly before the groin.

- Flat strokes, which are pulled from the transverse intergluteal cleft to the popliteal cavity.
- Flat strokes from the inner side of the thigh, starting below the patella and running around the medial malleolus.
- Bimanual stretching between the muscle bellies of the gastrocnemius muscle, from cranial to caudal, pulling in the direction of the Achilles tendon.

Comments

Therapists should look for the muscular imbalances that were caused by the structural changes. In the ischiocrural muscle group this especially applies to the short head of the biceps femoris, in the popliteal cavity, the popliteal muscle and the pes anserinus on the medial side of the knee joint.

3.3.6 Additional Disorders of the Musculoskeletal System and of the Skin

Humeroscapular Periarthritis

Definition

"Humeroscapular periarthritis" is used to describe various disorders of the shoulder, mostly pathological processes of the rotator cuff. Isolated osteoarthritis of the clavicular joints and of the shoulder joint (glenohumeral joint) may also be attributed to this pathology (▶ Fig. 3.5).

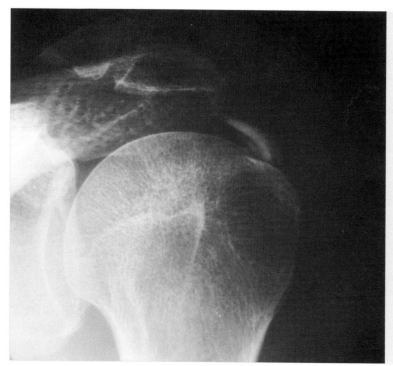

Fig. 3.5 Calcification in the rotator cuff of the shoulder joint with humeroscapular periarthritis (calcific tendinitis).

Disorders of the myocardium, lung, and abdominal organs can also cause shoulder pain. Degenerative changes of the lower cervical spine (C4–C6) are rarely responsible for humeroscapular periarthritis.

In terms of differential diagnosis, forms of plexus neuritis (rare) caused by viruses or *Borrelia* must be excluded.

In tendinopathy of the rotator cuff (the supraspinatus tendon is most often affected with necrobiotic, degenerative, and inflammatory changes of the tendon tissue), there is painful entrapment of the tendon in the space under the acromion caused by the humerus head hitting the roof of the shoulder (so-called impingement; Latin *impingere* = to strike).

Calcifications within this tendon tissue can spontaneously discharge into the neighboring bursa, causing severe pain.

Ruptures of the rotator cuff are incomplete and there are complete interruptions of the tendon tissue's continuity due to reduced tensile tissue strength and necrosis.

Extensive defects of the rotator cuff are the end stage of a disease that has developed over many years in many stages. For biochemical and biomechanical reasons this may lead to severe damage of the joint (rotator cuff arthropathy). The same pathological changes can develop on the long biceps tendon as on the rotator cuff, often in combination with other degenerative disorders of the shoulder.

Shoulder stiffness is a rare special form of humeroscapular periarthritis. It develops either spontaneously or after minor injuries of the shoulder ("frozen shoulder"). The disease progresses in stages and is usually reversible and belongs to the diseases described as complex regional pain syndrome (p. 94).

Findings

Increased turgor and muscle tone are located in the segments C4–C8, T1–T6, T12 and L2.

The entire shoulder girdle is also affected. The glenohumeral rhythm is disturbed, the shoulder is elevated, and the scapula is only slightly movable. The capsule has shrunk and the muscles are atrophic.

The entire region of the back has changed in structure. There are retractions and distensions of the tissue on the sacral bone, scapula, and upper arm. Dermis and hypodermis can barely be moved against each other.

Mobility is very limited and movement is extremely painful. A typical capsular pattern develops: restrictions in external rotation, abduction, and flexion. It becomes impossible to lift the arm above shoulder level.

Treatment Plan

Starting position: sitting.
- Small basic sequence, flat strokes over back and arm.

- Small basic sequence, first sequence, flat strokes over back and arm.
- Small basic sequence, first and second sequence, ventral side, flat strokes on the arm.
- Small basic sequence, first and second sequence, ventral side of the body, treatment of the upper arm, flat strokes of forearm and hand.
- Small basic sequence, first, second, and third sequence, treatment of the upper arm, ventral side of the body, flat strokes on forearm and hand.

Balancing strokes over the pectoral muscles, dorsal dispersion stroke, and flat strokes of the arms are applied at the end of each treatment session to support the venous backflow.

Additional Strokes

First Sequence (▶ Fig. 2.37, ▶ Fig. 2.38, ▶ Fig. 2.39)

▶ **From dorsal**
- When changing the direction, the intercostal strokes are also performed in the opposite direction from the spine along the lateral thoracic wall to the ventral axillary line in order to gently grasp the tissue there.
- The large balancing stroke starts in the ventral axillary line at the level of the sixth/seventh intercostal space and is flatly pulled around the lower angle of the scapula toward C7.
- Short strokes from the lower angle of the scapula to the spine at the level of segment T4.
- Flat transverse strokes over the spine beginning at the level of T6 under the angle of the left scapula and ending under the angle of the right scapula and then back again.
- Small, flat transverse strokes along the spine within the area of the long extensor spinae muscles from T12 to T7.

▶ **From ventral**
- In the ventral intercostal area a set of flat strokes are pulled, beginning at the dorsal axillary line through the intercostal spaces. These should start at the lowest ribs.

Second Sequence (▶ Fig. 2.46, ▶ Fig. 2.47, ▶ Fig. 2.48, ▶ Fig. 2.49)

▶ **From dorsal**
- Long downward stretching, along the edge of the latissimus dorsi muscle in the direction of the iliac crest.
- Prolonged upward stretching, beginning at the level of the sixth/seventh intercostal space, along the edge of the latissimus dorsi muscle in the direction of the axilla.
- Axillary stretching with elevated arm: the patient puts his or her arm on the therapist's shoulder. Connecting

transverse strokes are applied through the axilla to thoroughly loosen the axillary fold.

- A flat fan-shaped stroke is pulled transversely over the scapula toward the shoulder joint, starting at the outer edge of the scapula and ending at the lower edge of the spine of the scapula.
- Small, flat transverse strokes over the spine within the area of the long extensor spinae muscles, from T7 to T3 or C7.
- Flat transverse strokes from the inner side to the lateral edge of the scapulae, starting at the level of T7, ending at the spine of the scapula.
- Small hooks around the upper angle of the scapula followed by outlining the scapula with cutting strokes.

▶ **From ventral**
- The ventral edge of the trapezius muscle is pulled out starting from the cervical base, while pressing against it with the free hand.
- Strokes over the sternum, beginning at the xiphoid process pulling toward the jugular notch.
- Short hooks on the connection points between the ribs and sternum pulling from caudal to cranial.
- Short transverse strokes along the sternum. These start at the junction between the xiphoid process and the body of the sternum, along the area of the sternal angle. At the base of the second rib at the sternum, the strokes should become wider to just under the sternoclavicular joints.
- Short fanlike strokes on the suprasternal notch, beginning on the clavicle and ending on the dorsal edge of the sternocleidomastoid muscle.
- Short strokes on the interclavicular ligament.

▶ **On the arm**
- Bimanual soft stretching of flexor and extensor of the upper arm.

Comments

The focus of the treatment is always placed on the region of the scapula and axilla.
- If the adhesions of the tissue on the affected side have not yet loosened after application of the second sequence, treatment of the shoulder and axilla should be started on the unaffected side to trigger the consensual response again.
- The therapist must not work too soon in the tense tissue layers.
- In the course of treatment, the adhesions of the capsule and muscular septa are solved, pain subsides, and the joint is sufficiently prepared for physical therapy exercises.
- The sensitivity of the mammary glandular tissue must always be taken into consideration when applying strokes on the ventral side, so the therapist must work very carefully here. The exploratory strokes are long

and extensive when treating the upper arm. The loosening hooks are applied to the edges of the flexor and extensor muscles of the elbow and pulled toward the shoulder joint.
- On the scapula below the spine of the scapula there is a maximal point in T2. Strokes must be avoided in this region, since otherwise pain can be triggered in the region of the ulnar nerve. Therefore, the fan-shaped transverse strokes that run diagonally over the scapula are applied only when the tension in the tissue has decreased (very often after the administration of the third sequence).
- With inhibited movements of the arm, significant spots of pain can be considered and accurately palpated to determine their tension level:
  ○ Along the long biceps tendon
  ○ The delta origin
  ○ The origin of the biceps muscle in the crook of the elbow
  ○ The insertion of the triceps muscle, long head, on the joint capsule
- Treatment often ends at the crook of the elbow. The forearm and hand always recover with previously described segmental treatment.
- For all shoulder joint pain, the possibility of liver or gallbladder disease should be considered, which mainly projects in this section of the body at C3/C4 over the diaphragm.

Humeral Epicondylitis
Definition

Functional overexertion (microtraumas) and endogenous degeneration of the tendon's insertion structure are the causes of pain in the elbow in the lateral region, rarely also of the medial epicondyle. For differential diagnoses the supinator syndrome and peripheral nerve lesions must be considered as well as trigger points in the lower cervical syndrome (p. 64).

The treatment consists of elimination of pain-triggering mechanical factors, possibly through immobilization, local and systematic medicinal analgesic and anti-inflammatory therapy, and surgical treatments, which are rarely necessary due to the efficiency of CTM and other physical therapy treatment methods.

Findings

Segments affected are C3–C8; the focus very often lies at C6. Almost all thoracic segments are affected, probably because of cervical innervation of the latissimus dorsi muscle.

Increased tension is located in the area of the entire back, in the shoulder girdle, on the spinous processes of the thoracic vertebrae, and on the edge of the latissimus dorsi muscle up to the axillae.

There is an especially tender spot on the scapula just under the spine of the scapula in T2, which must be viewed and treated as the maximal point. Distensions can often be observed between the spinal column and the scapula of the affected side. Hardened connective tissue is found in the region of the deltoid and triceps muscles of the upper arm, as well as in the crook of the elbow, and in the forearm down to the wrist. Atrophy of the muscles develops increasingly the longer the illness.

Treatment Plan

Starting position: sitting.
- Small basic sequence, flat strokes over back and arms.
- Small basic sequence, first sequence, flat strokes over back and arm.
- Small basic sequence, first and second sequence, ventral side, flat strokes on the arm.
- Small basic sequence, first and second sequence, ventral side of the body, treatment of the upper arm, flat strokes of forearm and hand.
- Small basic sequence, first and second sequence, ventral side of the body, treatment of the upper arm and forearm, flat strokes on the hand.
- Small basic sequence, first, second, and third sequence, ventral side, treatment of arm.

Balancing strokes over the pectoral muscles, dorsal dispersion strokes, and flat strokes of the arms are applied at the end of each treatment session to support the venous backflow.

Additional Strokes

First Sequence (▶ Fig. 2.37, ▶ Fig. 2.38, ▶ Fig. 2.39)

▶ **From dorsal**
- When changing the direction, the intercostal strokes are also performed in the opposite direction, from the spine along the lateral thoracic wall to the ventral axillary line, in order to gently grasp the tissue there.
- The large balancing stroke starts in the ventral axillary line at the level of the sixth/seventh intercostal space and is flatly pulled around the lower angle of the scapula toward C7.
- Short strokes from the lower angle of the scapula to the spine at the level of segment T4.
- Flat transverse strokes over the spine, beginning at the level of T6 under the angle of the left scapula and ending under the angle of the right scapula and then back again.
- Small, flat transverse strokes along the spine within the area of the long extensor spinae muscles from T12 to T7.

▶ **From ventral**
- In the ventral intercostal area a set of flat strokes is pulled beginning at the dorsal axillary line through the intercostal spaces. These should start at the lowest ribs.

Second Sequence (▶ Fig. 2.46, ▶ Fig. 2.47, ▶ Fig. 2.48, ▶ Fig. 2.49)

▶ **From dorsal**
- Long downward stretching, along the edge of the latissimus dorsi muscle in the direction of the iliac crest.
- Prolonged upward stretching, beginning at the level of the sixth/seventh intercostal space along the edge of the latissimus dorsi muscle in the direction of the axilla.
- Axillary stretching with elevated arm: The patient puts his or her arm on the therapist's shoulder. Connecting transverse strokes are applied through the axilla to thoroughly loosen the axillary fold.
- A flat fan-shaped stroke is pulled transversely over the scapula toward the shoulder joint, starting at the outer edge of the scapula and ending at the lower edge of the spine of the scapula.
- Small, flat transverse strokes over the spine within the area of the long extensor spinae muscles from T7 to T3 or C7.
- Flat transverse strokes from the inner side to the lateral edge of the scapulae, starting at the level of T7, ending at the spine of the scapula.
- Small hooks around the upper angle of the scapula followed by outlining the scapula with cutting strokes.

▶ **From ventral**
- The ventral edge of the trapezius muscle is pulled out starting from the cervical base, while pressing against it with the free hand.
- Strokes over the sternum, beginning at the xiphoid process pulling toward the jugular notch.
- Short hooks on the connection points between the ribs and sternum, pulling from caudal to cranial.
- Short transverse strokes along the sternum. These start at the junction between the xiphoid process and the body of the sternum, along the area of the sternal angle. At the base of the second rib at the sternum, the strokes should become wider to just under the sternoclavicular joints.
- Short fanlike strokes on the suprasternal notch, beginning on the clavicle and ending on the dorsal edge of the sternocleidomastoid muscle.
- Short strokes on the interclavicular ligament.

▶ **On the arm**
- Bimanual soft stretching of flexor and extensor of the upper arm.

Comments

- The higher tension of the tissue on the affected side and the arm must especially be considered, if the disorder has persisted over a lengthy period. In this case, the unaffected side of the body and arm must be treated first.
- Long strokes are applied to the scapula and the axilla, whereby the hooks must be applied carefully.
- When the spinous processes of the thoracic spine become less sensitive, flat transverse strokes are applied from one side to the other side of the scapula edge.
- Special attention should be paid to the long biceps tendon in the crook of the elbow. The insertion of the biceps tendon can be palpated well on the pronated forearm next to the radial head.
- Locally palpate the originating tendons of the extensor muscles to determine their level of tension.

Irritated Joints

(See also Osteoarthritis, p.82).

Definition

Joints in the region of the knee and shoulder with metabolic disturbances are very sensitive to movement and have an extremely limited range of motion. Pain and joint effusions occur after minor injuries or even spontaneously. The capsule and the para-articular tissue are distended and mobility is limited.

These problems show an excellent and rapid response to treatment with CTM. Classical massage or kinesiotherapy is not indicated.

Findings in the Upper Extremity

Increased turgor and muscle tone are located in the segments C5–C8, T1–T8, L2.

▶ **Tense tissue on the posterior side of the body**
- Extending below the spine of the scapula into the posterior axillary wall
- At the lower angle of the scapula along the latissimus dorsi muscle toward the pelvic edge and along the axillary line extending under the axilla

▶ **On the anterior side of the body**
- Extending over the clavicle toward the shoulder joint,
- Below the clavicle on the sternoclavicular joint along the subclavius muscle
- Along the lower edge of the ribs extending toward the rectus abdominis muscle

▶ **On the arm**
- On the anterior part of the deltoid muscle extending to the upper arm

- Extending from the origin of the triceps brachii to the insertion of the elbow
- In the region of the flexor of elbow and hand, on the medial epicondyle of the upper arm, extending into the wrist

Treatment Plan for the Upper Extremity

Starting position: sitting, lateral position.
- Small basic sequence, flat strokes over back and arms.
- Small basic sequence, first sequence, flat strokes over rib cage and arms.
- Small basic sequence, first and second sequence, ventral side, flat strokes on the arms.
- Small basic sequence, first and second sequence, treatment of the upper arm, ventral side of the body, flat strokes on forearm and hand.
- Small basic sequence, first, second, and third sequence, ventral side, treatment of arm.

Balancing strokes over the pectoral muscles, dorsal dispersion strokes, and flat strokes of the arms are applied at the end of each treatment session to support the venous backflow.

Additional Strokes

First Sequence (▶ Fig. 2.37, ▶ Fig. 2.38, ▶ Fig. 2.39)

▶ **From dorsal**
- When changing the direction, the intercostal strokes are also performed in the opposite direction from the spine along the lateral thoracic wall to the ventral axillary line in order to gently grasp the tissue there.
- The large balancing stroke starts in the ventral axillary line at the level of the sixth/seventh intercostal space and is flatly pulled around the lower angle of the scapula toward C7.
- Short strokes from the lower angle of the scapula to the spine at the level of segment T4.
- Flat transverse strokes over the spine beginning at the level of T6 under the angle of the left scapula and ending under the angle of the right scapula and then back again.
- Small, flat transverse strokes along the spine, within the area of the long extensor spinae muscles, from T12 to T7.

▶ **From ventral**
- In the ventral intercostal area a set of flat strokes are pulled beginning at the dorsal axillary line through the intercostal spaces. These should start at the lowest ribs.

Second Sequence (▶ Fig. 2.46, ▶ Fig. 2.47, ▶ Fig. 2.48, ▶ Fig. 2.49)

▶ **From dorsal**
- Long downward stretching, along the edge of the latissimus dorsi muscle in the direction of the iliac crest.

- Prolonged upward stretching, beginning at the level of the sixth/seventh intercostal space along the edge of the latissimus dorsi muscle in the direction of the axilla.
- Axillary stretching with elevated arm: the patient puts his or her arm on the therapist's shoulder. Connecting transverse strokes are applied through the axilla to thoroughly loosen the axillary fold.
- A flat fan-shaped stroke is pulled transversely over the scapula toward the shoulder joint, starting at the outer edge of the scapula and ending at the lower edge of the spine of the scapula.
- Small, flat transverse strokes over the spine within the area of the long extensor spinae muscles, from T7 to T3 or C7.
- Flat transverse strokes from the inner side to the lateral edge of the scapulae, starting at the level of T7, ending at the spine of the scapula.
- Small hooks around the upper angle of the scapula followed by outlining the scapula with cutting strokes.

▶ **From ventral**
- The ventral edge of the trapezius muscle is pulled out starting from the cervical base, while pressing against it with the free hand.
- Strokes over the sternum, beginning at the xiphoid process pulling toward the jugular notch.
- Short hooks on the connection points between the ribs and sternum, pulling from caudal to cranial.
- Short transverse strokes along the sternum. These start at the junction between the xiphoid process and the body of the sternum, along the area of the sternal angle. At the base of the second rib at the sternum, the strokes should become wider to just under the sternoclavicular joints.
- Short fanlike strokes on the suprasternal notch, beginning on the clavicle and ending on the dorsal edge of the sternocleidomastoid muscle.
- Short strokes on the interclavicular ligament.

▶ **On the arm**
- Bimanual soft stretching of flexor and extensor of the upper arm.

Findings in the Lower Extremity

Increased muscle tone and turgor are located in the segments L1–L5 and S1–S3.

▶ **In the posterior part of the body**
- On the edges of the sacral bone (origin of the gluteus maximus muscle) pulling down to the ischiorectal fossa
- Under the edges of the pelvis in the region of the origin of the lesser gluteal muscle

▶ **In the anterior part of the body**
- From the anterior superior iliac spine extending into the groin

▶ **On the leg**
- Along the course of the iliotibial tract to the popliteal cavity
- Along the course of the adductors and the fascial tube of the sartorius muscle
- Around the knee joint
- On the outside of the calf
- Between the gastrocnemius heads toward the heel
- Along the edge of the anterior tibial muscle
- On the sole of the foot, on the inner edge of the foot, and over the metatarsophalangeal joints of the toes

Treatment Plan for the Lower Extremity

Starting position: sitting, lateral position.
- Small basic sequence, flat strokes over back and legs.
- Small basic sequence, treatment of the thigh on the unaffected side, flat strokes over the back and legs.
- Small basic sequence, treatment of the thigh on the affected leg from distal to proximal, treatment of the knee, flat strokes over the back and legs.
- Small basic sequence, treatment of the leg.

Balancing strokes over the pectoral muscles, dorsal dispersion stroke, and flat strokes of the legs are applied at the end of each treatment session to support the venous backflow.

Additional Strokes

Small Basic Sequence (▶ Fig. 2.27, ▶ Fig. 2.28, ▶ Fig. 2.29)

▶ **From ventral**
- Hooks to the sacral bone edges from caudal to cranial.
- Flat transverse strokes over the sacral bone from caudal to cranial.
- Hooks in the course of the first pelvic stroke.
- Small, flat transverse strokes along the spine within the area of the long extensor spinae muscles, from L5 to T12.
- Hooks and stretching stroke at the ischial tuberosity.
- Stretching stroke in the region of the lumbar triangle.

Small Basic Sequence in Lateral Position (▶ Fig. 2.33)

▶ **From dorsal**
- Small hooks around the greater trochanter.
- Flat balancing stroke, starting above the greater trochanter toward the ischial tuberosity.

Small Basic Sequence in Prone Position (▶ Fig. 2.33)

▶ **From dorsal**
- Short hooks along the intergluteal cleft pulling up from the lateral side.

▶ **On the leg** (▶ Fig. 2.70)
- Short hooks from the last third of the fascia lata in the shape of a fan toward the patella.
- The thigh stroke starts in the upper third of the thigh, on the lateral edge of the sartorius muscle, and ends shortly before the groin.
- Flat strokes, which are pulled from the transverse intergluteal cleft to the popliteal cavity.
- Flat strokes from the inner side of the thigh, starting below the patella and running around the medial malleolus.
- Bimanual stretching between the muscle bellies of the gastrocnemius muscle from cranial to caudal, pulling in the direction of the Achilles tendon.

Comments on the Upper and Lower Extremities

- The consensual mode of action of CTM is employed at the beginning of treatment on the unaffected extremity.
- When the adhesions around the shoulder joint loosen through application of the second and third sequences, the treatment of the arm is added.
- When the adhesions around the greater trochanter loosen after application of the small basic sequence, treatment of the affected leg is added.
- These treatments are applied from distal to proximal and should aim especially to promote arterial blood supply.
- Susceptibility to spasms must be taken into consideration with disturbances of the venous blood supply and tense tissue. It might be necessary to work only from the segment and not to move to the periphery with this technique. Careful administration is a prerequisite here so that the stimuli are not too strong.

Muscle Rheumatism (Fibromyalgia)

Definition

At least for therapists, this generic term can include myalgia with or without myogelosis or hardening of the muscles. Specific spots become painful to pressure (so-called tender points) in the diagnostic process due to overstrain or as symptoms of mental disorders.

Inflammatory forms of soft tissue rheumatism with muscular inflammation in connective tissue diseases, rheumatoid arthritis, and rheumatic polymyalgia must be distinguished through differential diagnostics. Some clinical pictures include myositis ossificans and para-articular ossification; for example, following endoprosthetic joint replacement, head trauma, or peripheral paralysis.

Treatment essentially depends on the location, extent, and stage of the disorder.

Highly acute myalgic centers must be approached first. Acute inflammatory pathological processes of this kind are contraindications for CTM.

Findings

Visible and palpable retractions and massive distensions can be observed in the region of the lumbar spine and pelvis. The tissue is hard to move, the muscles (e.g., the gluteal muscles) are hypertonic. When the lower extremity is affected, the tissue around the greater trochanter and along the iliotibial tract is palpable with increased tension.

When the shoulder girdle is affected, retractions and distensions can be detected especially between the spinal column and scapulae, which may be very sensitive during palpation. The patient also reports pain in the region of the neck, where the tissue is often very tense and seems to be swollen.

If the rheumatism extends into the arms, the tissue on the edges of the deltoid muscle is very tender and very poorly mobile, especially at the origin.

Treatment Plan for the Upper Extremity

Starting position: sitting or lateral position, supine position.
- Small basic sequence, flat strokes over back and arms.
- Small basic sequence, first sequence, flat strokes over back and arms.
- Small basic sequence, first and second sequence, ventral side, flat strokes on the arms.
- Small basic sequence, first and second sequence, ventral side of the body, treatment of the upper arm, flat strokes of forearm and hand.
- Small basic sequence, first, second, and third sequence, ventral side of the body, treatment of the upper arm and forearm, flat strokes on the hand.
- Small basic sequence, first, second, and third sequence, ventral side, treatment of arm.

Balancing strokes over the pectoral muscles, dorsal dispersion stroke, and flat strokes of the arms are applied at the end of each treatment session to support the venous backflow.

Additional Strokes

First Sequence (▶ Fig. 2.37, ▶ Fig. 2.38, ▶ Fig. 2.39)

▶ **From dorsal**
- When changing the direction, the intercostal strokes are also performed in the opposite direction, from the spine along the lateral thoracic wall to the ventral axillary line, in order to gently grasp the tissue there.
- The large balancing stroke starts in the ventral axillary line at the level of the sixth/seventh intercostal space and is flatly pulled around the lower angle of the scapula toward C7.
- Short strokes from the lower angle of the scapula to the spine at the level of segment T4.

- Flat transverse strokes over the spine, beginning at the level of T6 under the angle of the left scapula and ending under the angle of the right scapula and then back again.
- Small, flat transverse strokes along the spine, within the area of the long extensor spinae muscles, from T12 to T7.

▶ **From ventral**
- In the ventral intercostal area a set of flat strokes are pulled beginning at the dorsal axillary line through the intercostal spaces. These should start at the lowest ribs.

Second Sequence (▶ Fig. 2.46, ▶ Fig. 2.47, ▶ Fig. 2.48, ▶ Fig. 2.49)

▶ **From dorsal**
- Long downward stretching, along the edge of the latissimus dorsi muscle in the direction of the iliac crest.
- Prolonged upward stretching, beginning at the level of the sixth/seventh intercostal space, along the edge of the latissimus dorsi muscle in the direction of the axilla.
- Axillary stretching with elevated arm: the patient puts his or her arm on the therapist's shoulder. Connecting transverse strokes are applied through the axilla to thoroughly loosen the axillary fold.
- A flat fan-shaped stroke is pulled transversely over the scapula toward the shoulder joint, starting at the outer edge of the scapula and ending at the lower edge of the spine of the scapula.
- Small, flat transverse strokes over the spine, within the area of the long extensor spinae muscles, from T7 to T3 or C7.
- Flat transverse strokes from the inner side to the lateral edge of the scapulae, starting at the level of T7, ending at the spine of the scapula.
- Small hooks around the upper angle of the scapula followed by outlining the scapula with cutting strokes.

▶ **From ventral**
- The ventral edge of the trapezius muscle is pulled out starting from the cervical base, while pressing against it with the free hand.
- Strokes over the sternum, beginning at the xiphoid process pulling toward the jugular notch.
- Short hooks on the connection points between the ribs and sternum, pulling from caudal to cranial.
- Short transverse strokes along the sternum. These start at the junction between the xiphoid process and the body of the sternum, along the area of the sternal angle. At the base of the second rib at the sternum, the strokes should become wider to just under the sternoclavicular joints.
- Short fanlike strokes on the suprasternal notch, beginning on the clavicle and ending on the dorsal edge of the sternocleidomastoid muscle.
- Short strokes on the interclavicular ligament.

▶ **On the arm**
- Bimanual soft stretching of flexor and extensor of the upper arm.

Treatment Plan for the Lower Extremity

Starting position: sitting, lateral position, supine position.
- Small basic sequence, flat strokes over back and legs.
- Small basic sequence, first sequence, flat strokes over lower leg and foot.
- Small basic sequence, first sequence, treatment of thigh and knee, flat strokes over lower leg and foot.
- Small basic sequence, first sequence, treatment of thigh, knee, and lower leg and flat strokes on the foot.
- Small basic sequence, first sequence, treatment of the leg.

Balancing strokes over the pectoral muscles, dorsal dispersion stroke, and flat strokes of the legs are applied at the end of each treatment session to support the venous backflow.

Additional Strokes

Small Basic Sequence (▶ Fig. 2.27, ▶ Fig. 2.28, ▶ Fig. 2.29)

▶ **From dorsal**
- Hooks to the sacral bone edges from caudal to cranial.
- Flat transverse strokes over the sacral bone, from caudal to cranial.
- Hooks, in the course of the first pelvic stroke.
- Small, flat transverse strokes along the spine, within the area of the long extensor spinae muscles, from L5 to T12.
- Hooks and stretching stroke at the ischial tuberosity.
- Stretching stroke in the region of the lumbar triangle.
- Fanlike strokes in the upper respiratory angle: Fanlike strokes are flatly applied to the angle between the lowest rib and the spine. These should start on the lower edge of the rib cage and end with the last strokes along the spine (L3 to T12).

Small Basic Sequence in Lateral Position (▶ Fig. 2.33)

▶ **From dorsal**
- Small hooks around the greater trochanter.
- Flat balancing stroke, starting above the greater trochanter toward the ischial tuberosity.

Small Basic Sequence in Prone Position (▶ Fig. 2.33)

▶ **From dorsal**
- Short hooks along the intergluteal cleft pulling up from the lateral side.

▶ **On the leg** (▶ Fig. 2.70)

- Short hooks from the last third of the fascia lata, in the shape of a fan toward the patella.
- The thigh stroke starts in the upper third of the thigh, on the lateral edge of the sartorius muscle, and ends shortly before the groin.
- Flat strokes, which are pulled from the transverse inter-gluteal cleft to the popliteal cavity.
- Flat strokes from the inner side of the thigh, starting below the patella and running around the medial malleolus.
- Bimanual stretching between the muscle bellies of the gastrocnemius muscle, from cranial to caudal, pulling in the direction of the Achilles tendon.

Comments on the Upper and Lower Extremity

- The skin reaction is very lively during CTM treatment of muscle rheumatism. Intensive red discoloration is often followed by the development of welts. This indicates to the therapist that he or she should reconsider the technique and strokes through the tissue.
- The treatment of the iliotibial tract from the middle at first in the proximal direction, then in the distal direction, guarantees well-dosed support of the leg's blood supply. The adhesions of the tissue in the tract indicate an involvement of the kidney. The segments T8–T12, L1–L3 should be palpated well in the paravertebral region. Existing edemas in the legs are mobilized and dissolved through loosening hooks in the region of the tract.
- If the upper and lower extremities are affected, treatment is applied alternately: small basic sequence and treatment of the leg or small basic sequence with other sequences and treatment of the arm.
- CTM is not suitable during the acute stage of rheumatic and infectious arthritis. After the acute inflammatory symptoms have disappeared, however, the after effects can be carefully treated with CTM. The measures are then consistent with the treatment plan that is described in the sections on Osteoarthritis (p.82) and Irritated Joints (p.90).

Complex Regional Pain Syndrome

Definition

Complex regional pain syndrome is a spontaneous or post-traumatic disorder that is accompanied by inflammatory changes in peripheral parts of the extremities. Its pathogenesis is not yet fully understood (▶ Fig. 3.6).

The symptoms affect the skin, muscles, joints, and all adjoining parts.

The disorder goes through the stages of acute inflammation and dystrophy and can also reach the stage of

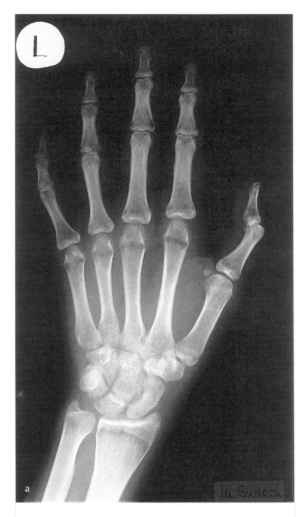

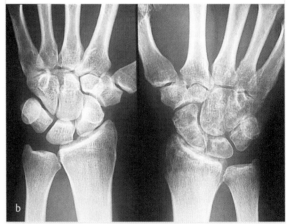

Fig. 3.6 Complex regional pain syndrome.
a Onset of complex regional pain syndrome of the left hand (increased radiolucency due to bone atrophy).
b Complex regional pain syndrome with typical spotty decalcification of carpal bones (see unaffected side on the left for comparison).

terminal atrophy. The disorder does not necessarily progress in stages but can also be lingering, which is why diagnosing the disease is often difficult.

Edematous swellings with livid discoloration of the skin develop, hot and cold temperatures of the distal parts of the body are detectable, and atrophy of the bones is radiologically detectable at the earliest after 8 weeks. Fibrous stiffness of joints develops only after the inflammatory changes have disappeared. Skin atrophy and the typical spotty decalcification of bone tissue are discernible in the radiographic image. The initially accelerated growth of skin appendages normalizes again. The end stage is marked by extensive muscular atrophy and contractures and is usually reached a year after the onset of the disorder. There is no longer pain in this stage.

Treatment focuses on the stage of the disorder and very different medicinal and physical measures can be considered. The main objective is to eliminate the pain.

The application of CTM is combined with well-dosed physical therapy exercises. Contrary to previous policy, CTM is started in the earliest stage. During hospitalization, CTM is applied every day; during outpatient treatment it is administered two to three times a week as long-term therapy.

Findings

Increased turgor and muscle tone are located in the segments C4–C8, T1–T12, and L1–L5. There is atrophy, especially in the distal parts of the body. In the stage of acute inflammation the extremity is warm to hot. The joints are poorly mobile; the swelling is located in the metacarpophalangeal or metatarsophalangeal joints of the foot or hand, extending into the phalanges.

In the stage of dystrophy the distal part of the extremity is swollen and also warm. In the stage of atrophy the extremity feels cold and the skin turns gray and dry.

Tissue changes observed in **dystrophy of the hand**:

▶ **On the posterior side of the body**
- Along the muscle fascia of the latissimus dorsi muscle, on the origin of the lower angle of the scapula down to the iliac crest
- In the lower section of the scapula along the spine of the scapula toward the shoulder joint extending into the deltoid and pectoral muscles

▶ **On the arm**
- On the triceps brachii, especially on the olecranon to the flexors of the elbow and the hand on the ulnar side of the forearm

▶ **On the anterior side of the body**
- On the lower edge of the rib cage along the rectus abdominis muscle
- In the intercostal area over the pectoralis major muscle and in the axilla

- Under and on the clavicle extending to the sternocleidomastoid muscle

Tissue changes observed in **dystrophy of the foot**:

▶ **On the posterior side of the body**
- The sacral bone and on the edges of the sacral bone

▶ **On the leg**
- Around the greater trochanter and along the iliotibial tract
- On the adductors extending over the dorsal side of the knee joints
- On the edge of the anterior tibial muscle, the peroneal muscle, around the malleolus mortise, and on the back of the foot

Treatment Plan for the Upper Extremity

Starting position: sitting, supine position.

The patient's arm is elevated (elbow higher than shoulder joint, hand higher than elbow).
- Small basic sequence, flat strokes over back and arm.
- Small basic sequence, first sequence, flat strokes over back and arm.
- Small basic sequence, first and second sequence, ventral side, flat strokes on the arm.
- Small basic sequence, first, second, and third sequence, ventral side, flat strokes on the arm.
- Small basic sequence, first, second, and third sequence, ventral side of the body, treatment of the upper arm, flat strokes of forearm and hand.
- Small basic sequence, first, second, and third sequence, ventral side, treatment of arm.
- Small basic sequence, first, second, and third sequence, ventral side, treatment of arm, treatment of face.

Balancing strokes over the pectoral muscles, dorsal dispersion stroke, and flat strokes of the arms are applied at the end of each treatment session to support the venous backflow.

Additional Strokes

Small Basic Sequence (▶ Fig. 2.27, ▶ Fig. 2.28, ▶ Fig. 2.29)

▶ **From dorsal**
- Hooks to the sacral bone edges from caudal to cranial.
- Flat transverse strokes over the sacral bone from caudal to cranial.
- Hooks, in the course of the first pelvic stroke.
- Small, flat transverse strokes along the spine within the area of the long extensor spinae muscles from L5 to T12.
- Hooks and stretching stroke at the ischial tuberosity.
- Stretching stroke in the region of the lumbar triangle.

- Fanlike strokes in the upper respiratory angle: fanlike strokes are flatly applied to the angle between the lowest rib and the spine. Starting on the lower edge of the rib cage and ending with the last strokes along the spine (L3 to T12).

First Sequence (▶ Fig. 2.37, ▶ Fig. 2.38, ▶ Fig. 2.39)

▶ **From dorsal**
- When changing the direction, the intercostal strokes are also performed in the opposite direction from the spine along the lateral thoracic wall to the ventral axillary line in order to gently grasp the tissue there.
- The large balancing stroke starts in the ventral axillary line at the level of the sixth/seventh intercostal space and is flatly pulled around the lower angle of the scapula toward C7.
- Short strokes from the lower angle of the scapula to the spine at the level of segment T4.
- Flat transverse strokes over the spine, beginning at the level of T6 under the angle of the left scapula and ending under the angle of the right scapula and then back again.
- Small, flat transverse strokes along the spine within the area of the long extensor spinae muscles from T12 to T7.

▶ **From ventral**
- In the ventral intercostal area a set of flat strokes are pulled beginning at the dorsal axillary line through the intercostal spaces. These should start at the lowest ribs.

Second Sequence (▶ Fig. 2.46, ▶ Fig. 2.47, ▶ Fig. 2.48, ▶ Fig. 2.49)

▶ **From dorsal**
- Long downward stretching along the edge of the latissimus dorsi muscle in the direction of the iliac crest.
- Prolonged upward stretching, beginning at the level of the sixth/seventh intercostal space, along the edge of the latissimus dorsi muscle in the direction of the axilla.
- Axillary stretching with elevated arm: The patient puts his arm on the therapist's shoulder. Connecting transverse strokes are applied through the axilla to thoroughly loosen the axillary fold.
- A flat fan-shaped stroke is pulled transversely over the scapula toward the shoulder joint, starting at the outer edge of the scapula and ending at the lower edge of the spine of the scapula.
- Small, flat transverse strokes over the spine within the area of the long extensor spinae muscles, from T7 to T3 or C7.
- Flat transverse strokes from the inner side to the lateral edge of the scapulae, starting at the level of T7, ending at the spine of the scapula.

- Small hooks around the upper angle of the scapula followed by outlining the scapula with cutting strokes.

▶ **From ventral**
- The ventral edge of the trapezius muscle is pulled out starting from the cervical base, while pressing against it with the free hand.
- Strokes over the sternum, beginning at the xiphoid process and pulling toward the jugular notch.
- Short hooks on the connection points between the ribs and sternum pulling from caudal to cranial.
- Short transverse strokes along the sternum. These start at the junction between the xiphoid process and the body of the sternum, along the area of the sternal angle. At the base of the second rib at the sternum, the strokes should become wider to just under the sternoclavicular joints.
- Short fanlike strokes on the suprasternal notch, beginning on the clavicle and ending on the dorsal edge of the sternocleidomastoid muscle.
- Short strokes on the interclavicular ligament.

▶ **On the arm**
- Bimanual soft stretching of flexor and extensor of the upper arm.

Comments on the Upper Extremity

The decision whether or not to apply CTM to an affected side depends on the findings. Otherwise, the therapist should wait for the consensual reaction triggered by processes of the autonomic nervous system when treating the unaffected side.
- When applying the small basic sequence the tissue's response must be closely observed. The other treatment sequences are only added when intensive reddening and a cutting sensation develop.
- The hooks to the spinal column are omitted in the first sequence. Only the intercostal strokes are applied in both directions while grasping at the axillary line.
- At the beginning of the second sequence, the unaffected side of the body is treated. When the tissue tension loosens, the strokes are administered to the affected side.
- The application of the facial treatment following the third sequence is very calming and relaxing. Treatment of the scapula and the axillary stretching are given special attention here. During the first 14 days no local treatment is administered to the hand or forearm, since no additional stimuli should be applied from the outside.
- The forearm and the hand are treated with flat strokes.
- If the periphery is treated after the various treatment sequences, the strokes of the small basic sequence and first sequence are applied only once or twice. Treatment focuses on the shoulder and upper arm.

- The swelling of the hand should visibly decrease and show better circulation. Otherwise, only intensive segmental strokes are applied to T3–T7, and the arm receives strokes only in the proximal direction.
- The bimanual stretching of the flexor and extensor of the hand and elbow should loosen the adhesions between the muscle septa, thus supporting the metabolism. If the affected arm cannot be elevated high enough in the initial sitting position, the patient is treated in the lying position and the arm is relieved through elevation.
- When applying strokes on the hand, it is very important that both the dorsal and palmar interosseous muscles are stroked from distal to proximal. Remember to stretch the palm from palmar to dorsal. Carefully drawing the skin of the interdigital web spaces to both sides with the thumbs supports flexion of the finger at the metacarpophalangeal joints.

Treatment Plan for the Lower Extremity

Starting position: lateral position, supine position.
The affected leg is elevated (knee higher than the hip joint, foot higher than the knee joint).
- Small basic sequence, flat strokes over the back and leg.
- Small basic sequence, first sequence, ventral side of the body, flat strokes over the leg.
- Small basic sequence, first sequence, ventral side of the body, treatment of the thighs, flat strokes on the lower leg.
- Small basic sequence, first sequence, ventral side of the body, treatment of thigh and knee, flat strokes over the lower leg and foot.
- Small basic sequence, first sequence, ventral side of the body, treatment of the thigh, knee and lower leg, flat strokes on the foot.
- Small basic sequence, first sequence, treatment of the leg.

Balancing strokes over the pectoral muscles, dorsal dispersion stroke, and flat strokes of the legs are applied at the end of each treatment session to support the venous backflow.

Additional Strokes

Small Basic Sequence (▶ Fig. 2.27, ▶ Fig. 2.28, ▶ Fig. 2.29)

▶ **From dorsal**
- Hooks to the sacral bone edges from caudal to cranial.
- Flat transverse strokes over the sacral bone from caudal to cranial.
- Hooks in the course of the first pelvic stroke.
- Small, flat transverse strokes along the spine within the area of the long extensor spinae muscles from L5 to T12.

- Hooks and stretching stroke at the ischial tuberosity.
- Stretching stroke in the region of the lumbar triangle.
- Fanlike strokes in the upper respiratory angle: fanlike strokes are flatly applied to the angle between the lowest rib and the spine. These should start on the lowest edge of the rib cage and end with the last strokes along the spine (L3 to T12).

Small Basic Sequence in Lateral Position (▶ Fig. 2.33)

▶ **From dorsal**
- Small hooks around the greater trochanter.
- Flat balancing stroke, starting above the greater trochanter toward the ischial tuberosity.

Small Basic Sequence in Prone Position (▶ Fig. 2.33)

▶ **From dorsal**
- Short hooks along the intergluteal cleft pulling up from the lateral side.

First Sequence (▶ Fig. 2.37, ▶ Fig. 2.38, ▶ Fig. 2.39)

▶ **From dorsal**
- When changing the direction, the intercostal strokes are also performed in the opposite direction, from the spine along the lateral thoracic wall to the ventral axillary line, in order to gently grasp the tissue there.
- The large balancing stroke starts in the ventral axillary line at the level of the sixth/seventh intercostal space and is flatly pulled around the lower angle of the scapula toward C7.
- Short strokes from the lower angle of the scapula to the spine at the level of segment T4.
- Flat transverse strokes over the spine, beginning at the level of T6 under the angle of the left scapula and ending under the angle of the right scapula and then back again.
- Small, flat transverse strokes along the spine, within the area of the long extensor spinae muscles, from T12 to T7.

▶ **From ventral**
- In the ventral intercostal area a set of flat strokes are pulled from the dorsal axillary line through the intercostal spaces. These should start at the lowest ribs.
- Bimanual strokes, from dorsal on the lower edge of the rib cage to the medioclavicular line and from the pelvic edge to the anterior superior iliac spine. These strokes are performed bimanually, first on one side of the body then on the other.
- Short hooks along the rectus sheath from the symphysis up to the navel.
- Short strokes, like rays, pulling toward the navel.

- Bimanual strokes crossing over the abdominal walls starting in the dorsal region and ending at the opposite edge of the rectus abdominis muscle.

▶ **On the leg** (▶ Fig. 2.70)
- Short hooks from the last third of the fascia lata in the shape of a fan toward the patella.
- The thigh stroke starts in the upper third of the thigh, to the lateral edge of the sartorius muscle, and ends shortly before the groin.
- Flat strokes, which are pulled from the transverse intergluteal cleft to the popliteal cavity.
- Flat strokes from the inner side of the thigh, starting below the patella and running around the medial malleolus.
- Bimanual stretching between the muscle bellies of the gastrocnemius muscle from cranial to caudal, pulling in the direction of the Achilles tendon.

Comments on the Lower Extremity

- The tissue's response must be closely observed during the application of the small basic sequence. The small basic sequence is applied three or four times. Only when intensive reddening and a cutting sensation develop should the lower extremity be included in the treatment.
- At the beginning the treatment is performed only on the unaffected leg.
- Strokes on the tract are applied from distal to proximal (carefully watch for disturbances in circulation). The hooks start in the middle of the thigh. Treat the region of the tract intensively with the flat and cutting stroke technique.
- The sole of the foot should receive particular attention when the foot is being treated. It is treated with strong strokes from the heel to the metatarsophalangeal joints. The medial and lateral edges are given special attention with longitudinal strokes and small hooks from plantar to dorsal.
- The toes are treated the same way as the fingers.

Scar Treatment

Definition

The treatment of scars depends on the location and dimensions of the scar, but also on the stage of scar formation. Changes of subcutaneous tissue without lesion of the dermis can be considered to be the same as a real scar.

The treatment of scars with CTM should start soon after the wound has healed. Initially the center must not be touched. The therapist slowly works through the small basic sequence and periphery with the goal of improving the blood supply of the scarring tissue and preventing hardened scars. Although more difficult, the therapy of older scars is not completely hopeless.

Special caution must be applied when treating scars on the neck—for example, after thyroid gland surgery—or in the segment areas of particularly sensitive organs such as the heart.

Burn scars can be loosened up with a good prognosis. Starting with the small basic sequence, possibly supplemented with the other treatment sequences, the therapist works toward the scar.

Hardened scars are also slowly loosened with small hooks. Painful scars caused by syringe abscesses are treated in the same manner.

If a scar is retracted deeply and adheres to the periosteum, CTM will remain ineffective. Surgery scars, which trigger dysfunctions due to adhesions, can be carefully loosened after brief segmental preparation.

If there is no peristalsis after an appendectomy, constipation (p. 149) is treated in a lightly dosed form without exercises. When the elevated abdominal tension decreases, the scar itself is treated after strokes have been applied to the edges of the pelvis (small basic sequence in lateral position). Usually normal peristalsis is regained once the adhesions are loosened.

Findings

> Therapists must draw their own conclusions when palpating the tissue involved, since this text cannot define the area of the body where the scar is located.

Care should be taken to note the segmental relations of organs. An adhering scar is always a source of irritation. In new scars the adhesions lie between the skin and hypodermis, in older scars they lie correspondingly deeper between hypodermis and muscular fascia.

Treatment Plan

Starting position: sitting, lateral position, supine position, prone position.
- Small basic sequence, flat strokes over the back from caudal toward cranial.
- Small basic sequence, with necessary additional treatment sequences.
- Small basic sequence with section sequences and treatment of the extremities.

Balancing strokes over the pectoral muscles, dorsal dispersion stroke, and flat strokes of the legs and/or arms are applied at the end of each treatment session to support the venous backflow.

Additional Strokes

Since they cannot be listed here individually, the therapist is advised to use the additional strokes of the small basic sequence (p. 34) and of the individual section sequences.

▶ **Special remarks**
- Depending on the location of the scar, include the additional section sequences after the small basic sequence and then work locally on the scar.
- Short hooks toward and away from the scar. The surrounding tissue is held back with the free hand, if necessary, so that the traction needed for the response of the autonomic nervous system in the tissue can be generated.
- Transverse stretching along the course of the muscles.
- The short hooks must not be applied with strokes that are raised too high.
- Special attention should be paid to the tissue response around the scar area.
- Treatment of complex regional pain syndrome with CTM is a long-term therapy. At the beginning, treatment should be performed on a daily basis; afterward, treatments can be reduced to two or three times a week.
- The patient and therapist need to have much patience and mutual trust.
- It must be ensured that the patient rests after treatment.

Comments

- Depending on the location of the scar, the additional section sequences are included after the small basic sequence and then work is done locally on the scar, scar tissue permitting.
- Special attention should be paid to the tissue response around the scar area.
- Initially, the short hooks must be applied with strokes that are not raised too high.

Scleroderma

Definition

Progressive scleroderma is an immunological inflammatory systemic disease of the connective tissue that affects the general skin and also internal organs. It progresses chronically or in bouts and is incurable.

With *circumscribed scleroderma* or morphea, which in itself can be an indication for CTM, there are demarcated, sclerosing, rarely individually developing skin changes, often on the elbow and above the knee, occasionally on the face or above the forehead ("linear scleroderma").

In its pathogenesis circumscribed scleroderma is closely related to generalized scleroderma. It differs in its distribution and its often much more favorable course. If there are no signs of active inflammation, CTM is indi-

cated with the goal of loosening and improving the blood supply of the surrounding connective tissue.

Findings

Skin and hypodermis of the affected area are rock-hard and immobile. Wrists and ankles can be restricted in their mobility.

Increased turgor and muscle tone in the tissue can be found throughout the entire body:
- In the paravertebral region of the spinal column
- Above the sacral bone, the edges of the sacral bone, on the rounding of the buttocks
- On the iliotibial tract, especially in the region of the greater trochanter
- On the adductors and in the popliteal cavity
- On the muscle septa of the gastrocnemius muscle, especially on the lateral head
- On the muscle septa of the deltoid muscle, extending from the lateral side to the scapula and the axilla
- On the medial and lateral edge of the scapula
- On the trapezius muscle, in the neck and shoulder area
- On the upper arm, the muscle septa of the triceps brachii, the flexors of the hand and of the elbow
- On the edge of the latissimus dorsi muscle
- Along the muscle edges of the abdominal wall
- In the region of the anterior superior iliac spine extending to the groin
- On the edges of the sartorius muscle, on the edge of the tibia along the anterior tibial muscle
- Around the malleolus mortise, along the outer edge of the foot, over the metatarsophalangeal joints of the toes extending in the medial direction
- Over the clavicle, on the edges of the pectoralis major muscle and deltoid muscle
- On the inner side of the upper arm, along the muscle septa to the crook of the elbow and the inner side of the hand

Treatment Plan

Starting position: Sitting, supine position, prone position.
- Small basic sequence, flat strokes over the back from caudal toward cranial.
- Small basic sequence, first sequence, flat strokes over rib cage and arms.
- Small basic sequence, first and second sequence, ventral side, flat strokes on the arms.
- Small basic sequence, first, second, and third sequence, ventral side, flat strokes on the arms.
- Small basic sequence, first, second, and third sequence, facial treatment, flat strokes on the arms.

Balancing strokes over the pectoral muscles, dorsal dispersion stroke, and flat strokes of the legs and/or arms are applied at the end of each treatment session to support the venous backflow.

Additional Strokes

The additional strokes are taken over from the small basic sequence (p. 34) and the additional section sequences in the affected areas.

▶ **Special remarks**
- It should be ensured that the cutting sensation develops when CTM is applied. Should the patient feel blunt pressure, the therapist must apply flat strokes over the entire torso and wait until slight reddening develops in the tissue.
- CTM intensifies the blood supply in the tissue, the metabolism is elevated, and the mobility between the skin layers is improved.
- Not only does the patient feel subjectively better, there is also an objective improvement of the pathological processes.
- If the pathology affects the lower extremity, a focus is placed on intensive application of the small basic sequence and treatment of the leg.
- If the upper part of the body is affected, the intensity of the treatment is shifted toward the first and second sequences with treatment of the arm.
- With this pathology the treatment is a long-term therapy, in which the patient and therapist must have much patience and mutual trust.
- Pauses in treatment should be scheduled.
- The treatment should be properly coordinated with the concomitant physical therapy. It must be ensured that the patient rests after treatment.

Comments

It must be ensured that the patient experiences a cutting sensation. Should the patient perceive the treatment as blunt pressure, the therapist should apply flat strokes over the entire torso instead.
- CTM intensifies the blood supply in the tissue, the metabolism is elevated, and the mobility between the skin layers is improved.
- Not only does the patient feel subjectively better, there is also an objective improvement of the pathological processes.
- If the lower extremity is affected, perform the small basic sequence three times a week (including the iliotibial tract and trochanter area).
- If the upper part of the body is affected, the small basic sequence should be performed three times a week, then adding the first sequence and, depending on the individual findings, also second and third sequences with treatment of the head/face.
- Longer series of treatment should be planned.

Pressure Ulcer

Definition

Decubitus ulcers (Latin *decubare* = to lie down) are also called pressure ulcers, which are liable to develop as a consequence of long periods of immobility in patients who are weak and bedridden.

These lesions are found on those sites of the body where continuous pressure is applied: for example, on the sacral bone, the trochanters, the elbows, the heels, the malleoli, the scapulae, and in rare cases also on the back of the head.

This continuous pressure leads to severe circulatory disturbances and in the end to necrosis (death of tissue) of the skin, the extent of which can range from the size of a coin to two palms' width. In the deeper layers they can even reach the bone. Severe permanent suppuration and life-threatening infections can be the consequence.

Thorough care of the patient, especially frequent repositioning of the body, can prevent these types of complications. CTM is also a tried and proven method of improving the blood supply of skin areas at risk (prevention) or the surrounding areas. In severe cases tissue necroses must be surgically removed and the condition must be corrected with plastic surgery.

Findings

The tension is locally increased in the tissue around the pressure ulcer. The tissue shows adhesions under the pelvic edges, on the sacral bone, and around the area of the trochanter. The therapist palpates the segmental body areas and adapts the treatment accordingly.

Treatment Plan

Starting position: prone position, lateral position.
- Small basic sequence, flat strokes over the rib cage from caudal toward cranial.
- Small basic sequence, treatment of the thigh, flat strokes on lower leg and foot.
- Small basic sequence, treatment of thigh, lower leg, and foot.
- Small basic sequence with additional section sequences and the upper extremity.

Balancing strokes over the pectoral muscles, dorsal dispersion stroke, and flat strokes of the legs and/or arms are applied at the end of each treatment session to support the venous backflow.

Additional Strokes

- The tissue tension is locally increased around the ulcer. The therapist will apply the necessary strokes from the small basic sequence (p. 34) and the additional section sequences according to the status of the illness.

▶ **Special remarks**
- The pressure spots must be relieved when positioning the patient. The therapist will coordinate this as well as possible with the nursing staff and develop a positioning plan together.
- The therapist will increasingly place emphasis on treatment of the condition after administering the small basic sequence and any additional section sequences necessary.
- The wound edges of the pressure ulcer are grasped with short strokes and long flat strokes are applied around the wound edges.
- Treatment of pressure ulcers is a long-term treatment. Patience and trust are again absolutely essential here.
- It must be ensured that the patient rests thoroughly after the treatment.
- Patients with pain in the heel, who have been bedridden for a long time, are treated in supine position:
  ○ Careful pulling strokes are applied to the Achilles tendon.
  ○ The heel is to be treated.
  ○ Pulling strokes are applied on the sole of the foot.

Comments

The wound edges of the pressure ulcer are hooked with short strokes and long flat strokes are applied around the wound edges.

When positioning the patient it must be ensured that the pressure spots are relieved. The therapist will coordinate this as well as possible with the nursing staff and develop a positioning plan together with them.

3.4 Neurological Diseases

Roland Schiffter, Rauthgundis Gleich von Muenster

Neurological diseases are a significant area of indication for CTM. The object of treatment here is to improve motor functions, specifically muscles, and the organs innervated by the autonomic nervous system.

3.4.1 Selected Diseases

Cerebral Lesions

Definition

Disturbances of motor functions in cerebral lesions usually result in hemiplegia, more specifically spastic hemipareses, which is most frequently caused by a stroke. The majority are cerebral infarctions (ca. 85%) (▶ Fig. 3.7); significantly less frequent are hemorrhages (15%) (▶ Fig. 3.8), which damage or destroy the cells of the motor cortex or their process, the pyramidal pathways, in the brain, which leads to contralateral paralysis. Cerebral lesions are often combined with deficits of unilateral sensory functions and/or unilateral visual impairment (hemianopsia) or speech impairment (aphasia) if the left side

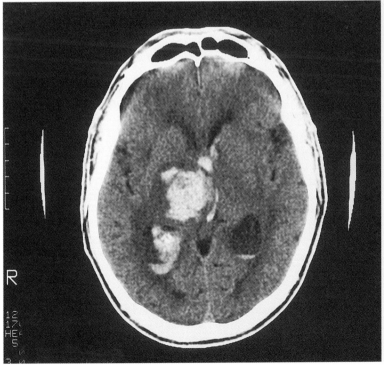

Fig. 3.7 Hemorrhage in a cerebral mass in the area of the brainstem with infiltration into the ventricular system.

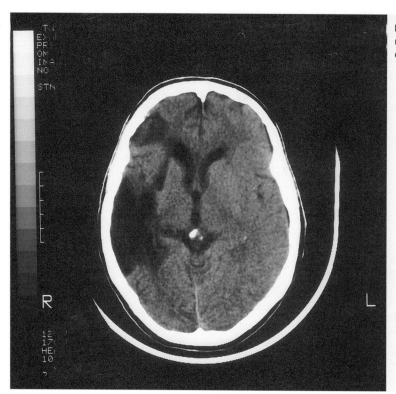

Fig. 3.8 Large cerebral infarction on the right side caused by occlusion of the middle cerebral artery.

of the brain is damaged. Hemiparesis may affect the face, arm, or leg, depending on which area of the brain (or with cerebral infarctions, what part of the vessels) is specifically affected.

Other causes of such spastic hemipareses are brain injuries caused, for example, by traffic or work accidents (cerebral contusion and hemorrhage). Epidural and subdural hematomas, which are usually surgically removed by a neurosurgeon, can also cause hemipareses.

Less frequent, but still very important are tumors of the brain. In many cases, people who have had brain tumors, brain injuries, or surgery often continue to be at risk of having epileptic seizures, which can also occur during connective tissue massage.

Spastic muscle cramps are especially easy to influence with CTM. The muscle spasm is a springy firm muscle resistance that can be felt when passively moving the extremity. It is always caused by damage to the pyramidal pathway and can also affect the muscles of the back, shoulder, and pelvis.

Central regulatory disturbances of blood vessels, so-called vasomotor disturbances, in the region of the paralyzed extremities are also suitable targets of connective tissue massage.

Findings

Changes in the mobility of skin and muscle tissue must be palpated individually by the therapist and considered when developing the treatment plan.

Treatment Plan

Starting position: lateral position, lying on the affected side, prone position, supine position, sitting.

Once the circulation has stabilized (this is usually the case after two or three sessions), the therapist continues to work on the sitting patient.

- Small basic sequence on the unaffected side, flat strokes on both legs.
- Small basic sequence on both sides of the body, flat strokes on both legs.
- Small basic sequence, first sequence on the unaffected side, treatment of the thigh, flat strokes on both legs.
- Small basic sequence, first sequence on both sides, second sequence on the unaffected side, treatment of thigh and knee, flat strokes on both legs and both arms.
- Small basic sequence, first and second sequence on both sides, ventral side, treatment of leg, treatment of arm on the unaffected side, flat strokes on both arms.
- Small basic sequence, first and second sequences, ventral side, treatment of leg and arm on the affected side.
- Small basic sequence, first, second, and third sequence, ventral side, treatment of leg and arm on the affected side, facial treatment.

Balancing strokes over the pectoral muscles, dorsal dispersion stroke, and flat strokes of the legs and arms are applied at the end of each treatment session to support the venous backflow.

Additional Strokes

Small Basic Sequence

► **From dorsal** (► Fig. 2.33)
- Small hooks toward the edges of the sacral bone.
- Short hooks along the intergluteal cleft pulling up from the lateral side.
- Flat transverse strokes over the sacral bone.
- Hooks along the course of the large pelvic stroke and around the greater trochanter.
- Small, flat transverse strokes within the area of the long extensor spinae muscles, from L5 to T12, after the hooks to the spinal column.

► **From ventral** (► Fig. 2.35)
- Bimanual strokes, beginning simultaneously from dorsal on the lower edge of the rib cage to the medioclavicular line and from the pelvic edge to the anterior superior iliac spine. These strokes are performed bimanually, first on one side then on the other.
- Bimanual strokes crossing over the abdominal walls, starting in the dorsal region and ending at the opposite edge of the rectus abdominis muscle.

First Sequence

► **From dorsal**
- The intercostal strokes are also pulled in the opposite direction from the spinal column to the lateral thorax wall to the ventral axillary line and hooked in there gently.
- The large balancing stroke starts in the ventral axillary line at the level of the sixth/seventh intercostal space and is flatly pulled around the lower angle of the scapula toward C7.
- Flat transverse strokes over the spine, beginning at the level of T6 under the left scapula and ending under the right scapula.
- Small, flat transverse strokes along the spine, within the area of the long extensor spinae muscles, from T12 to T7.

► **From ventral** (► Fig. 2.39)
- In the ventral intercostal area a set of flat strokes are pulled beginning at the dorsal axillary line through the intercostal spaces. These should start at the lowest ribs.

Second Sequence (► Fig. 2.45, ► Fig. 2.46, ► Fig. 2.47, ► Fig. 2.48)

► **From dorsal**
- Long downward stretching.
- Prolonged upward stretching.
- Axillary stretching with cutting strokes on the arm that rests on the therapist's shoulder. Connecting transverse strokes are applied in the region of the anterior serratus muscle to thoroughly loosen the dorsal and ventral axillary fold.

- A flat fan-shaped stroke is pulled transversely over the scapula toward the shoulder joint, starting at the outer edge of the scapula and ending at the lower edge of the spine of the scapula.
- Small, flat transverse strokes are applied over the spine, within the area of the long extensor spinae muscles, from T7 to C7 (► Fig. 2.48 [1]).
- Small hooks around the angle of the scapula followed by outlining the scapula with cutting strokes along the same course (► Fig. 2.48 [3]).

► **From ventral** (► Fig. 2.49)
- The ventral edge of the trapezius muscle is pulled out starting from the cervical base up to the level of the shoulder, while pressing against it with the free hand.
- Flat strokes along the sternum, beginning at the xiphoid process, to the jugular notch.
- Short hooks on the connection points between the ribs and sternum, pulling from caudal to cranial.

► **On the arm** (► Fig. 2.45)
- Bimanual soft stretching of flexor and extensor of the upper arm in the lateral direction. Flat strokes along the muscle bellies of the biceps and triceps brachii to the proximity of the elbow.

► **On the leg** (► Fig. 2.66, ► Fig. 2.67, ► Fig. 2.68, ► Fig. 2.69, ► Fig. 2.70)
- Short strokes from the last third of the fascia lata, in the shape of a fan toward the patella.
- The thigh stroke, starting in the upper third of the thigh along the lateral edge of the sartorius muscle and ending shortly before the groin.
- Strokes from the inner side of the thigh, starting below the patella and running around the medial malleolus.
- Bimanual stretching between the muscle bellies of the gastrocnemius muscle from top to bottom, pulling in the direction of the Achilles tendon.

Comments

- The strokes must be applied flatly in patients with spastic paresis. The hooks must not create too strong a stimulus, since this may increase the spasm.
- The spasm is reduced on the affected side due to the consensual effect triggered at the beginning through treatment on the unaffected side of the patient's body. It is possible that the patient may no longer be able to walk after treatment. Since this reaction is only temporary it should not alarm the therapist.
- The reactions of the autonomic nervous system over the spinal cord from the paravertebral and lateral area explain why CTM has different effects in the deep mobile layers of the skin. Several lateral strokes in the first and second sequences stimulate the areas of the shoulder and arm that are connected over the cervical spinal cord. Strokes applied to the paravertebral area

influence the organs that are connected to these segments.

- When determining the findings, preexisting distensions or retractions in the lumbar and sacral area must be noted, which may indicate existing constipation (p. 149) or involvement of the bladder (p. 160) and which should then be included in the treatment plan.
- CTM must be applied with extreme care after surgical procedures for brain tumors or injuries, where a predisposition to epileptic seizure may remain. The reactions of the patient must be carefully observed. It must be noted that CTM has a great impact on the ascending, afferent sensory nervous system and this effect may trigger an epileptic seizure. Accordingly, a good way to start treatment is to apply the small basic sequence longer and then gradually go to the additional section sequences.
- The bladder should be emptied before each treatment, since CTM stimulates the activity of the organs and especially the kidneys.
- In the further course of treatment the strokes are fully applied to the torso only once or twice and treatment of the leg and/or arm is emphasized. When applying strokes to the hand, special attention should be given to treatment of the thumb.
- With existing hypertension.

Parkinson Disease

Definition

The symptoms of Parkinson disease targeted by connective tissue massage include increased muscle tone (also called rigor) and frequent symptoms of the autonomic nervous system. Parkinson disease symptoms are caused by degenerative cell break-up in the so-called black nucleus ("nucleus niger") of the brain and a deficiency in the transmitter (dopamine) in the area of the other extrapyramidal ganglia cells. In addition to these motor cell formations, cells of the autonomic nervous system, especially parent cells of the sympathetic nervous system, are often destroyed so that there are also dysfunctions of the autonomic nervous system in addition to motor disorders.

The cause of Parkinson disease is unknown. The clinical picture is characterized by a gradual reduction of facial motor or psychomotor functions (facial expressions and gestures) as well as a slow "freezing" of spontaneous motor functions—that is, the motivation for movements, and general mobility, especially additional movements of the arms. These symptoms, called hypokinesia or akinesia, affect all striated muscles. Those suffering from the disease appear to be stiff, as though "frozen," walk with tiny steps and the body bent forward, and speak quietly, monotonously, and without modulation.

The second symptom is the rigor already mentioned: an increase in muscle tone that manifests as a stiff, doughlike resistance of the body muscles during whole range of motion movement. It especially affects the muscles of the neck and extremities, but also other muscles, including those of the pelvic floor (disturbances in urination). The rigor can also be cramplike and painful. The goal of CTM is again to loosen the muscle tension that occurs with these motor dysfunctions according to the same principle as with spasm.

The tremor, shaking, and trembling of hands, feet, head, abdomen, and lower jaw, which is especially noticeable at rest, is considered the third symptom but is only detectable in about one-half to two-thirds of cases. Like the rigor and akinesia, the tremor at rest increases with mental tension, excitation, joy, or fear. It is predominantly the psychomotor function that is disturbed here, so that it is important to generate a relaxed atmosphere during therapy.

The orthostatic "asympathetic" susceptibility to blackouts, which occurs particularly when getting up and standing, is of therapeutic significance when looking at the symptoms of the autonomic nervous system.

Improvement of the gastrointestinal passage is another treatment goal of CTM. This is accomplished over cutaneous visceral reflexes. Cooperation with the physician is of utmost importance here, and increased attention is required when the patient gets up after the massage (risk of collapse).

The allegedly increased flow of saliva seen in many patients with Parkinson disease is not a symptom of the autonomic nervous system, but rather a consequence of akinesia and rigor of the muscles of the throat and mouth so that saliva is rarely automatically swallowed and runs out of the "rigid mouth opening".

Findings

- The skin and subcutaneous tissue of the torso, arms, and legs are less easy to slide against each other.
- Increased tension is found in three locations: The tissue in the angle between the iliac crest and spinal column; on the trochanter; and on the iliotibial tract. The muscle fibers show massive adhesions within themselves and are only slightly stretchable. The movement sector of the joints is significantly limited.

Treatment Plan

Starting position: sitting or lateral position, prone position, supine position.
- Small basic sequence, flat strokes over back and legs.
- Small basic sequence, first sequence, flat strokes over back and legs.
- Small basic sequence, first and second sequence, ventral side, flat strokes over arms and legs.
- Small basic sequence, first, second, and third sequence, ventral side, flat strokes over arms and legs.
- Small basic sequence, first, second, and third sequence, ventral side, facial treatment, flat strokes over both arms and legs.

Balancing strokes over the pectoral muscles, dorsal dispersion stroke, and flat strokes of the legs and arms are applied at the end of each treatment session to support the venous backflow.

Additional Strokes
Small Basic Sequence
▶ **From dorsal (▶ Fig. 2.27)**
- Hooks from caudal to cranial, along the course of the first pelvic stroke.
- Fanlike strokes are flatly applied to the respiratory angle between the lowest rib and the spinal column, starting on the lower edge of the rib cage and ending with the last strokes along the spinal column (T12 to L3).

▶ **From ventral (▶ Fig. 2.35)**
- Bimanual strokes, beginning from dorsal on the lower edge of the rib cage to the medioclavicular line and from the pelvic edge to the anterior superior iliac spine.
- Bimanual strokes crossing over the abdominal walls, starting in the dorsal region and ending at the opposite edge of the rectus abdominis muscle.
- The liver stroke is applied in the ventral region at the level of the medioclavicular line on the right lower edge of the rib cage in the dorsal direction with a flat hand, at first only lightly, then gradually more intensively until just before the spinal column.
- Short hooks on the lower edge of the rib cage, loosening the origins of the abdominal muscles.

First Sequence
▶ **From dorsal (▶ Fig. 2.37)**
- The intercostal strokes are also pulled in the opposite direction from the spinal column to the lateral rib cage wall to the ventral axillary line and hooked in there gently.
- The intercostal strokes are followed by a stroke from the lower angle of the scapula to the spinal column at the level of T4.
- Flat transverse strokes over the spinal column, beginning at the level of T6 under the left scapula and ending under the right scapula.
- Small, flat transverse strokes along the spinal column, within the area of the long extensor spinae muscles, from T12 to T7.

▶ **From ventral (▶ Fig. 2.39)**
- In the ventral intercostal area a set of flat strokes are pulled through the intercostal spaces, beginning at the dorsal axillary line at the lowest rib.

Second Sequence (▶ Fig. 2.46)
▶ **From dorsal (▶ Fig. 2.47, ▶ Fig. 2.48)**
- Long downward stretching.
- Prolonged upward stretching.

- Flat fan-shaped strokes are pulled transversely over the scapula toward the shoulder joint. Beginning with the stroke on the outer scapula and ending on the lower edge of the spine of the scapula.
- Small, flat transverse strokes over the spine within the area of the long extensor spinae muscles from T7 to C7.
- Flat transverse strokes from the inner side to the lateral edge of the scapulae, starting at the level of T7 and ending at the level of the spine of the scapula.
- Short hooks around the angle of the scapula followed by outlining the scapula with cutting strokes along the same course.

Comments
- CTM is applied primarily to the torso in this Parkinson disease. The rotation of the torso should be supported and the range of motion of the extremities should be increased.
- Facial treatment should relax the facial muscles, preventing or alleviating the reduction of facial expressions.
- Akinesia and disturbances in innervation of the autonomic nervous system may cause disturbances in the digestive tract and the bladder. Thus, the therapist must note distensions or retractions in the lumbar and sacral region during diagnostics, which indicate involvement of organs—for example constipation (p. 149) or disorders of the bladder (p. 160).
- The risk of collapse mentioned in the medical section when changing the patient's position should be taken into consideration in any case.
- CTM and physical therapy can complement each other very well, but the patient must be allowed to rest after CTM. Over a longer period CTM is applied twice a week. From time to time a break is taken from treatment.

Multiple Sclerosis
Definition
Synonym: Multiple sclerosis is also known as encephalomyelitis disseminata.

Multiple sclerosis is a frequent disease of the central nervous system that is associated with attacks of almost randomly distributed small inflammatory foci in the brain and spinal cord, which cause destruction of or interruptions in the white matter—that is, the nervous pathways. Accordingly, the symptoms are diverse but also characteristic. In summary, multiple sclerosis is a disease with small foci, multiple foci, and a relapsing-remitting form and is generally progressive. It especially affects young people starting at the age of 25 and occurs in women more frequently than in men. The attacks, with an increase then a decrease of symptoms, usually last for 2–5 weeks. They can occur several times a year or repeatedly after symptom-free intervals of years.

Typical symptoms include sudden visual impairments in one eye (hazy vision, veiled vision), double vision, dizziness, prickling and numb sensations in one of the extremities or one-half of the body, minor hemiplegia or paralysis in both legs, so-called ataxia with clumsy excessive movements and gait disturbances, or disturbances of urination. All of these and other symptoms develop episodically in 3 out of 4 cases, while primarily chronic courses are rare. Relapsing-remitting multiple sclerosis often gives way to a chronic development with continuous worsening.

The cause of multiple sclerosis is unknown. It is an autoimmune disease, in which a malfunction of the immune system triggers autoimmune antibodies against the body's own myelin—the nerve conduction substance of nervous pathways—and this key structure is destroyed in the inflammatory foci. Drug therapy corresponds to this concept. During an attack the patient receives high-dose cortisones, and after some time immune modulators such as interferon beta or Copaxone (Copolymer 1; glatiramer acetate) or immunoglobulin infusions.

Indications for CTM are muscle spasms and their consequences (pain) and disturbances of the gastrointestinal passage with constipation. Treatment with CTM is especially indicated if there are already partial or complete symptoms of paraplegia or the patients are unable to walk or are bedridden. This includes vasomotor deficits in the legs and circulatory dysregulation, which can also be positively influenced by CTM. Even the mentally relaxing effect of connective tissue massage alone can be an indication for these often still young and severely disabled people.

Findings

Specific findings cannot be described because the effects of the pathology are very variable. The therapist determines the findings for each case individually.

Treatment Plan

Starting position: sitting, lateral position, prone position, supine position.
- Small basic sequence, flat strokes over back and legs.
- Small basic sequence, first sequence, flat strokes on the legs.
- Small basic sequence, first and second sequence, ventral side, flat strokes on the legs.
- Small basic sequence, first and second sequence, ventral side of the body, treatment of the thighs, flat strokes on lower leg and foot.
- Small basic sequence, first and second sequence, ventral side, treatment of the leg, flat strokes on the arms.
- Small basic sequence, first and second sequence, ventral side of the body, treatment of the leg, treatment of the upper arm, flat strokes of forearm and hand.
- Small basic sequence, first and second sequence, ventral side, treatment of leg and arm.

- Small basic sequence, first, second, and third sequence, ventral side, treatment of leg and arm.
- Small basic sequence, first, second, and third sequence, ventral side, treatment of leg and arm, treatment of face.

Balancing strokes over the pectoral muscles, dorsal dispersion stroke, and flat strokes of the legs and arms are applied at the end of each treatment session to support the venous backflow.

Additional Strokes

Depending on the respective findings these can be found in Chapter 2 (p.20) (small basic sequence, first and second sequence) and are then integrated into the treatment plan. The goal is to improve the functions of the tissue and its reactions.

Comments

- When administering CTM the therapist should pay particular attention to the physical and psychological reactions of the patient. It may be that only flat strokes can be applied to avoid increasing the tone of the presently increased spasm.
- CTM must not be applied during attacks. The patient should remain quiet during that time. A focus will then be placed on achieving relaxation through physical therapy.
- If CTM is not tolerated, the therapist should consult with the physician.
- Susceptibility to constipation (p.149) and bladder (p.160) evacuation disturbances must also be taken into consideration here. When recording the findings a note should be made of existing distensions or retractions in the lumbar and sacral area and the treatment plan supplemented accordingly.

CTM must be regarded as long-term therapy and should be properly coordinated with physical therapy. It must be ensured that the patient has adequate rest after CTM.

Paraplegia
Definition

The considerations for multiple sclerosis are also applicable for pathologies of incomplete or complete paraplegia of other etiology.

The goals of therapy include:
- Loosening of spasms
- Avoiding contractures and alleviating pain
- Supporting the activity of the stomach, intestines, and bladder, including on the one hand the prevention of intestinal spasms with diffuse abdominal complaints, and on the other the helpful effects in avoiding symptoms of ileus or urinary retention

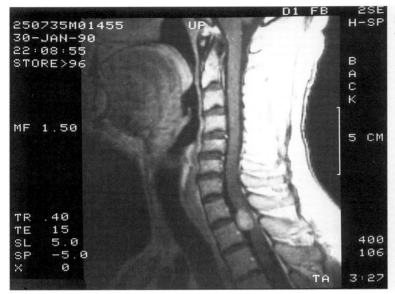

Fig. 3.9 Spinal meningioma at T2 as the cause of paraplegia.

Therapy is once again based on the cutaneous visceral reflexes that can be triggered by CTM.

The most frequent causes of paraplegic symptoms are severe accidents, tumors of the spinal cord including metastases (▶ Fig. 3.9), and inflammations as well as late stages of multiple sclerosis. Younger people are often affected.

Patients with high paraplegia due to injuries in the cervical part of the spinal cord are especially in need of therapy. Arms, legs, and torso are paralyzed and insensitive; there are also severe disturbances in the regulation of the autonomic nervous system, since the sympathetic and parasympathetic pathways in the spinal cord are interrupted.

Quite often there are also critical disturbances of the autonomic nervous system with outbreaks of sweating, increased blood pressure, and other symptoms, especially when an overfilled bladder is overlooked.

Asympathetic blackouts are a particular danger for these patients because the interruption of the sympathetic spinal pathways causes denervation of all vessels located from the neck down and accordingly they can no longer constrict sufficiently. Close collaboration is again necessary between patients, physicians, and therapists, and all parties involved should draw on the experience of paraplegia centers.

Findings

- The therapist finds changes in mobility between the skin and hypodermis and between the hypodermis and muscle fascia, which must be palpated individually.
- The therapist must be attentive for adhesions in the paravertebral tissue, since they may indicate disturbances in the organs.

- The extremities in the distal parts show disturbances in the blood supply; sometimes they also show sensory deficits.

Treatment Plan

Starting position: lateral position, prone position, supine position, and sitting.
- Flat strokes in the areas above the lesion along the cleavage lines of the dermis.
- Flat strokes in the areas above the lesion along the cleavage lines of the dermis.
- Small basic sequence, flat strokes over rib cage, legs, and arms.
- Small basic sequence, first sequence, flat strokes over rib cage and arms.
- Small basic sequence, first sequence, ventral side, treatment of the leg, flat strokes on the arms.
- Small basic sequence, first and second sequence, ventral side, treatment of leg and arm.
- Small basic sequence, first, second, and third sequence, ventral side, treatment of leg and arm.
- Small basic sequence, first, second, and third sequence, ventral side, facial treatment, treatment of leg and arm.

Balancing strokes over the pectoral muscles, dorsal dispersion stroke, and flat strokes of the legs and arms are applied at the end of each treatment session to support the venous backflow.

Additional Strokes

The additional strokes are not described here in detail as they should be selected depending on the findings in the tissue and the possible mobility. They can be found in Chapter 2 (p. 20) (small basic sequence, first and second sequence) and are then integrated into the treatment plan.

Comments

- When applying CTM with flat strokes in the area of the body above the lesion, the therapist should watch carefully for light reddening. Only when this reddening develops are the paralyzed parts of the body included in the treatment.
- This reaction in the innervated parts of the body tells the therapist that there was a connection through the autonomic nervous system and the technique of CTM may then be applied to the paralyzed parts of the body. It is expected that the constantly repeated light stimulus will trigger the cutaneous visceral reflex and subsequently stimulate the activity of the liver, lung, heart, kidney, bladder, and intestines.
- The blood pressure may increase and respiratory function, urination, and defecation may be affected. The tissue is better suffused and the supply of nutrients is improved by the treatment, especially in transition from flat strokes to the CTM technique.
- Areas that are at risk of developing pressure ulcers, such as the ischial tuberosity, spinous processes of the spinal column, over the sacral bone, over the trochanters, in the region of the scapulae, on the elbow, and on the heels, must be especially closely observed.
- The physician must be informed immediately about any changes of the skin (p. 24).
- When recording the findings a note should be made of existing distensions or retractions in the lumbar and sacral area that could indicate constipation or disturbances of bladder evacuation. This must be taken into consideration when developing the treatment plan (p. 27).
- With increased blood pressure.

Since the patient should rest after CTM, physical therapy using special techniques must be coordinated with the application of CTM.

If the patient has frequent spasms it must be decided whether CTM is not better performed before physical therapy.

Connective tissue massage must be regarded as long-term therapy.

Polyneuropathies

Definition

Polyneuropathies are acute or chronic diseases of the entire peripheral nervous system, though the longest nervous fibers—those toward the feet—are affected first and most severely. Causes include toxins, metabolic disorders, or infections that are found throughout the body but specifically damage peripheral nerves.

The symptoms are characteristic and start with prickling, weakness, numbness, and paresthesia in the region of the toes on both sides; later, pain also frequently develops at rest (in bed at night), especially with diabetic polyneuropathies, which have a prickling burning character.

Depending on the cause, these paresthesias swiftly or very slowly ascend toward the knee and thigh (with a stockinglike distribution). The fingertips are also affected and the disturbances ascend toward the torso. Finally, pareses and muscular atrophy develop that similarly ascend from distal to proximal and affect the muscles of the torso and respiratory system, which can be life-threatening as a result of respiratory paralysis. Constipation and urinary retention will be noted before this.

Such a course is rather rare. It does occur in acute polyradiculitis—inflammation of nerve roots in Guillain–Barré syndrome—which is immunologically communicated. Primary chronic, slowly worsening diabetic polyneuropathies are much more frequent, making up about one-third of all polyneuropathies.

One-third of polyneuropathies are triggered by alcohol abuse; the rest are caused by chronic poisoning with medications, organic solvents, heavy metals, and other substances as well as some pathogens such as *Borrelia*.

In addition to sensory deficits accentuated in the distal area and possible pain and paralysis with a flaccid muscle tone and increasing atrophy of muscles and skin, sympathetic denervation also plays a key role. The skin on the feet is dry because the sweat glands no longer secrete, and is bluish in color because the blood vessels in the skin can no longer be constricted and regulated.

Connective tissue massage can reduce these symptoms, alleviate the pain and improve the blood supply as well as trigger effects that stimulate the circulation.

Additional indications for CTM are disturbances of the gastrointestinal passage and/or weakness of the urinary bladder.

Acute, swiftly ascending Guillain–Barré syndrome is a contraindication for CTM in the early phase.

Findings

- There is reduced blood supply of the extremities, especially in the distal parts. The tissue is edematous and has a livid discoloration.
- The skin and hypodermis are segmentally stuck to each other on the torso and extremities and can be moved and lifted only to a limited extent.
- These adhesions are especially found in the region under the pelvic crests, on the edges of the sacral bone and on the sacral bone, around the trochanters and along the iliotibial tract, and on the muscle septa of the gastrocnemius muscle and of the ischiocrural group. When the upper extremity is affected, the adhesions are especially found in the region of the rotators on the upper arm and on the scapula.

Treatment Plan

Starting position: sitting or lateral position, prone position, supine position.
- Small basic sequence, flat strokes over back and legs.

- Small basic sequence, treatment of the thigh, flat strokes on both legs.
- Small basic sequence, first sequence, treatment of the thigh, flat strokes on both legs.
- Small basic sequence, first and second sequence, ventral side, treatment of leg.
- Small basic sequence, first and second sequence, ventral side of the body, treatment of the leg, treatment of the upper arm, flat strokes on forearm and hand.
- Small basic sequence, first, second, and third sequence, treatment of arm and leg.

Balancing strokes over the pectoral muscles, dorsal dispersion stroke, and flat strokes of the legs and arms are applied at the end of each treatment session to support the venous backflow.

Additional Strokes

Small Basic Sequence (▶ Fig. 2.27, ▶ Fig. 2.28, ▶ Fig. 2.29)

▶ **From dorsal**
- Hooks to the sacral bone edges from caudal to cranial.
- Flat transverse strokes over the sacral bone from caudal to cranial.
- Hooks, in the course of the first pelvic stroke.
- Small, flat transverse strokes along the spine within the area of the long extensor spinae muscles from L5 to T12.
- Hooks and stretching stroke at the ischial tuberosity.
- Stretching stroke in the region of the lumbar triangle.
- Fanlike strokes in the upper respiratory angle: fanlike strokes are flatly applied to the angle between the lowest rib and the spine. These should start at the lower edge of the rib cage and end with the last strokes along the spine (L3 to T12).

Small Basic Sequence in Lateral Position (▶ Fig. 2.33)

▶ **From dorsal**
- Small hooks around the greater trochanter.
- Flat balancing stroke, starting above the greater trochanter toward the ischial tuberosity.

Small Basic Sequence in Prone Position (▶ Fig. 2.33)

▶ **From dorsal**
- Short hooks along the intergluteal cleft pulling up from the lateral side.

▶ **From ventral**
- Bimanual strokes, from dorsal on the lower edge of the rib cage to the medioclavicular line and from the pelvic edge to the anterior superior iliac spine. These strokes are performed bimanually, first on one side then on the other.

- Short hooks along the rectus sheath from the symphysis up to the navel.
- Short strokes, like rays, pulling toward the navel.
- Bimanual strokes crossing over the abdominal walls, starting in the dorsal region and ending at the opposite edge of the rectus abdominis muscle.

First Sequence (▶ Fig. 2.37, ▶ Fig. 2.38, ▶ Fig. 2.39)

▶ **From dorsal**
- When changing the direction, the intercostal strokes are also performed in the opposite direction from the spine along the lateral thoracic wall to the ventral axillary line in order to gently grasp the tissue there.
- The large balancing stroke starts in the ventral axillary line at the level of the sixth/seventh intercostal space and is flatly pulled around the lower angle of the scapula toward C7.
- Short strokes from the lower angle of the scapula to the spine at the level of segment T4.
- Flat transverse strokes over the spine, beginning at the level of T6 under the angle of the left scapula and ending under the angle of the right scapula and then back again.
- Small, flat transverse strokes along the spine within the area of the long extensor spinae muscles from T12 to T7.

▶ **From ventral**
- In the ventral intercostal area a set of flat strokes are pulled beginning at the dorsal axillary line through the intercostal spaces. These should start at the lowest ribs.

Second Sequence (▶ Fig. 2.46, ▶ Fig. 2.47, ▶ Fig. 2.48, ▶ Fig. 2.49)

▶ **From dorsal**
- Long downward stretching, along the edge of the latissimus dorsi muscle in the direction of the iliac crest.
- Prolonged upward stretching, beginning at the level of the sixth/seventh intercostal space, along the edge of the latissimus dorsi muscle in the direction of the axilla.
- Axillary stretching with elevated arm: the patient puts his or her arm on the therapist's shoulder. Connecting transverse strokes are applied through the axilla to thoroughly loosen the axillary fold.
- A flat fan-shaped stroke is pulled transversely over the scapula toward the shoulder joint, starting at the outer edge of the scapula and ending at the lower edge of the spine of the scapula.
- Small, flat transverse strokes over the spine within the area of the long extensor spinae muscles from T7 to T3 or C7.
- Flat transverse strokes from the inner side to the lateral edge of the scapulae, starting at the level of T7 and ending at the spine of the scapula.

- Small hooks around the upper angle of the scapula followed by outlining the scapula with cutting strokes.

▶ **From ventral**
- The ventral edge of the trapezius muscle is pulled out starting from the cervical base, while pressing against it with the free hand.
- Strokes over the sternum, beginning at the xiphoid process pulling toward the jugular notch.
- Short hooks on the connection points between the ribs and sternum pulling from caudal to cranial.
- Short transverse strokes along the sternum. These start at the junction between the xiphoid process and the body of the sternum, along the area of the sternal angle. At the base of the second rib at the sternum, the strokes should become wider to just under the sternoclavicular joints.
- Short fanlike strokes on the suprasternal notch, beginning on the clavicle and ending on the dorsal edge of the sternocleidomastoid muscle.
- Short strokes on the interclavicular ligament.

▶ **On the arm**
- Bimanual soft stretching of flexor and extensor of the upper arm.

▶ **On the leg** (▶ Fig. 2.70)
- Short hooks from the last third of the fascia lata in the shape of a fan toward the patella.
- The thigh stroke starts in the upper third of the thigh, on the lateral edge of the sartorius muscle, and ends shortly before the groin.
- Flat strokes, which are pulled from the transverse intergluteal cleft to the popliteal cavity.
- Flat strokes from the inner side of the thigh, starting below the patella and running around the medial malleolus.
- Bimanual stretching between the muscle bellies of the gastrocnemius muscle, from cranial to caudal, pulling in the direction of the Achilles tendon.

Comments

- The therapist first works with flat strokes. The therapist should always make sure that the traction of the tissue causes a "cutting" sensation. The flat strokes on the extremities must be applied patiently over a sufficiently long period.
- Only when minor reddening develops—the body reporting the connection through the autonomic nervous system—should treatment with the flat technique of CTM be started in the distal parts of the body. Initially the strokes should be applied from proximal to distal, and later in both directions.
- The stretchability of the muscles is severely reduced due to the pain and the metabolic disturbances.

Therefore, origins and insertion points of the muscles must be carefully palpated and, if necessary, loosened.
- Since the pathology and the ascending nature of the paralysis also affects the activity of the gastrointestinal tract and bladder, the therapist should watch for existing distensions or retractions in the lumbar and sacral region during diagnostics and integrate them into the treatment plan (see Chapter 2).

During inpatient treatment the patient receives CTM every day, in outpatient care three times a week. If successful, treatment may be reduced to twice a week.

The effect of CTM is based on long-term application. It is advisable to have intervals without treatment in between and then to start anew.

Nerve Root Lesions

Definition

Isolated individual nerve root lesions are primarily caused by slipped disks. A smaller fraction are caused by tumors or shingles or other rare processes close to the spinal column. Acute and chronic slipped disks and protrusions must be distinguished in terms of three very different types of pain:
- Receptor pain caused by irritation of bone and cartilaginous membrane and soft tissue directly caused by the tissue pressing on the nucleus pulposus
- Muscle pain of segmental back muscles due to cramps through reflexes (also a type of receptor pain)
- Neuralgia (nerve pain), caused by irritation and contusion of the nerve root itself or of the posterior root of the nerve pair

In neuralgia (sciatica, brachialgia) (▶ Fig. 3.10, ▶ Fig. 3.11), the pain is exactly projected to the sensory territory supplied by this nerve—that is, into the appropriate segmental dermatome—but, of course, also into the myotome and sclerotome, because muscles and periosteum or perichondrium (meaning the coating of bone and cartilage) also possess sensory innervation and are subject to the segmental structure.

The types of pain therefore differ on a fundamental level. The receptor pain is felt where the pain receptors are irritated locally; the location of irritation and pain are thus identical.

The neuralgic pain caused by the irritation of sensitive pain-conducting nervous structures in the posterior roots or peripheral nerves is felt where this nerve cable has its sensory territory. The patients can indicate into which areas the pain is radiating. These radicular projection areas are shown in ▶ Fig. 3.10 and ▶ Fig. 3.11.

Radicular pain occurs more frequently in legs than in arms, because lumbosacral slipped disks are correspondingly more frequent. It is often difficult to distinguish radicular pain from other types of pain in arms or legs. A

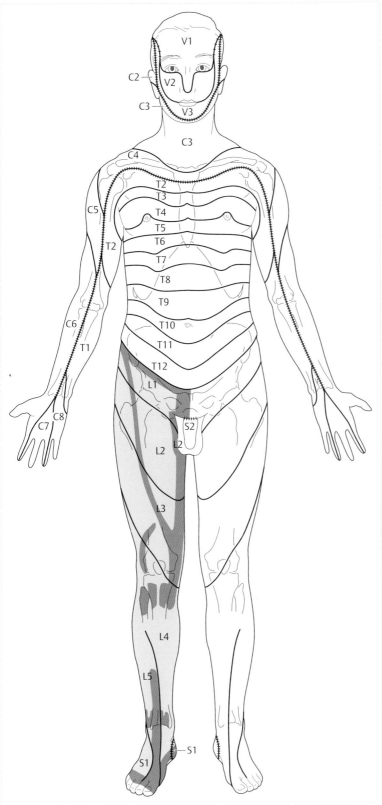

Fig. 3.10 Sciatica on the right. Affected: T12, L1–L5, S1.

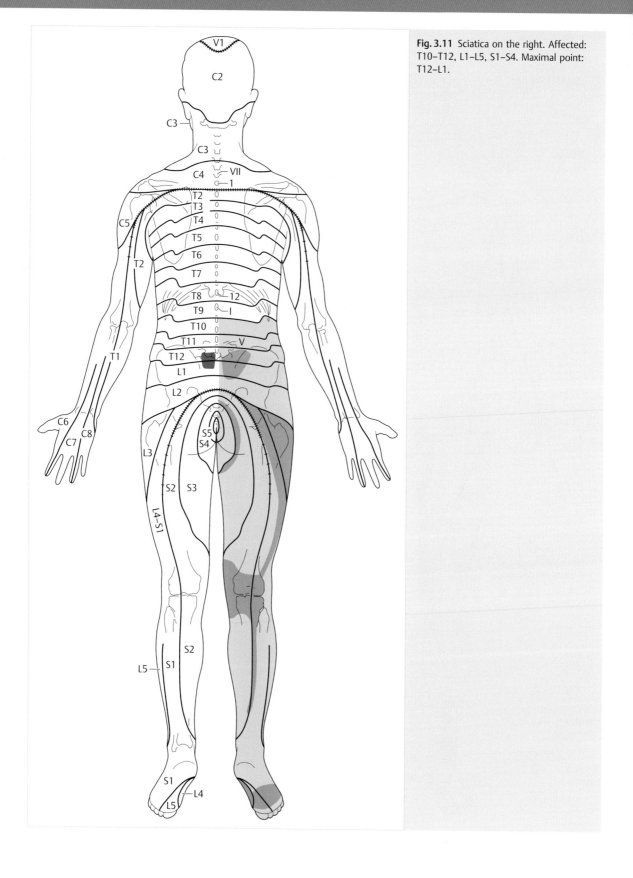

Fig. 3.11 Sciatica on the right. Affected: T10–T12, L1–L5, S1–S4. Maximal point: T12–L1.

comprehensive interview and description of the patient regarding the extent of pain and an exact neurological examination are essential here.

In the region of the leg, the pain is also slightly projected from the hip joint, but over a shorter distance, into the surrounding area, especially into the groin and into the lateral part of the thigh. Pain in the knee joint is projected toward the thigh and also the tibial edge. The full set of available clinical and technologically aided neurological and orthopedic diagnostic instruments must be employed here for differential diagnostics. The most frequent radicular pain in the region of the arms is caused by irritation of the C6 nerve root (i.e., toward the thumb/index finger); of the C7 nerve root with projected pain toward the middle finger, but also toward the part of the pectoral muscle that belongs to C7 or that part of C7 of the lower shoulder muscles (especially latissimus dorsi); and the projection of pain from C8 toward the little finger.

The pain is often projected primarily into the area of the myotome; at the same time, prickling paresthesia or even numbness develops in the area of the dermatome. If the posterior root is damaged—that is, with defective conduction—the pain slowly subsides and gives way to numbness in the dermatome. Parts of the anterior root are also often damaged and pareses in the myotome develop with muscular atrophy. Simultaneously, the corresponding proprioceptive muscle reflexes are weakened or eliminated. Differential diagnosis with respect to shoulder joint–related pain can also be difficult, and the orthopedist and the neurologist should collaborate closely here.

In the region of the leg, with the complex of so-called sciatica, the following nerve root lesions caused by slipped disks must be taken into account:

- With L4 nerve root lesions the pain is projected toward the knee joint and medial side of the lower leg where numbness can develop; the patellar tendon reflex as well as the quadriceps reflex are weakened or eliminated. Ultimately pareses and atrophy of the quadriceps muscles on the thigh and of the anterior tibial muscle (i.e., the dorsal flexor of the foot) may develop.
- L5 and S1 are most frequently affected by nerve root lesions, which comprise the actual sciatic syndrome.
  - In the L5 pain projection the pain radiates from the sacral area over the lateral part of the thigh to the front in the direction of the tibial edge and great toe; if the nerve root damage progresses, the L5 strip to the great toe also goes numb and pareses of the great toe and later also the little toe dorsal flexor develop.
  - In compression of the S1 nerve root the pain is projected into a so-called general strip, meaning the lateral side of the thigh and lower leg toward the small toe, whereas the patient often reports numbness on the lateral side of the foot; the Achilles tendon reflex will then probably be weak or eliminated and,

ultimately, paresis of the dorsal flexor of the foot develops through paralysis and atrophy of the triceps surae muscle. L5 or S1 pain is often also projected into the groin, because the L5/S1 sclerotome includes parts of the femoral head and pubic bone. Most nerve root lesions caused by the intervertebral disk can be identified by clinical assessment alone, but CT or MRI of the cervical or lumbar spine can also be helpful if there is any doubt.

The majority of intervertebral disk-related nerve root lesions or afflictions are treated conservatively with local heat application, physical therapy, and especially CTM. Intervertebral disk surgery is necessary in only about 10% of cases: for example, with progressive paralysis or with therapy-resistant pain syndromes.

CTM is appropriate and very successful in these pain syndromes because it promotes relaxation of the tense back muscles and also has a positive influence on the entire muscular structure and function due to its nature as a "whole body therapy."

Diagnostic and treatment concepts for these pathologies still differ between orthopedists and neurologists. Orthopedists often treat with analgesic injections and are more likely to employ surgical measures. Neurologists favor physical therapy and thus also connective tissue massage.

Findings in Lesions of the Cervical Spine

The changes in turgor and muscle tone are located in segments C4–C8, T1–T12 and manifest themselves in the following regions of the body:

- Along the course of the latissimus dorsi muscle down to the pelvic edge, especially on the lower angle of the scapula
- In the dorsal angle between rib cage and upper arm, along the upper arm and forearm, especially on the ulnar side of the forearm
- On the anterior side of the torso along the clavicle, proximally above and distally below the clavicle
- Traveling along the anterior delta portion over the upper arm to the axilla

With the relief posture the scapula is elevated and shows adhesions in its muscular formation. If the disorder persists for a longer period, atrophy due to inactivity can develop, especially in the hand and arm.

Treatment Plan

Starting position: sitting, supine position.
- Small basic sequence, flat strokes over the back from caudal toward cranial.
- Small basic sequence, first sequence, flat strokes over rib cage and arm.

- Small basic sequence, first and second sequence, ventral side, flat strokes over rib cage and arm.
- Small basic sequence, first and second sequence, ventral side, treatment of the upper arm, flat strokes on forearm and hand.
- Small basic sequence, first, second, and third sequence, ventral side, treatment of arm.

Balancing strokes over the pectoral muscles, dorsal dispersion stroke, and flat strokes of the arms are applied at the end of each treatment session to support the venous backflow.

Additional Strokes

First Sequence

▶ **From dorsal (▶ Fig. 2.38, ▶ Fig. 2.39)**
- The intercostal strokes are also pulled in the opposite direction from the spinal column to the lateral rib cage wall toward the ventral axillary line and hooked in there gently.
- The large balancing stroke starts in the ventral axillary line at the level of the sixth/seventh intercostal space and is flatly pulled around the lower angle of the scapula toward C7.

▶ **From ventral**
- Flat strokes are applied over the ventral intercostal spaces starting at the lowest ribs.

Second Sequence

▶ **From dorsal (▶ Fig. 2.45, ▶ Fig. 2.46, ▶ Fig. 2.48)**
- Long downward stretching.
- Prolonged upward stretching.
- Bimanual axillary stretching. If the patient is able to place his or her arm at the level of the therapist's shoulder, the dorsal and ventral axillary folds are carefully loosened with connecting transverse strokes in the region of the serratus muscle.
- Flat transverse strokes from the inner side to the inner side of the scapulae, starting at the level of T7, ending at the spine of the scapula.
- Short hooks around the angle of the scapula followed by outlining the scapula with cutting strokes along the same course.
- The flat fan-shaped stroke is pulled transversely over the scapula toward the shoulder joint, starting at the outer edge of the scapula and ending at the lower edge of the spine of the scapula.

▶ **From ventral**
- The ventral edge of the trapezius muscle is pulled out starting from the cervical base, while pressing against it with the free hand.
- Short hooks on the insertion points of the ribs toward the sternum from caudal to cranial.

Comments

- If a painful maximal point is palpated on the scapula at the level of the spine of the scapula, involvement of the liver and gallbladder must be taken into consideration.
- With persistent, chronic complaints in the left arm, consider involvement of the heart.
- Apply a rolled-up hot pack to the dorsal areas of the body along T3–T7. Head, neck, rib cage, and arms are treated from the segments that are located there.
- The focus of the treatment lies in first and second sequences, since the upper extremity includes the innervation of the autonomic nervous system in segments T5–T7.

Segment reflexes with diseases of the liver and gallbladder may cause the pain to project into the area of the right shoulder. For this reason the T7/T8 dermatomes should be included in such cases with the application of flat strokes, which has proven to be useful. However, it must be kept in mind that only a disease of the liver or gallbladder can cause pain in the shoulder. If such a connection is assumed, the organ must be examined by an internist.

Findings in Lesions of the Lumbar Spine

- Visible and palpable changes in tension differ greatly in localization and duration of the disorder. In addition to all lumbar and sacral segments, sections in T10–T12 are also affected.
- The entire leg is usually tender. Muscle tensions are also located on the healthy side in the area of T10–T11, which may be caused by relieving or faulty postures.
- A maximal point can be found at the level of T12–L1 on the unaffected side.
- In L3/L4 over the greater trochanter, an intensive point of pain can be located that is characteristic of tension caused by reflexes, which extends from the lateral side of the thigh to the lower leg. The tissue shows massive adhesions and is difficult to mobilize.

▶ **Location of notable tissue changes**
- Under the edges of the pelvis, in the lesser gluteal muscles
- Around the trochanter
- At the origin of the pelvitrochanterian muscles
- Along the course of the iliotibial tract, on the edges of the adductor muscles

Treatment Plan

Starting position: Lateral position, lying on the affected side, supine position, sitting.
- Small basic sequence, flat strokes over back and legs.
- Small basic sequence, first sequence, flat strokes on the legs.

- Small basic sequence, first sequence, treatment of the thigh, flat strokes over the lower leg and foot.
- Small basic sequence, first sequence, treatment of the leg.

Balancing strokes over the pectoral muscles, dorsal dispersion stroke, and flat strokes of the legs are applied at the end of each treatment session to support the venous backflow.

Additional Strokes

Small Basic Sequence

▶ **From dorsal** (▶ Fig. 2.27, ▶ Fig. 2.28, ▶ Fig. 2.29)
- Hooks to the edges of the sacral bone from caudal to cranial.
- Flat transverse strokes over the sacral bone, elevating from caudal to cranial.
- Hooks in the course of the first pelvic stroke from caudal to cranial.
- Small, flat transverse strokes over the spine within the area of the long extensor spinae muscles, from L5 to T12.
- Hooks and stretching stroke at the ischial tuberosity.
- Stretching stroke in the lumbar triangle.

▶ **On the leg** (▶ Fig. 2.68a)
- Short strokes from the last third of the fascia lata, in the shape of a fan toward the patella.
- The thigh stroke starts in the upper third of the thigh, on the lateral edge of the sartorius muscle, and ends shortly before the groin.
- Short hooks, which are pulled from the transverse intergluteal cleft to the popliteal cavity.
- Strokes from the inner side of the lower leg, starting below the patella and running around the medial malleolus.
- Bimanual stretching between the muscle bellies of the gastrocnemius muscle from cranial to caudal, in the direction of the Achilles tendon.

Comments

- It may be impossible to start with the flat technique of CTM because the traction in the skin tissue is perceived by the patient as too painful due to severe tension. In this case, the therapist should start with flat strokes along the back, especially in the pelvic area.
- Over the maximal point at T12–L1 on the unaffected side, occasionally sensations extend into the affected leg along the ischial nerve down to the sole of the foot. The patient describes this as prickling, stitching, or burning. Balancing strokes are applied when such sensations occur. The hardening of the tissue, probably caused by reflexes, is distinctively palpable.
- Severe adhesions of the tissue can be found in this area and down to the pelvic crests. In such cases the first pelvic stroke must be applied in both directions. The

therapist applies flat strokes to the tissue around the trochanter in an arch and grasps with short strokes. Strokes along the edges of the sacral bone toward the intergluteal cleft relax the tissue and relieve the ischial nerve.
- The focus of the treatment is to apply the small basic sequence and to treat the ischial nerve root.
- In minor cases the affected leg recovers through the segmental reaction to CTM. In chronic cases treatment of the leg is given special attention, focusing especially on the thigh.
- Initially, flat long strokes along the iliotibial tract in the middle of the thigh are applied; the therapist continues in the proximal direction to include the area of the trochanter to the anterior superior iliac spine. Palpable relaxation of the thigh is achieved and thus relief of the entire leg.

CTM should be performed after physical therapy and the patient should rest afterward.

Pareses of Individual Peripheral Nerves

Plexus pareses in the arm—simultaneous damage of several nerves in the arm, with sensory disturbances and pain—must be mentioned here. These are often caused by accidents, especially traffic accidents (to motorcyclists). Other causes are malignant tumors (e.g., from the area of the pulmonary tip) which grow into the plexus. Such plexus pareses must then be treated according to their cause. The remaining healing is still painful and also causes faulty posture of the spinal column and muscle tension in the back, so that there is an indication for CTM. The indication for CTM lessens in pareses of individual peripheral nerves located more distally in the region of the arm. Frequently encountered lesions of individual nerves, for instance the radial nerve, due to injuries of the upper arm or of the median nerve in the context of so-called carpal tunnel syndrome on the wrist, are rarely treated with CTM.

In the region of the legs, plexus lesions are often caused by the invasion of malignant tumors into the plexus area. Again, during healing (after surgery and radiotherapy) the areas affected with pain and muscular atrophy can be improved with CTM. Pareses of individual peripheral nerves, for instance the femoral nerve or the ischial nerve, are rarer. When they have healed to stable, possibly painful states, CTM can be very helpful here.

However, the focus of treatment will probably be physical therapy.

Findings

Since in pareses of individual nerves CTM is not applied during the illness but rather during healing of the affected area, it is not possible to determine findings and an appropriate treatment plan.

The therapist will determine the visible and palpable findings on the torso and affected extremities and allocate distensions, retractions, adhesions, and reduced mobility of tissue layers to segment-associated organs and develop a treatment plan.

Treatment

The treatment always starts with the small basic sequence, which is followed by necessary treatment of additional sections and the extremities.

Additional Strokes

Small basic sequence and additional section sequences: see Chapter 2.

Comments

The goal of the treatment is to improve the blood supply and to stimulate the metabolism in those areas where the defects are located on the affected extremity. See the statements in the Principles of CTM section of Chapter 2.

After surgery: for example, treatment of scars (p. 98).

Although, as mentioned above, the indication for CTM is less in the early stage, it should be noted that any CTM that is applied, beginning with the small basic sequence and the following additional section sequences, can improve the blood supply and circulation in the extremities, nerves, and vessels.

Given this and also that CTM has a mentally relaxing and calming effect, consideration should be given to whether to apply CTM immediately after an accident.

Good timing between CTM and physical therapy is vital for their success. An appropriate amount of time for rest must be allowed after CTM.

Muscle Diseases

Definition

Muscle diseases that are diagnosed and treated within the scope of neurology are categorized into two large groups:
- Acute or subacute muscle inflammation (polymyositis and dermatomyositis), which cannot be considered for treatment with connective tissue massage. This method can only be applied after the acute inflammation has healed in an attempt to improve subsequent states of affected tissue.
- CTM is indicated in the degenerative muscle diseases—so-called muscular dystrophies. These often affect children and young adults with progressive flaccid paralysis and muscular atrophy, where connective tissue massage can have an alleviating effect; it does not stop the process, of course.

Connective tissue massage is not indicated in myasthenia, which is an immunologically communicated block of the nerve/muscle transmission point.

Findings

These clinical pictures may be associated with changing findings. When palpating the body, the therapist realizes that skin layers cannot easily be moved against each other in certain spots. The reduced stretchability of the muscles is notable.

Accentuated changes of turgor and muscle tone are located in the following parts of the body:
- Dorsally on the lower legs
- Ventrally and laterally on the thighs
- Under the pelvic crests
- On the sacral bone and on the edges of the sacral bone
- Dorsally and ventrally along the edge of the lower ribs and around the scapula
- In the angle between the arm and lateral edge of the scapula
- In the region of the neck, radiating to the clavicle

Treatment Plan

Starting position: sitting, lateral position, prone position, supine position.
- Small basic sequence, flat strokes over back and legs.
- Small basic sequence, treatment of the thigh, flat strokes on the back, lower leg, and foot.
- Small basic sequence, first sequence, treatment of the thigh and lower leg, flat strokes over the foot.
- Small basic sequence, first and second sequence, ventral side, treatment of the leg, flat strokes on both arms.
- Small basic sequence, first and second sequence, ventral side, treatment of the leg, upper arm, and forearm.
- Small basic sequence, first, second, and third sequence, ventral side, treatment of arm and leg.

Balancing strokes over the pectoral muscles, dorsal dispersion stroke, and flat strokes of the legs and/or arms are applied at the end of each treatment session to support the venous backflow.

Additional Strokes

Small Basic Sequence

▶ **From dorsal** (▶ Fig. 2.27)
- Flat transverse strokes over the sacral bone, ascending from caudal to cranial.
- Hooks in the course of the first pelvic stroke from caudal to cranial.

First and Second Sequence

▶ **From dorsal** (▶ Fig. 2.35, ▶ Fig. 2.37, ▶ Fig. 2.38, ▶ Fig. 2.39)
- Fan-shaped flat strokes in the area between the lowest rib and the spinal column.
- With the patient in a lying position, bimanual strokes on one side, beginning simultaneously on the lower edge of the rib cage to the medioclavicular line and

from the pelvic edge to the anterior superior iliac spine. First on one side, then on the other side of the body.

- The intercostal strokes are also pulled in the opposite direction from the spinal column to the lateral rib cage wall up to the anterior axillary line and hooked in there.
- The large balancing stroke coming from the ventral axillary line at the level of the sixth/seventh intercostal space is pulled flatly around the lower angle of the scapula toward C7.
- Flat transverse strokes from inner side to the lateral edge of the scapulae, starting at the level of T7 and ending at the level of the spine of the scapula.
- Crossing over the scapula toward the shoulder joint is done in the third sequence.

▶ **On the leg** (▶ Fig. 2.70)
- A long flat stroke beginning in the upper third of the thigh, along the lateral edge of the sartorius muscle, ending at the superior iliac spine.
- Bimanual stretching between the muscle bellies of the gastrocnemius muscles from the middle of the calf from top to bottom down to the Achilles tendon.

Comments

- Since the muscles show significant loss in muscle tone the therapist must hold the tissue with his or her free hand, if necessary, while applying the strokes in order to guarantee traction and thus an adequate stimulus. Applying resistance that is too strong, however, could also generate artificial tension and subsequently distort the intensity of the stimulus applied through the traction.
- The strokes are applied to the arms and legs until minor reddening becomes visible. Only then is CTM applied to the extremities in flat technique.
- Soft and persisting bimanual stretching of the muscles of the thigh and lower leg are repeatedly integrated into the treatment.

CTM is regarded as long-term therapy, but it is advisable to impose pauses of 3 to 4 weeks and then start anew.

If possible, physical therapy should be applied before CTM, since the patient must rest after each treatment.

3.4.2 Headaches

Headaches are a common complaint in many people who are not necessarily ill in the stricter sense. Nevertheless, if headaches become persistent and excruciating, treatment is necessary. The "headache" syndrome is within the competence of neurologists. Headaches can be caused acutely by meningitis, chronically by large brain tumors, in older people by vasculitis (so-called cranial arteritis), and also by sinusitis, eye diseases, and many other factors.

Three groups of headaches in particular can be considered for treatment with connective tissue massage:
- Tension headaches
- Migraines
- Cervical headaches in the occiput region, with changes of the cervical spine

The most frequent type of headaches are tension headaches and—defining the syndrome in the broad sense—migrainelike headaches or migraine itself.

Tension Headaches

Definition

Tense, pressing, pulling pain and/or diffusely stinging pain are characteristic of this type of headache, which usually starts in the occiput region or the neck and radiates extensively on both sides to the temples, the roof of the skull, and the forehead and even the area of the eyes. Many patients describe the pain as being as though they were wearing a rubber cap or swimming cap that is too tight, or like having a tight ring around the head. The pain is often already present in the morning and then decreases and increases in waves; it can last for days, then disappear again or become chronic in the long term. Actual headache "attacks" are not typical.

The previous description "vasomotor headaches" is obsolete nowadays because the pain almost certainly has less to do with cramps or other disorders in the region of vascular muscles and is rather caused by contraction of the head and neck muscles. Electromyography provides evidence of tense muscles near the head.

As described in the opening chapters, with mental stress, frustration, or high levels of stress of any kind, a syndrome with increased sympathetic tone develops, which is in general accompanied by preparedness of the muscles for action—fight or flight—and therefore with a more or less persistent muscle contraction or tension. If this continues, the muscle tension causes pain. The underlying conflict or triggering stressful situation must be analyzed, discussed, and, if possible, solved.

This means that such headaches have a broadly or even predominantly psychosomatic cause. Psychosomatic muscle pain (p. 123) is described further in a separate section below; in this section it is mentioned only for differential diagnostic discrimination from other types of headaches. When the neck and head muscles are tense, this is obviously a particularly promising indication for connective tissue massage. In conjunction with an informative conversation with the patient and solution of the underlying conflicts, this treatment is especially effective and gentle.

In these cases, CTM reduces the muscle tone and thus alleviates the pain in the region of neck and shoulder. The involvement of the vascular muscles, which cannot be ignored (i.e., the vasomotor aspect of headaches), can also be improved by this treatment.

Findings

Changes in turgor and muscle tone are distributed over the entire back and are located in segments C1–C8, T1–T12, L2, L4, S1 (▶ Fig. 3.12, ▶ Fig. 3.13).

The connection between increased tissue tone and the allocated organs like the liver, gallbladder, stomach, lungs, and heart, should be taken into consideration. There are retractions and distensions; the skin and subcutaneous tissue are difficult to move against each other. The chest seems to be ironclad. Particularly stubborn adhesions in certain tissue areas are palpated in the following areas:

- On the sacral bone, especially in the lower part
- In the paravertebral region of the lower ribs
- Between the scapulae
- On the lateral side of the scapulae, extending into the upper arms
- Along the latissimus dorsi muscle (C7) extending to the axilla
- Along the edge of the trapezius muscle (descending part)
- On the back of the head, in the region of the short neck muscles
- In the area of the anterior side of the body on the costal arches
- On the pectoralis major muscle and deltoid muscle
- On the edges of the sternocleidomastoid muscle

Treatment Plan

Starting position: sitting or lateral position, supine position, prone position.
- Small basic sequence, flat strokes over the back from caudal toward cranial and vice versa.
- Small basic sequence, first sequence, flat strokes over the back.
- Small basic sequence, first and second sequence, ventral side of the body, flat strokes over the arms.
- Small basic sequence, first and second sequence, ventral side of the body, treatment of the upper arm, flat strokes of forearm and hand.
- Small basic sequence, first, second, and third sequence, ventral side, treatment of arm.
- Small basic sequence, first, second, and third sequence, ventral side, facial treatment, treatment of arm.
- Small basic sequence, first, second, and third sequence, ventral side, facial treatment, treatment of the head, flat strokes on both arms.

Balancing strokes over the pectoral muscles, dorsal dispersion stroke, and flat strokes of the arms are applied at the end of each treatment session to support the venous backflow.

Additional Strokes

Small Basic Sequence

▶ **From dorsal** (▶ Fig. 2.27)
- Small hooks to the sacral bone edges from caudal to cranial.
- Hooks along the course of the first pelvic stroke from caudal to cranial.
- Small, flat transverse strokes over the spinal column within the long erector spinae muscle from L5 to T12.
- Stretching stroke in the lumbar triangle.
- Fan-shaped flat strokes on the angle between the lower edge of the rib cage and the spinal column, T12 to L3.
- Bimanual strokes on the lower edge of the rib cage, beginning from dorsal toward the medioclavicular line and on the pelvic edge toward the anterior superior iliac spine (▶ Fig. 2.35). This set of strokes is performed bimanually, first on one side and then on the other side of the patient in supine position.

First Sequence

▶ **From dorsal** (▶ Fig. 2.38, ▶ Fig. 2.39, ▶ Fig. 2.40)
- The intercostal strokes are also pulled in the opposite direction from the spinal column to the lateral rib cage wall to the ventral axillary line and hooked in there gently.
- Flat strokes over the spinal column, beginning at the level of T6 under the angle of the left scapula and ending under the angle of the right scapula.
- Small, flat transverse strokes along the spine within the area of the long extensor spinae muscles from T12 to T7.

▶ **From ventral**
- In the ventral intercostal area a set of flat strokes are pulled, beginning at the dorsal axillary line through the intercostal spaces. These should start at the lowest ribs.

Second Sequence

▶ **From dorsal** (▶ Fig. 2.46, ▶ Fig. 2.48)
- Short strokes from the lower angle of the scapula to the spine at the level of T4.
- Small, flat transverse strokes over the spine, within the area of the long extensor spinae muscles, from T7 to C7.
- Short hooks around the angle of the scapula followed by outlining the scapula with cutting strokes along the same course.
- Long downward stretching.
- Prolonged upward stretching.

▶ **From ventral** (▶ Fig. 2.49)
- The ventral edge of the trapezius muscle is pulled out starting from the cervical base, while pressing against it with the free hand.

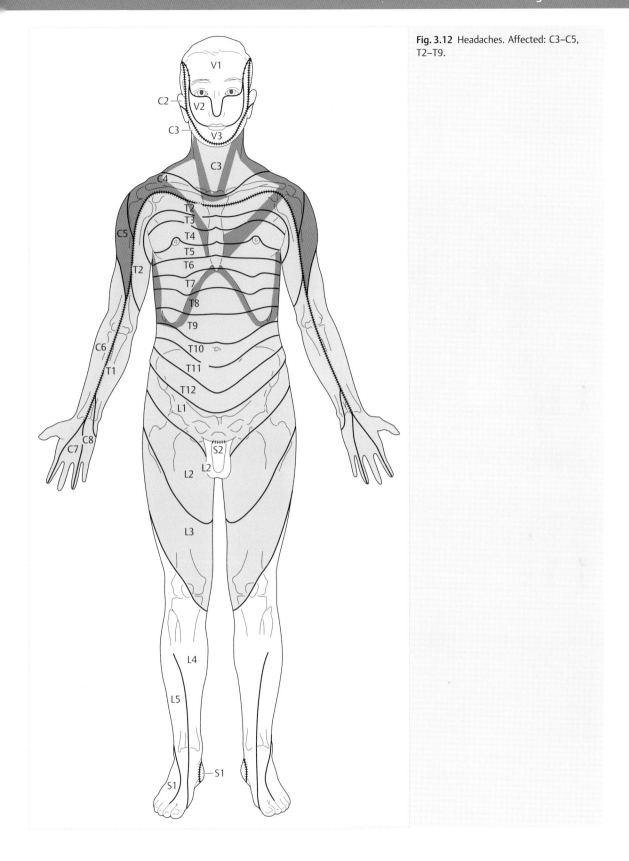

Fig. 3.12 Headaches. Affected: C3–C5, T2–T9.

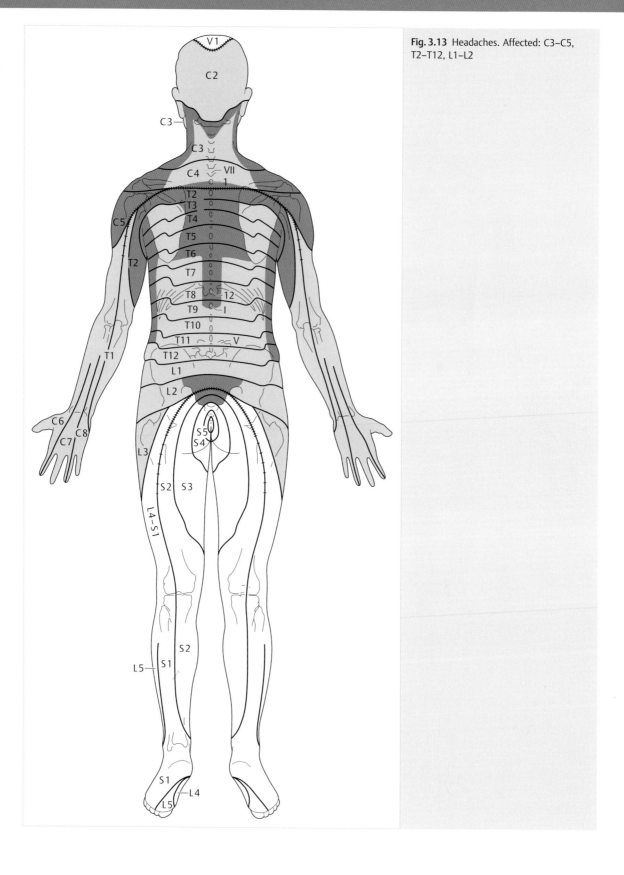

Fig. 3.13 Headaches. Affected: C3–C5, T2–T12, L1–L2

- Strokes along the sternum beginning at the xiphoid process to the jugular notch.
- Short hooks on the connection points between the ribs and sternum from caudal to cranial.
- After the third sequence, flat fanlike strokes are pulled transversely over the scapula toward the shoulder joint, beginning with the stroke on the outer scapula and ending on the lower edge of the spine of the scapula.

Comments

- Only the small basic sequence is applied during the first three to four sessions. After the usual dispersion stroke, the patient lies in prone position and flat strokes are applied from caudal to cranial over the entire back and from the axillae over the lateral rib cage.
- While work is being done in the region of the sacral bone, the pressure in the head may decrease. The therapist therefore applies these additional strokes during the small basic sequence.
- In the additional treatment sequences, the skin reaction and the traction of the fingertips in the connective tissue are repeatedly checked.
- Flat strokes on the lateral part of the scapula toward the shoulder joint loosen the tense tissue between the scapulae so that the inner edge of the scapula can be pulled upward with cutting strokes.
- The transverse strokes between the scapulae and pulling out the scapula under the medial edge toward the spinal column can have a releasing effect on the pressure in the head. This stroke is repeated several times in the second sequence.
- After facial treatment the therapy is continued on the scalp by applying hooks along the hairline and the back of the head. Raised fingertips of the entire hand apply circular movements on the scalp along the cranial sutures. The adhering tissue is loosened especially in the region of the ear and temple.
- The application of a rolled-up hot pack in the T3–T7 sections of the rib cage over the right side can be beneficial for the blood supply of the tissue and subsequently the metabolic reaction.
- If the patient reports feelings of discomfort during CTM, such as an increase in head pressure, nausea, or heart palpitations, the therapist can regulate this by repeating the strokes in the small basic sequence and applying the large balancing stroke (▶ Fig. 2.38) at the level of the sixth/seventh intercostal space that is flatly pulled around the lower angle of the scapula toward C7. However, the therapist should also check his or her technique. The position of the fingers may have been raised too high, making the traction through the tissue too strong; the strokes would therefore be too intense through the tissue, which was still tense. Alternatively, the therapist might have gone ahead too quickly to the next treatment sequence.

- Physical therapy and CTM should be coordinated. The patient must rest after CTM.
- Headache patients are long-term patients. Patient and therapist must have much patience and endurance. The therapist must convince the patients so that they keep coming back for treatment. The general goal is mental and muscular relaxation.
- The sensitivity of the task within CTM highlights the importance of collaboration between therapists and neurologists.

Migraine

Definition

Migraine is a genetic disposition of the vascular system to abnormally excessive constriction and dilation; inflammatory reactions in the vascular walls and the occurrence of pain-inducing substances also play important roles. The general mechanism involves the blood vessels, though the pathogenesis of this clinical picture is still unclear.

In classical migraine, the actual pain attack is often preceded by a so-called aura, a preliminary phase during which neurological symptoms develop. Twinkling and flickering are seen on one side of the visual field of both eyes, either on the right or on the left. Flashing light effects develop with dancing, circulating, spikelike misperceptions and, in the end, a temporary loss of vision may develop on this half of the visual field (hemianopsia). Temporary double vision rarely develops; expect unilateral paresthesia in the arm and leg, or more rarely temporary hemiplegia.

Subsequently, pressing, tense headaches develop and quickly intensify, typically starting at the opposite side and remaining accentuated there. After varying time this pain gives way to a throbbing, pulsating pain. This is accompanied by nausea and often retching or vomiting, irritability, and sensitivity to light and noise.

If possible, patients should rest in a darkened room. The syndrome has often disappeared on waking after sleep. Migraine attacks can last 1–2 days.

Women most frequently develop migraines during menstruation. In other cases, stress, unresolvable conflicts, and psychological tension are usually triggering factors of migraine attacks.

The headaches themselves are obviously a vascular headache, because the blood vessels of the head are also supplied with nerve endings that are sensitive to pain, and pain is especially felt in the vessels of the scalp and meninges. Involvement of the actual cerebral vessels triggers the neurological symptoms described above.

Migraine is generally treated with medication: for example, with a beta-receptor blocker or a calcium antagonist and during the attack with aspirin-containing preparations or modern triptans. These are considerations for the neurologist.

CTM can be applied as additional treatment quite effectively during pain-free intervals.

For differential diagnosis the physician must also consider so-called cluster headaches as well as chronic paroxysmal hemicrania. These are less suitable for CTM treatments.

In the facial area, neuralgia of the trigeminal nerve with its flashlike attacks into the territory of one or more trigeminal branches must be considered. CTM is also not indicated for this disease.

Findings, Treatment Plan, Additional Strokes

See the section Tension Headaches (p. 117).

Comments

The causes of migraine described at the beginning of this section must be watched for by the therapist when considering treatment with CTM.

Methodically determined findings are registered and constantly updated. It may very well be that treatment can only be started by applying flat strokes to the patient who is in the horizontal position.

The following aspects must be noted in general when treating migraine with CTM:
- The more carefully treatment is started and continued in the additional section sequences, the more likely it is to have an alleviating, curative effect.
- The strokes in the paravertebral area and between the scapulae must be applied with care, since the stimuli are transferred to the autonomic nervous system over the shortest route and can contribute to improvement, but also to worsening of the condition.
- When treating the face, the therapist should start with the unaffected half first. It is assumed that the consensual effect has a preparatory effect for the application of CTM on the affected side.
- Application of a rolled-up hot pack is indicated. It is applied first over the sacral bone and then continued in the angle between the lower edge of the ribs and spinal column. The rolled-up hot pack is also applied to the ventral side of the body, on the lower edge of the ribs, and on the origins of the ribs on the sternum.
- The opportunity to stop a migraine attack may present itself if the patient is currently in treatment and can correctly assess and evaluate the course of the migraine.

The following strokes can then be applied (▶ Fig. 2.11):
- Pulling out several times over the lower sacral bone and rib cage edges.
- Soft and flat balancing strokes on the pectoral muscles.
- Balancing strokes above the clavicle.
- Flat transverse strokes between the scapulae to the level (T2) of the spine of the scapula.
- Repeat lower rhomboid strokes and strokes over the rib cage edge.

- Apply the "rake" several times from the neck over the spine of the scapula to the shoulder joint and between the scapulae to the lower edge of the rib cage.
- The large balancing stroke starts in the ventral axillary line at the level of the sixth/seventh intercostal space and is flatly pulled around the lower angle of the scapula toward C7.
- Physical therapy and CTM should be coordinated appropriately. The patient must rest after CTM.

Cervical Headaches

Definition

Cervical or cervicogenic headaches or upper cervical spine syndrome are highly controversial and dubious terms, just as so-called cervical spine syndromes are highly over-rated. In particular, the practices of "manual medicine" must be critically mentioned here.

The pathogenesis of headaches that can be triggered by the cervical spine has two possible explanations. Osseous changes in the two top cervical segments can occasionally cause irritations of the top cervical roots that exit here, which then cause neuralgic pain in their territory exclusively in the occiput area. This so-called occiput neuralgia is rare and may only be diagnosed if the headaches have an attacklike neuralgic character, if they occur mainly on one side, and if they are exclusively detectable in the area supplied by the C2 nerve root.

Pain caused by muscle tension and contractions in the area between the upper cervical spine and back of the head are more frequent. Blunt and movement-dependent pain is possible that is accentuated in the neck, although proof must be provided for relevant osseous changes in the upper cervical spine and for palpable and detectable muscle tension to make such a diagnosis.

There is a blurred border or transitional zone to tension headaches (p. 117) with this syndrome, which may present with similar symptoms to tension headaches.

Pain throughout the skull and in the forehead cannot be triggered by the cervical spine from a pathophysiological perspective and such headaches are definitely not caused by degenerative changes of the medial or lower cervical spine.

Any form of muscle tension and pain in the neck and back of the head is a promising field of application for connective tissue massage.

Findings, Treatment Plan, Additional Strokes

See the relevant section on tension headache (p. 117).

Comments

- See the section on tension headache (p. 117).
- It appears that the tension in the muscle decreases when the pressure on cervical spine structures is reduced and the mobility of the cervical spine is improved.

- It is advisable to collaborate with the attending physician, review the findings of the radiographic scan and appropriately coordinate physical therapy with CTM.

3.4.3 Psychosomatic Syndromes

Psychogenic pain is a controversial and difficult issue. Neurophysiological explanations can be derived for pain and muscle tensions, which are generally described as psychosomatic.

Psychosomatic disorders are disturbances of physical wellbeing and function that develop for psychological reasons. Chronic unresolved conflicts and stress at work, in the family, or in relationships that cannot be resolved satisfactorily are usually at the heart of the problem. Thorough examination often also detects a local physical trigger, mostly harmless. Equally often, patients with similar complaints and medical histories can be found in the patient's milieu (i.e., role models).

As discussed in the opening chapters, every form of mental stress leads to increased sympathetic tone and more or less generalized muscle tension. If mental stress becomes chronic, because no solution can be found, the muscle tension persists and will become painful over time. In many cases, some form of work-related stress or other external factors will play an additional role in relation to the region of the pain.

Psychosomatic Pain in Neck and Shoulder

Definition

Similar to tension headaches, this condition is in the broader sense psychologically related chronic tension of the shoulder and neck muscles. Degenerative changes of the cervical spine are frequently accused of being the culprits, but often these are only insignificant ancillary findings or there is no important reason why the psychologically related pain has manifested where it has and not in some other region of the body.

Many physicians are satisfied with radiographic findings and do not evaluate the history.

Psychosomatic pain in the neck and shoulder due to chronic muscle tension often affects people who have to work in a sitting position with head and torso leaning forward (secretaries, people who work constantly with a computer, etc.).

Another group comprises people who are highly susceptible to tension and tension headaches.

A third group includes people with a depressive disposition. They "hang their head" or come in with "hanging shoulders": as has already been mentioned, depression causes a reduction of muscle tone and in this constellation spraining and stretching pain develops in the region of the neck and shoulder if the depression lasts for any lengthy period.

All of these patients must of course receive psychological counseling and, if necessary, psychotherapeutic treatment. Co-treatment with physical therapy, however, is equally important and connective tissue massage is an excellent option.

Findings, Treatment Plan, Additional Strokes

See the section on tension headache (p. 117).

Comments

See the section on tension headaches (p. 117).

The fact that psychosomatic pain in the neck and shoulder develops secondarily, that is, it develops due to the patient's body posture and mental state, must be considered in the treatment.

The task of CTM is to make the muscles stretchable and ready to work again. The patient should be offered a posture training program. It should be kept in mind that headache patients are long-term patients. Again, good collaboration by everyone involved is vital here.

Psychosomatic Back Pain

Psychosomatic factors in back pain may play a role even more frequently in the lumbar area than in the region of the cervical spine. Here also degenerative changes of the lumbar spine, which regularly occur in every older person, are widely over-rated. It must be carefully assessed orthopedically and neurologically whether the pain is actually triggered by these osseous changes or by a slipped disk or only an intervertebral disk protrusion, and whether psychosomatic factors aggravate the situation. Very often both pathogeneses can be found: organic causes in the region of the lumbar spine as well as typical mental and psychosomatic constellations can be found. Again, two groups must be distinguished:

- Ambitious, aspiring persons with a predisposition to "aggressive self-assertion" and the need to "show backbone." These people often have limited opportunities to vent and are chronically frustrated, being continuously "on the edge" with muscles tensed and remaining in this state until the muscle tension starts to hurt. In men, "macho" characters can often be seen who have a need to permanently demonstrate power and who present themselves in a "victory pose" that often competes with reality.
- The second group comprises people who have a depressive disposition, who "let everything droop." They have a weak muscle tone and therefore suffer from stretching and spraining pain in the region of the back.

Patients with psychosomatic back pain often use very extravagant expressions ("as if some crazy fire is burning in my back," "pain like stabs of a sword"); they have the constant impression that their back is "breaking." Attempts to obtain pensions and benefits or other nonmedical reasons may also play a large role in such cases.

It is important for therapy that the therapist who performs connective tissue massage, which is very helpful and curative in these cases, also generates a supportive environment for the therapy. The therapist must be relaxed himself or herself, must signal positive attentiveness, and should never play down or doubt the complaints reported by the patient. The therapist must take the patient seriously as a person and help to lead this person out of their dead end without their losing face.

Findings, Treatment Plan, Additional Strokes

See statements on lesion of the lumbar spine (p. 67).

Comments

See comments on lesions of the lumbar spine (p. 67) in the section on Sciatica and Chronic Lumbar Syndrome.

CTM is performed in accordance with a treatment plan that will alleviate the complaints: it is the task of all of those involved in the patient's treatment to determine the cause of the complaints. The physician must perform a good diagnosis; the psychotherapist must determine the patient's mental disposition; and the physical therapist must take care of the patient's body posture.

CTM loosens and improves the blood supply of muscular structures, which plays a significant role here.

3.5 Disorders in Internal Medicine

Axel Gehrke, Michael Weber, Rauthgundis Gleich von Muenster

3.5.1 Disorders of the Heart

The complaints and performance of a patient with heart disease determine the therapeutic considerations before CTM is applied, whether as sole or as concomitant physical therapy, especially when it comes to hyperthermal procedures. The function of the heart is always in unison with the circulation: therefore, therapists have very simple yet valuable functional tests at their disposal, such as taking the pulse and measuring blood pressure, which help to evaluate the patient's physical condition and endurance.

With heart diseases in particular, the therapist must examine the patient to correctly evaluate the patient's current condition, even if an attending physician has provided a diagnosis.

Advanced heart disease can cause pain or shortness of breath even while the patient is undressing. Chronic cardiac insufficiency that is becoming more severe is easy to detect because of cardiac cachexia and cyanosis. Edema in the legs, congested cervical veins, and ascites indicate a worsening of right-sided heart failure, while massive pulsations of the arteries are typical of aortic insufficiency. In such cases, the patient should present to the attending physician again. In any case the measurement of blood pressure and heart rate before and after treatment is mandatory, because it is the only way to evaluate therapeutic success and the risk level that can be expected from an additional therapeutic measure.

Disorders of the musculoskeletal system that can exclusively or additionally imitate heart problems must be included as targets of successful treatment, irrespective of the actual presence of organic heart problems. Occasionally muscle tension caused by reflexes, myotendinosis, or fibromyalgic disturbances that originate in the cervical and thoracic spine can trigger such extensive pain in the chest that patients are sent to the hospital with suspected angina pectoris or myocardial infarction.

Disorders of the gastrointestinal tract can also lead to severe chest pain imitating heart problems as a result of the interconnection of the organs with the autonomic nervous system.

CTM may have both direct and indirect effects on the autonomic nervous system. Among other effects, the regulation of the arterial blood pressure and the blood supply to internal organs can be influenced. When taking the changes in the soft tissue into account, such as agonizing meteorism, CTM often achieves astonishing results in respect of the alleged angina pectoris, which is in fact a symptom of Roemheld syndrome.

Before each application of CTM, even with ascertained coronary heart disease, it should be determined whether the current complaints are also triggered or intensified by physical exertion. Pain that only occurs during rest or not associated with physical exertion more likely indicates an extracardiac etiology, which can be treated with CTM and physical therapy.

The pain typically caused by angina pectoris has a segmental structure. It is an intense and brief pain that quickly disappears when the patient adopts a relief posture. By contrast, functional complaints last for hours or days and can easily drive patients into depression, since they do not see any way to escape the situation. Nitrates could help here for differential diagnosis. They are usually prescribed to patients with true angina pectoris and always alleviate the pain. Their effectiveness is only minor or absent with functional heart problems and their use is frequently discontinued due to the development of headaches.

Painful spots that are exactly located by the patient in the region of the chest, such as in the middle of the left pectoral muscle or in the region of the descending part of the right trapezius muscle, are maximal points. They signal reflexes in the segment, which can be influenced well by CTM and methods of physical and rehabilitative medicine.

Coronary Heart Disease

Definition

Coronary heart disease is characterized by a disproportion of the heart's oxygen supply and oxygen consumption. Stenoses causing reduction of less than 50% in the vascular linear diameter generally do not have any hemodynamic relevance. Only more severe stenoses lead to signs of insufficient blood supply during exertion. In progressive cases the blood supply is usually no longer adequate to ensure the supply of the myocardium. Depending on the extent of coronary stenosis, the patient experiences attacks of angina pectoris or myocardial infarction.

In addition to arteriosclerosis, sudden physical or psychological strains, excessive metabolic deviations, hypertension, or extreme changes in heart rate can trigger the complaints.

Severe thoracic and pulmonary disorders, which lead to a permanent arterial oxygen pressure (PO_2) of under 60 mm Hg, can trigger coronary insufficiency and even an infarction, if there are corresponding preexisting changes in the coronaries. For differential diagnosis, a stress ECG allows exact evaluation of the range of coronary performance.

Occasionally there is generalized pain, mostly in the left shoulder, arm, and hand, which can develop into a postinfarction syndrome or even become a complex regional pain syndrome. It is advisable to include the left arm in the treatment, if these complaints become apparent. The complaints usually improve when working the tense parts of the body in the region of the heart and applying careful stretching strokes to the left axilla.

Findings

Changes in turgor and muscle tone are located in segments C3–C4, C8, T1–T9 (▶ Fig. 3.14, ▶ Fig. 3.15).

▶ **Tissue changes on the posterior side of the body**
- Between the spinal column and left scapula, which appear as bulges (myocardial damage)
- Retractions on the left scapula
- Adhesions in the tissue between the upper arm, axilla, and rib cage on the left side
- Retractions in the left intercostal area and on the lateral side on the edge of the rib cage along the latissimus dorsi muscle

Maximal points are palpated below the spine of the scapula on the left and on both sides at the level of the inferior angle of the scapula close to the spinal column.

▶ **On the anterior side of the body**
- Retractions on the lower costal arch; these are more accentuated on the left than on the right side.
- Hardening on the origin of the anterior serratus muscle on the costal arches.

- Accentuated tenderness close to the costosternal joints of the second to fifth ribs. Special attention must be given here to distensions.
- Pain radiating into the arm, especially into the little finger, indicates C8.

Maximal points are palpated in the middle of the pectoralis major muscle on both sides of the rib cage, in the trapezius muscle under the bulge of the descending part on the left side, and in the origin of the rectus abdominis muscle in the region of the lower costal arch.

Treatment Plan

Starting position: sitting or lateral position, supine position.
- Small basic sequence, flat strokes over the back.
- Small basic sequence, first sequence on the right side of the rib cage, flat strokes over the back.
- Small basic sequence, first sequence on both sides of the rib cage, second sequence on the right side of the rib cage, flat strokes over the back and along the right arm.
- Small basic sequence, first and second sequence, on both sides of the rib cage, ventral side, flat strokes on the right arm.
- Small basic sequence, first and second sequence, ventral side, flat strokes on both arms.
- Small basic sequence, first and second sequence, ventral side, treatment of the right arm, flat strokes on the right forearm and hand and whole left arm.
- Small basic sequence, first and second sequence, ventral side, treatment of the right arm, treatment of the left upper arm, flat strokes on the left forearm and hand.
- Small basic sequence, first, second, and third sequence, ventral side, treatment of the right arm and treatment of the left arm.

Balancing strokes over the pectoral muscles, dorsal dispersion stroke, and flat strokes of the arms are applied at the end of each treatment session to support the venous backflow.

Additional Strokes

Small Basic Sequence

▶ **From dorsal** (▶ Fig. 2.27, ▶ Fig. 2.29)
- Hooks to the sacral bone edges from caudal to cranial.
- Hooks along the course of the first pelvic stroke from caudal to cranial.
- Small, flat transverse strokes along the spine within the area of the long extensor spinae muscles, from L5 to T12.
- Stretching in the lumbar triangle (▶ Fig. 2.29).
- Small, flat transverse strokes along the spine, within the area of the long extensor spinae muscles, from L5 to T12.

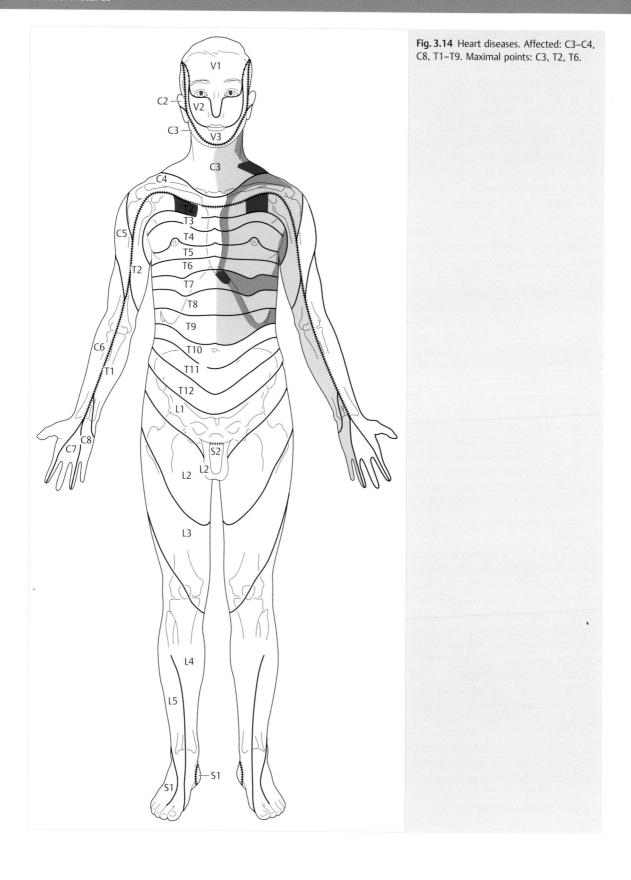

Fig. 3.14 Heart diseases. Affected: C3–C4, C8, T1–T9. Maximal points: C3, T2, T6.

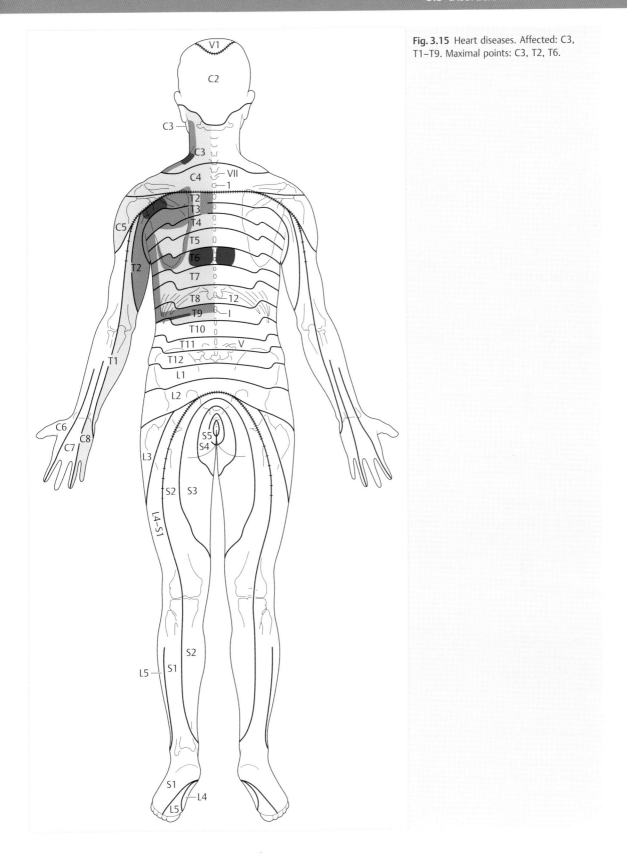

Fig. 3.15 Heart diseases. Affected: C3, T1–T9. Maximal points: C3, T2, T6.

▶ **From ventral** (▶ Fig. 2.35)

- Bimanual strokes, starting from the dorsal side. At the same time, the therapist pulls on the lower edge of the rib cage toward the medioclavicular line and on the pelvic edge toward the anterior superior iliac spine. These strokes are performed bimanually, first on one side then on the other.
- Bimanual strokes crossing over the abdominal walls, starting in the dorsal region and ending at the opposite edge of the rectus abdominis muscle.
- Balancing strokes on the pectoral muscles and strokes on the ventral pelvis and abdomen (▶ Fig. 2.32).

First Sequence

▶ **From dorsal** (▶ Fig. 2.39)

- The intercostal strokes are also pulled in the opposite direction from the spinal column to the lateral chest wall up to the ventral axillary line and hooked in there gently.
- A stroke from the lower angle of the scapula to the spinal column at the level of T4, which is started on the right side of the body.
- Flat transverse strokes over the spinal column, beginning at the level of T6 under the angle of the right scapula and ending under the angle of the left scapula.

▶ **From ventral**

- In the ventral intercostal area a set of flat strokes are pulled beginning at the dorsal axillary line through the intercostal spaces. These should start at the lowest ribs.

Second Sequence

▶ **From dorsal** (▶ Fig. 2.39, ▶ Fig. 2.46, ▶ Fig. 2.48)

- The large balancing stroke starts in the ventral axillary line at the level of the sixth/seventh intercostal space on the right side of the body and is flatly pulled around the lower angle of the scapula toward C7.
- Long downward stretching.
- Prolonged upward stretching.
- Small, flat transverse strokes over the spinal column within the long erector spinae muscle from T7 to T3.
- Flat transverse strokes from the inner edge to the inner edge of the scapulae, starting at the level of T7 and ending at the level of the spine of the scapula.

▶ **From ventral** (▶ Fig. 2.49)

- The ventral edge of the trapezius muscle is pulled out starting from the cervical base up to the level of the shoulder, while pressing against it with the free hand.
- Strokes along the sternum, beginning at the xiphoid process to the jugular notch.
- Short hooks on the connection points between the ribs and sternum from cranial to caudal.
- The therapist works on the right side of the body with small fanlike strokes on the medial clavicular

angle toward the suprasternal notch, starting with the first stroke on the clavicle, ending with the last one on the dorsal edge of the sternocleidomastoid muscle. These strokes are then transferred to the left side of the rib cage.

- After the third sequence (▶ Fig. 2.47) a flat fan-shaped stroke is applied transversely over the scapula toward the shoulder joint, starting at the outer border of the scapula and ending at the lower border of the spine of the scapula.

Comments

- The acute conditions of heart disease must have disappeared: CTM may be started about 6 weeks after the cardiac event.
- The additional sequences are first applied to the right side of the body and then transferred to the left side.
- The treatment is performed with the patient lying down when edemas of the leg are diagnosed. Flat strokes on the legs from distal to proximal support the venous backflow.
- The small basic sequence is more often applied with flat strokes on the rib cage until the segmental adhesions are reduced in T1–T9. After the small basic sequences strokes are applied bimanually to the lower edge of the sacral bone. Only then does the first sequence follow, which is initially pulled up only on the right side, while light strokes are applied to the left side.
  The left angle between the pelvic crest and spinal column and between the spinal column and lower edge of the rib cage is only added after the eighth to ninth treatment session.
- When the tension in the tissue subsides, the first sequence is also transferred to the left side. The same applies to the second sequence.
- Flat strokes can be enough to treat the arm, since the tension has been normalized through the segmental treatment of the torso.
- Ventral treatment is started on the right side of the rib cage and moved to the left side once the tension in the tissue becomes less. Initially omit the left pectoral muscle when applying the flat dispersion strokes and only apply strokes to the infra- and supraclavicular areas.
- When treatment is in its advanced phase, a rolled-up hot pack is applied along the sternocostal joints, on the pectoral muscle, and on the edge of the trapezius muscle.
- CTM is always administered after physical therapy, since the patient must rest after the treatment.

Functional Heart Complaints

Definition

These are complex syndromes with heart palpitations or tachycardia, tightness, and anxiety, or pain in the region of the heart that are accompanied by fear, excitation, and restlessness and where no organic reason can be found in the heart.

In addition to metabolic disorders, deficiencies, intoxications, and endocrine disorders, consideration must be given to psychovegetative or psychosomatic causes. A chronic unresolved conflict, or sometimes a recent event, could be at the root of things; these root causes must be investigated and the patient counseled, and, if necessary, psychotherapeutic treatment should be provided. Beta-blocking agents can be considered as medicinal treatment.

Changes in the spinal column are very rarely the cause. CTM can be very helpful as an additional therapy.

Findings

- See Coronary Heart Disease (p. 125).
- The palpable changes in the skin are located in the heart segments, not only in the dermatomes, but also in the myotomes and sclerotomes C8–T8. Localized painful spots can be palpated on the costovertebral joints.
- The tension of the tissue cannot be distinctively palpated on the left side of the body. This immediately provides the therapist with information that the heart complaints are of a functional nature.

Treatment Plan, Additional Strokes

See Coronary Heart Disease (p. 125).

Comments

- See Coronary Heart Disease (p. 125).
- The accentuated observation of the left side of the body is no longer a focus after the findings have changed. Additionally, the costovertebral joints are palpated and mobilized through techniques of manual therapy if a block is detected.

Cardiac Arrhythmia

Definition

Repolarization and conduction disturbances must be identified here. They are characterized by tachycardia with a persisting heart rate of over 100 beats per minute, by bradycardia with a heart rate of less than 50 beats per minute, and by extrasystoles caused by premature or delayed heart actions. Supraventricular and ventricular cardiac arrhythmia and irregular conduction with atrial fibrillation can accompany all cardiac disorders.

Most of these symptoms are also observed in people with a healthy heart and are usually hemodynamically irrelevant. It would therefore be wrong to alarm a patient because of an incidental finding. In the case of drug therapy, however, it is appropriate to attempt to assist the effects using CTM and a targeted physical therapy program.

Findings

- See Coronary Heart Disease (p. 125).
- The diagnostics surprisingly show minor cardiac findings on the left side of the body. There are adhesions of the tissue in the region of the whole thorax.

Treatment Plan, Additional Strokes, Comments

See Coronary Heart Disease (p. 125).

Congenital and Acquired Valvular Heart Disease

Definition

The spectrum of valvular heart disease has changed significantly because of antibiotic therapy. While they were mostly acquired through rheumatic fever in the past, the majority of valvular heart diseases nowadays are caused by congenital anomalies or degenerative valvular processes. The mitral valve prolapse syndrome is also part of this group.

Congenital and acquired defects can have a stable course over years or even decades. Sudden exertion or severe psychological strain can lead to sudden changes in the course of the illness. Particularly dreaded are acute bacterial valve infections with swift destruction of the valve itself. These syndromes in particular require thorough medical observation and treatment. The stress must be reasonable and well dosed and, if necessary, heart medication must be prescribed.

Surgical correction of acquired and congenital defects often leads to an impressive increase in performance. However, the full level of performance is regained in only a few cases. The reason for this relates mainly to problems after surgery, such as skeletal complaints after thoracotomy, residual gradients of artificial heart valves, and the reversibility of changes in the pulmonary vessels and myocardium. Aortic valve replacement usually leads to better surgical results than mitral valve replacement.

CTM can be applied here together with physical therapy measures. Pain in the operated thorax and accompanying incorrect respiration are favorably influenced.

Findings, Treatment Plan, Additional Strokes

See Coronary Heart Disease (p. 125).

Comments

- See Coronary Heart Disease (p. 125).
- In the course of treatment, strokes in the first and second sequences are applied to both sides. Special attention is needed here when applying the flat dispersion strokes and ensuring that the patient rests after treatment.

- In addition to the general cardiac findings, attention must be paid to edemas in the arms and legs. Edemas in the legs are addressed by intensively working on the iliotibial tract.
- Treatment of leg edemas is performed in lateral or supine position.
- Flat strokes on the legs are applied after the small basic sequence and first sequence. Treatment of the legs with additional strokes follows afterward.

Heart Transplantation

Patients with massive, therapy-resistant heart failure today undergo heart transplantation under certain circumstances.

A patient with a heart transplant will never regain normal performance. The decisive mechanism for increasing cardiac output, increase of the heart rate under exertion, is lost through this surgery, because the transplanted heart is not yet innervated by the autonomic nervous system. Extracardiac pain after surgery due to the wide retraction of the thorax during surgery as well as in later rehabilitation plays a major role in these patients. CTM together with physical therapy measures can be used with good chances for successful treatment.

Findings, Treatment Plan, Additional Strokes

See Coronary Heart Disease (p. 125).

Comments

- See Coronary Heart Disease (p. 125).
- Physical therapy treatment with respiratory therapy and straightening of the rib cage are in the forefront after thoracotomy due to heart surgery.
- CTM is applied in accordance with the treatment plan and particular attention is paid to the second sequence with additional strokes to the intercostal spaces and the origins of the abdominal muscles.

3.5.2 Circulatory Diseases

Hypertension

Definition

In accordance with the recommendations of the World Health Organization (WHO) an arterial blood pressure of up to 140/90 mm Hg is considered normal. Pathological values are given from 160/95 mm Hg, if this value has been measured several times at rest.

The cause of hypertension is unknown in approximately 80% of cases. Genetic factors are involved as well as environmental factors, stress, and obesity. Additionally, many disorders of the kidneys and adrenal glands (e.g., pheochromocytoma, Cushing syndrome), as well as

hyperfunction of internal secretory glands such as hyperthyroidism, can trigger secondary hypertension.

Hypertensive patients are often unaware of the disorder for many years. Headaches, nosebleeds, and reduced performance are frequent symptoms. The course of the illness depends on the quality of antihypertensive therapy and the extent of organ damage already developed.

The chances for successful application of CTM must be seen as relatively small, especially when organ damage has already developed. Treatment with CTM is justified before the disorder develops, especially in the presence of borderline hypertension or concomitant functional imbalances triggered by the autonomic nervous system.

Findings

Increased turgor and muscle tone are located in the segments T2–T9. The maximal point can be palpated on the dorsal side at the level of the superior angle of the scapula next to the spinal column.

Treatment Plan

Starting position: lateral position, sitting.
- Small basic sequence, flat strokes over the back.
- Small basic sequence, first sequence, flat strokes over the back.
- Small basic sequence, first and second sequence, ventral side.

Balancing strokes over the pectoral muscles and dorsal branching end each treatment session.

Additional Strokes

Small Basic Sequence

▶ **From dorsal** (▶ Fig. 2.27)
- Small, flat transverse strokes along the spine within the area of the long extensor spinae muscles from L5 to T12.
- Fanlike strokes in the upper respiratory angle.

▶ **From ventral** (▶ Fig. 2.35)
- Bimanual strokes starting from dorsal. At the same time, the therapist pulls on the lower edge of the rib cage toward the medioclavicular line and on the pelvic edge toward the anterior superior iliac spine. These strokes are performed bimanually, first on one side then on the other.
- The liver stroke.
- Balancing strokes on the pectoral muscles and strokes on the ventral pelvis and abdomen (▶ Fig. 2.32).

First Sequence

▶ **From dorsal** (▶ Fig. 2.37, ▶ Fig. 2.39)
- The intercostal strokes are also pulled in the opposite direction from the spinal column to the lateral chest

wall up to the ventral axillary line and gently hooked in there.

- Small, flat transverse strokes along the spine within the area of the long extensor spinae muscles from T12 to T7.
- Flat transverse strokes over the spinal column, beginning at the level of T6 under the angle of the left scapula and ending under the angle of the right scapula, then pulled back to the starting point.

▶ **From ventral**
- In the ventral intercostal area a set of flat strokes are pulled beginning at the dorsal axillary line through the intercostal spaces. These should start at the lowest ribs.

Second Sequence

▶ **From dorsal (▶ Fig. 2.45, ▶ Fig. 2.46, ▶ Fig. 2.48)**
- Long downward stretching.
- Prolonged upward stretching.
- Axillary stretching with elevated arm.
- Small, flat transverse strokes over the spine within the area of the long extensor spinae muscles from T7 to T3.
- Set of flat strokes from the lower angle of the scapula to the spine at the level of segment T4.
- Short hooks around the angle of the scapula followed by outlining the scapula with cutting strokes along the same course.
- Flat transverse strokes from the inner side to the lateral edge of the scapulae, starting at the level of T7 and ending at the level of the spine of the scapula.

▶ **From ventral (▶ Fig. 2.49)**
- The ventral edge of the trapezius muscle is pulled out starting from the cervical base, while pressing against it with the free hand.
- Strokes along the sternum, beginning at the xiphoid process to the jugular notch.
- Short hooks on the insertion points of the ribs toward the sternum from caudal to cranial.
- Short transverse strokes along the sternum. These start at the junction between the xiphoid process and the body of the sternum, along the area of the sternal angle. At the base of the second rib at the sternum, the strokes should become wider to just under the sternoclavicular joints.
- Short fanlike strokes working along the medial clavicular angle toward the suprasternal notch. These start with the first stroke on the clavicle, ending with the last one on the dorsal edge of the sternocleidomastoid muscle.
- Strokes toward the interclavicular ligament.
- After the third sequence (▶ Fig. 2.47), a flat fan-shaped stroke is applied transversely over the scapula toward the shoulder joint, starting at the outer border of the scapula and ending at the lower border of the spine of the scapula.

Comments

- CTM is started when the patient's general health allows for the increase in stress.
- The treatment is applied with the patient lying down and continued in sitting position after the fifth or sixth CTM session, if the circulation has stabilized by then. The patient's face may redden during treatment: this response documents the success of the stimulation.
- Stimulating strokes are not applied. The small basic sequence is targeted with intensive balancing strokes.
- Physical therapy–assisted cardiovascular training is recommended in addition to CTM.
- CTM is performed after physical therapy. It should be concluded with adequate and controlled rest after treatment.

Hypotension, Orthostatic Dysregulation

Definition

A low blood pressure of under 110/70 mm Hg should only be regarded as a disorder when it is associated with complaints. These may differ greatly from person to person.

Typical symptoms include paleness, tinnitus, nausea, sweating, collapse, and prickling and numbness in the extremities. Incipient orthostatic dysregulation presents itself as dimmed vision and flickering in the eyes when getting up too rapidly and the sudden onset of nausea.

In rare cases organic disorders cause chronic hypotension: for example, malignancies, latent internal hemorrhages, cirrhosis of the liver, hypothyroidism, and adrenal insufficiency.

Depression or psychosomatic disorders are frequently causes.

The effects of certain medications such beta-blocking agents, calcium antagonists, diuretics, and antihypertensive drugs must be considered. Since this is essentially a constitutional problem, the course is usually benign. All therapeutic and rehabilitative measures, CMT, physical therapy, and hydrotherapy must be employed and additional psychotherapeutic assistance can be considered.

Especially during puberty, the circulatory system often experiences imbalances between growth and blood pressure stabilization. This results in orthostatic dysregulation, which manifests especially when changing position from lying or sitting to standing. The blood pressure drops sharply due to insufficient sympathetic counter-regulation. Diffuse dizziness, dimmed vision, and even blackouts can follow.

Treatment with drugs is rarely indicated; cardiovascular training, CTM, and appropriate consultation are usually sufficient.

Findings

Retractions on the edges of the sacral bone, pelvis, and lumbar spine area as well as distensions on the sacral bone must be noted. The tissue is doughy; the skin layers have reduced mobility and are difficult to lift.

Treatment Plan

Starting position: sitting, prone position, supine position.
- Small basic sequence, flat strokes over the back from caudal toward cranial.
- Small basic sequence, first sequence, flat strokes over the back in both directions.
- Small basic sequence, first and second sequence, ventral side, flat strokes over the front and back of the body.
- Small basic sequence, first, second, and third sequence, ventral side, flat strokes over the front and back of the body.

Balancing strokes over the pectoral muscles, dorsal dispersion stroke, and flat strokes of the arms are applied at the end of each treatment session to support the venous backflow.

Additional Strokes

Small Basic Sequence

▶ **From dorsal** (▶ Fig. 2.27)
- Hooks pulled to the sacral bone edges from caudal to cranial.
- Flat transverse strokes pulled over the sacral bone from caudal to cranial.
- Hooks pulled along the course of the first pelvic stroke from caudal to cranial.
- Small, flat transverse strokes over the spine within the area of the long extensor spinae muscles from L5 to T12.
- Fanlike strokes in the upper respiratory angle.

▶ **From ventral** (▶ Fig. 2.35)
- Bimanual strokes, starting from the dorsal side. At the same time, the therapist pulls on the lower edge of the rib cage toward the medioclavicular line and on the pelvic edge toward the anterior superior iliac spine. These strokes are performed first on one side then on the other side of the body.
- Short hooks along the rectus sheath from the symphysis to the level of the navel.
- Bimanual strokes crossing over the abdominal walls, starting in the dorsal region and ending at the opposite edge of the rectus abdominis muscle.
- The liver stroke.

First Sequence

▶ **From dorsal** (▶ Fig. 2.39)
- The intercostal strokes are also pulled in opposite direction from the spinal column to the lateral chest wall up to the ventral axillary line and hooked in there gently.

- Small, flat transverse strokes along the spine within the area of the long extensor spinae muscles, from T12 to T7.
- Flat transverse strokes over the spinal column, beginning at the level of T6 under the angle of the left scapula and ending under the angle of the right scapula.

▶ **From ventral**
- In the ventral intercostal area a set of flat strokes are pulled beginning at the dorsal axillary line through the intercostal spaces. These should start at the lowest ribs.

Second Sequence

▶ **From dorsal** (▶ Fig. 2.46, ▶ Fig. 2.48)
- Long downward stretching.
- Prolonged upward stretching.
- Flat transverse strokes from the inner side to the lateral edge of the scapulae, starting at the level of T7 and ending at the level of the spine of the scapula.
- Set of flat strokes from the lower angle of the scapula to the spine at the level of segment T4.
- Flat transverse strokes over the spinal column, beginning at the level of T6 under the angle of the left scapula and ending under the angle of the right scapula.

▶ **From ventral** (▶ Fig. 2.35)
- The ventral edge of the trapezius muscle is pulled out starting from the cervical base, while pressing against it with the free hand.
- Short hooks on the insertion points of the ribs toward the sternum from caudal to cranial.
- Strokes over the sternum, beginning at the xiphoid process and ending at the suprasternal notch.
- Short transverse strokes along the sternum. These start at the junction between the xiphoid process and the body of the sternum, along the area of the sternal angle. At the base of the second rib at the sternum, the strokes should become wider to just under the sternoclavicular joints.
- Short fanlike strokes work along the medioclavicular angle toward the suprasternal notch. The first set of strokes start on the clavicle, the last set of strokes end on the dorsal edge of the sternocleidomastoid muscle.
- Strokes toward the interclavicular ligament.
- After the third sequence, flat fanlike strokes are pulled transversely over the shoulder blade toward the shoulder joint.

Comments

The patient's behavior is the decisive indication for the therapist, as it demonstrates to what extent the stress caused by CTM can be tolerated.

Physical therapy and CTM should complement each other. Resting afterward is an important part of the treatment.

3.5.3 Disorders of the Lungs and Respiratory Tract

Disorders of the respiratory tract including the nose and paranasal sinuses lead to functional deficits in gas exchange in the lungs, which, depending on the level of severity of the disorder, can subjectively be seen as shortness of breath, and objectively as an imbalance of the respiratory muscles as well as reduced oxygen saturation of the blood.

CTM is highly relevant, especially when treating chronic bronchial asthma and chronic obstructive bronchitis, but also with pulmonary emphysema and pulmonary fibrosis. Various complaints such as coughing and shortness of breath, which may also have an impact on the quality of sleep, can be favorably influenced by CTM.

An exact physical examination is indispensable (cyanosis, dyspnea) to evaluate the application of CTM. Before therapy the shape of the chest and level of ventilation must be determined by measuring the chest circumference and the range of respiration. The therapeutic procedures are determined on the basis of the mobility of the diaphragm and findings on percussion and auscultation.

Optimal treatment leads to significant improvement resulting from a positive influence on the blood pressure and reduction of congestion of the liver as well as various varicose symptom complexes. To document the progress, pulmonary function tests in a closed system (body plethysmography) are advisable at the beginning of treatment and every 2 years.

The success of the therapy should be regularly monitored through simple pulmonary function tests (spirometry). The evaluation of physical status (the breathing pattern, heart rate, and blood pressure) should be made through simultaneous physical therapy.

Disorders of the respiratory organs usually require a combination of pharmacological and physical therapy. The purpose of physical therapy is to normalize respiration. Together with other measures of physical therapy, such as CTM, dysfunctions of the mucosae can be corrected and constricting muscle tones of the bronchial muscles loosened.

This particularly applies to deforming disorders of the chest, as they can disturb the movements of respiration. CTM combined with physical therapy can frequently improve costo-abdominal respiration. This effect can be intensified by methods of hydrotherapy and thermotherapy, especially by enhancing a patient's resilience through so-called "refrigeration" with washing and cooling stimuli. Through targeted positioning, physical therapy supports the draining of secretions, and respiratory therapy promotes maintenance of the elasticity of the thorax.

Chronic hoarseness, pharyngitis, and tracheal dry cough affect the upper respiratory tracts and are triggered by inhalation of particulate matter or smoke as well as chronic irritation of the trachea.

Chronic cough or shortness of breath often causes complaints in the neck and shoulders. Differential diagnoses are absolutely necessary here for further evaluation.

During childhood there frequently occur typical respiratory tract disorders, especially laryngitis and tracheitis. Children who have acquired little or no immunity often suffer from viral infections. As with allergic rhinitis (hay fever), there are hardly any visible and palpable findings.

Acute Bronchitis

Definition

Acute bronchitis is triggered by an infection of the lower respiratory tract. In addition to drug therapy, nursing and physical measures are important: fresh air or moisturized ambient air from a cold vapor humidifier, which is also suitable for simultaneous administration of inhalable medications, such as secretolytic or anti-inflammatory medications as well as locally effective antibiotics.

Cold baths to stimulate deep respiration and respiratory exercises in combination with CTM are important aids, especially for patients who suffer frequent relapses.

Findings

Changes in muscle tone and turgor are located in the segments C3–C8 and T1–T12.

There is a maximal point on each side of the spine at the level of the spine of the scapula.

The following tissue sections in particular show increased muscle tone:

▶ **On the posterior side of the body:**
- On both sides of the spinal column at the level of the thoracolumbar junction
- In the intercostal spaces and on both lower edges of the rib cage
- Laterally along the latissimus dorsi muscle from the iliac crest to under the axilla
- In the paravertebral region between the scapulae, ascending to the cervical spine at the level of C3/C4

▶ **On the anterior side of the body:**
- From the lower edge of the rib cage ascending into the epigastric angle
- Along the sternum, especially on the cartilaginous joints of the ribs to the sternum
- On the base and along the sternocleidomastoid muscle insertion point
- On the anterior part of the deltoid muscle overlapping the pectoral muscle
- Above and under the clavicle

Treatment Plan

Starting position: sitting, lateral or supine position.
- Small basic sequence, flat strokes over the rib cage from caudal toward cranial.

- Small basic sequence, first sequence, flat strokes over the rib cage.
- Small basic sequence, first and second sequence, ventral side.
- Small basic sequence, first and second sequence, ventral side of the body, treatment of the upper arm, flat strokes of forearm and hand.
- Small basic sequence, first, second, and third sequence, ventral side, treatment of arm.

Balancing strokes over the pectoral muscles, dorsal dispersion stroke, and flat strokes of both arms are applied at the end of each treatment session to support the venous backflow.

Additional Strokes

Small Basic Sequence

▶ **From dorsal** (▶ Fig. 2.27)
- Fanlike strokes in the upper respiratory angle
- Stretching in the lumbar triangle (▶ Fig. 2.29)

▶ **From ventral** (▶ Fig. 2.35)
- Bimanual strokes starting from dorsal. At the same time, the therapist pulls on the lower edge of the rib cage toward the medioclavicular line and on the pelvic edge toward the anterior superior iliac spine. This set of strokes is first performed bimanually, first on one side then on the other side of the patient in the lying position.
- Balancing strokes on the pectoral muscles and strokes on the ventral pelvis and abdomen (▶ Fig. 2.32).

First Sequence

▶ **From dorsal** (▶ Fig. 2.39)
- The intercostal strokes are also pulled in the opposite direction from the spinal column to the lateral chest wall up to the ventral axillary line and hooked in there gently.
- Small, flat transverse strokes along the spine, within the area of the long extensor spinae muscles, from T12 to T7.
- Flat transverse strokes over the spinal column, beginning at the level of T6 under the angle of the left scapula and ending under the angle of the right scapula.

▶ **From ventral**
- In the ventral intercostal area a set of flat strokes are pulled beginning at the dorsal axillary line through the intercostal spaces. These should start at the lowest ribs.

Second Sequence

▶ **From dorsal** (▶ Fig. 2.46, ▶ Fig. 2.48)
- Long downward stretching.
- Prolonged upward stretching.

- Set of flat strokes from the lower angle of the scapula to the spine at the level of segment T4.
- Flat transverse strokes from the inner side to the lateral edge of the scapulae, starting at the level of T7 and ending at the level of the spine of the scapula.

▶ **From ventral** (▶ Fig. 2.35)
- The ventral edge of the trapezius muscle is pulled out starting from the cervical base, while pressing against it with the free hand.
- Short hooks on the insertion points of the ribs toward the sternum from caudal to cranial.
- Strokes over the sternum, beginning at the xiphoid process and ending at the suprasternal notch.
- Short transverse strokes along the sternum. These start at the junction between the xiphoid process and the body of the sternum, along the area of the sternal angle. At the base of the second rib at the sternum, the strokes should become wider to just under the sternoclavicular joints.
- Short fanlike strokes work along the medial clavicular angle toward the suprasternal notch, starting the first set of strokes on the clavicle and ending the last set of strokes on the dorsal edge of the sternocleidomastoid muscle.
- Strokes toward the interclavicular ligament.
- After the third sequence, flat fanlike strokes are pulled transversely over the shoulder blade toward the shoulder joint.

Comments

- Treatment with CTM may be started if the patient has no fever and the patient's general health allows for effective administration of CTM.
- The set of strokes in the small basic sequence is executed intensively, hooking in the stimulating strokes only with a minor cutting sensation; ischium, lumbar triangle.
- In the first and second sequences the hooks on the spinal column are omitted, since stimuli applied close to the spinal column evoke reactions which are too strong.
- In the second sequence, axillary stretching is performed intensively by working on the edge of the latissimus dorsi muscle.
- The ventral side of the torso is treated carefully at the beginning.
- In the further course of ventral torso treatment, the arms are positioned at the level of the head; if necessary, padding is provided and a cushion is placed under the lumbar spine.
- The origins of the abdominal muscles on the lower edge of the ribs, the course of the rectus abdominis muscle, and the insertion points of the abdominal muscles on the symphysis should receive heat applications after CTM. Special attention should be paid here to respiration and movements of the rib cage.

- In the further course, heat is applied to the sternum, to the costosternal joints, and on the insertion points of the sternocleidomastoid muscle.
- Heat is applied in the rib cage region after CTM of the respiratory angle, on the lower edge of the rib cage, on the medial and lateral edges of the scapula, along the trapezius muscle, descending part, and the region of the neck.
- When working on the third sequence, particular attention is paid to the tension in the tissue, since the phrenic nerve arises from the medial cervical segments (C3–C4), which innervates the diaphragm.
- Physical therapy and CTM should complement each other. It should be ensured that the patient rests properly after therapy.

Chronic Bronchitis

Definition

The nomenclature of this disorder is inconsistent. Synonyms include bronchial syndrome, spastic bronchitis, emphysema bronchitis, and obstructive respiratory tract syndrome.

Chronic bronchitis is a disorder of the bronchi during which there is persisting cough and sputum for at least 3 months in two consecutive years. This may cause early exertional dyspnea.

The following circumstances are also relevant for the development of chronic bronchitis: recurring infections of the bronchi, bronchopneumonia, disturbances of pulmonary ventilation through limitations of diaphragm and pleural function, disturbances of thoracic statics (scoliosis, especially kyphoscoliosis), and primary disorders of the lungs such as tuberculosis, silicosis, or sarcoidosis.

Functionally similar changes are caused by the so-called irritable bronchial system. Bronchial obstruction is increased by various enzymes (proteases, histamine, serotonin, prostaglandins) and also by exogenous allergens. A constitutional disposition, aging of tissue, and exogenous pollutants (e.g., from chronic nicotine abuse) are also suspected factors. The influences of environmental pollution are of increasing significance.

The evaluation depends on the clinical picture (cough, sputum, dyspnea) but must be quantified in any case by extensive pulmonary function tests.

Special attention must be paid to the detection of incipient, manifest, or even decompensated chronic pulmonary heart disease with load on the right heart. There are realistic chances of preventing or delaying progression of the disease through early rehabilitation.

Findings

- See Bronchial Asthma (p. 137).
- The adhesions are located between the hypodermis and muscular fascia and the tissues are difficult to move against each other.

Treatment Plan, Additional Strokes, Comments

See Bronchial Asthma (p. 137).

Spastic Bronchitis

Definition

This special form of bronchitis mainly occurs in adolescents and children. Due to its similarity to an asthma attack it is also called "asthmatic bronchitis."

There is a congenital or acquired propensity toward spastic reactions of the bronchial muscles, especially of the bronchioles, causing massive contractions of these muscles during episodes of inflammation of the bronchial mucosa, mostly virus related. This results in a predominantly expiratory dyspnea with overdilation up to the development of emphysema of the lungs. The simultaneous lack of oxygen due to insufficient ventilation causes shortness of breath, hypoxemia, and even cyanosis. In severe stages the hepatic circulation is congested, resulting in congestive hepatopathy.

An attempt is made to loosen the mucus with secretolytics and to facilitate coughing it up with physical therapy measures. When the acute process has subsided, respiratory exercises and CTM follow to help to relax thoracic stiffness caused by overdilation.

Findings, Treatment Plan, Additional Strokes, Comments

See Bronchial Asthma (p. 137).

Pleurisy

Definition

The pleura is the moist, smooth lining of the lung and inner chest wall. Its task is to allow friction-free movement of the lungs during respiration.

Inflammation of the pleura is called pleurisy. Causes include tuberculosis, bacterial purulent infections or (abacterial) rheumatoid disorders.

With so-called dry pleurisy, the patient suffers from pain related to breathing; pleural friction can be heard on auscultation.

An abacterial or purulent effusion often develops in the pleural cavity. When this mechanically affects the lung and heart, the effusion must be removed through thoracentesis.

Antibiotic treatment is given if a susceptible pathogen can be detected. CTM can be employed only after the acute stage has subsided.

Findings, Treatment Plan, Additional Strokes, Comments

See Acute Bronchitis (p. 133).

Pneumonia (Inflammation of the Lung)

Definition

Pneumonia develops either from purulent bronchitis or primarily in a pulmonary lobe. The cause may be a bacterial or viral infection (▶ Fig. 3.16, ▶ Fig. 3.17).

During the acute stage, treatment of the pneumonia with antibiotics is started, if a susceptible pathogen can be detected.

As with pleurisy, CTM may only be used after the acute stage has subsided (i.e., after approximately 6 weeks) to stabilize the circulation and prevent atrophy of the connective tissue in the corresponding segments.

Findings, Treatment Plan, Additional Strokes, Comments

See Acute Bronchitis (p. 133).

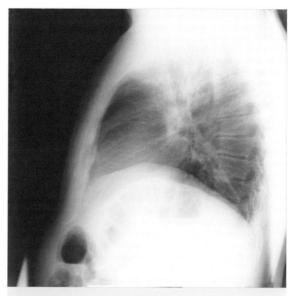

Fig. 3.16 Lobar pneumonia of the right upper pulmonary lobe.

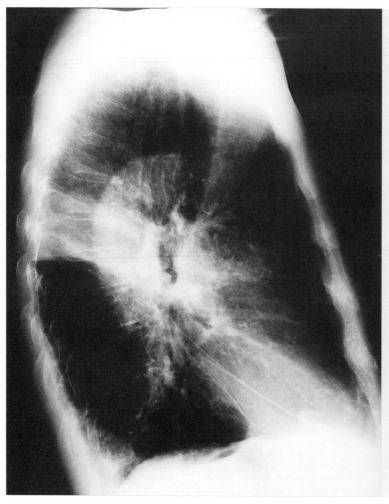

Fig. 3.17 Pneumonia.

Cystic Fibrosis

Definition

Cystic fibrosis is a hereditary metabolic disorder in which all mucous glands are altered in such a way that they produce only a thick, viscous secretion. The ducts of all glands producing digestive enzymes are obstructed. Due to the initially continuing production of secretion despite the clogging of the glands, the glands themselves develop cystic distension. This causes severe digestive insufficiency in the intestines.

A thick, viscous secretion is also produced in the bronchial glands, causing the unobstructed bronchial dispersion stroke to dilate and bulge (bronchiectasia).

Secondary symptoms often include the development of purulent bronchitis and pneumonia, possibly also pulmonary emphysema or atelectasis. For this reason, therapy of bronchiectasia is at the forefront of the treatment. In addition to secretolytics, fermentative decongestants, and antibiotics if necessary, special breathing exercises are performed regularly, especially in the morning, to facilitate a productive cough and CTM is given to stimulate respiration and to support the often insufficient intestinal peristalsis.

Early implementation of dietetic, medicinal, physical, and physical therapy measures significantly increases the chance of affected children reaching adulthood.

Findings, Treatment Plan, Additional Strokes

See Acute Bronchitis (p. 133).

Comments

- See Acute Bronchitis (p. 133).
- Treatment of constipation (p. 149) should be included in the treatment plan to support the frequently insufficient intestinal peristalsis.

Bronchiectasia

Definition

This usually irreversible dilation of the bronchi with acute and chronic inflammation in the region of the bronchial wall and the surrounding pulmonary tissue has both congenital and acquired causes—for example, after whooping cough, bronchitis, pleural fibrosis or injuries in the region of the lungs. The typical clinical finding is the abundant sputum, which settles in a glass in three layers after standing for some time. Hippocratic nails and clubbed fingers are also sometimes found. Concomitant episodes of chronic bronchitis are relevant for the course of the illness.

The prognosis has been improved over the years thanks to effective antibiotics and physical therapy. Such physical therapy measures as postural drainage and vibrations for the discharge of bronchiectasia as well as CTM can be applied with significant benefit.

The treatment plan for acute bronchitis is used for treatment with CTM and will be individually adapted depending on the intensity of the disorder.

Findings, Treatment Plan, Additional Strokes, Comments

See Acute Bronchitis (p. 133).

Bronchial Asthma

Definition

Bronchial asthma is a variable and reversible obstruction of the respiratory tract due to inflammation and hyperresponsiveness of the airways. Spasms of the bronchioles and mucosal edemas lead to a reduction of the width of the respiratory tract.

Airborne impurities (inhalation allergens) that are commonly present in the home or at work (e.g., moldy dusts, dust from bedding, pet hair, grass pollen, etc.) are known triggering factors. Food allergens can also cause asthma attacks. Elevated responsiveness to specific (allergenic) or unspecific (inhaled) stimuli is a characteristic symptom.

The cause of the illness cannot be exactly determined because triggering factors are often not detectable or may be hidden by several clinical pictures. Mucosal swelling and spasms of the smallest bronchi are the underlying causes of an acute asthma attack, which leads to difficulty in expiration and often also to wheezing coughs. Repeated asthma attacks or those that become chronic eventually lead to overdilatation and lung dysfunction (emphysema) and secondary cardiac insufficiency (pulmonary heart disease).

Treatment should first identify the triggering allergen and then ensure that the patient is no longer exposed to it. Further measures must be applied to calm the faulty and excessive reflexes triggered by the autonomic nervous system. Connective tissue massage can help considerably in this.

In children, bronchial asthma triggers symptoms similar to those seen in spastic bronchitis. Mental and emotional stress can lead to such attacks more strongly in predisposed children than in adults. As with spastic bronchitis the leading finding is a cramplike contraction of the smooth muscles of the bronchioles due to the allergenic stimulus; in some the stimulus may be wholly psychological.

The physical pulmonary findings are the same as for spastic bronchitis in children, adolescents, and adults. Accordingly, the same therapy is applied and air spas in the (high) mountains or by the sea (on islands) are especially suited for this purpose. Building up the immune system, cold showers or washing followed by an intensive rub down, sleeping with a window open, regular exercise with respiratory training, and CTM are often successful during attack-free intervals, but the avoidance or elimination of social factors with mental components that can promote asthma is also important. Physical therapy and CTM should help the patient with asthma to relax the "barrel-shaped thorax" and attempt to provide relief to the congestion of the pulmonary circulation.

Findings

In addition to increased turgor and muscle tone located in segments C3–C5 and T1–T12, segments L1–L2 are also affected. The adhesions in the tissue segments are wider and more visible than in other pulmonary diseases (▶ Fig. 3.18, ▶ Fig. 3.19).

The maximal points are located in T3 on each side of the spinal column.

The following tissue areas are particularly elevated with tension:
- Above the sacral bone and in the paravertebral area of the lumbar spine
- From the anterior superior spines extending to the groin and along the pelvic crests
- In the angle between the spinal column and lower costal arch

In the ventral region of the rib cage the lower ribs bulge severely, especially in children. The abdomen is rock-hard and the abdominal respiration is consequently impaired. The tissue behind the clavicle is retracted deeply within. There is elevated tension of tissue in the sternal angle, in the region of the pectoral and deltoid muscles.

Distensions can be found on the edges of the scapula and around C7. Characteristic postural features of asthma patients are a round back and elevated shoulders.

Treatment Plan

Starting position: sitting, lateral, or supine position.
- Small basic sequence, flat strokes over the rib cage from caudal toward cranial.
- Small basic sequence, first sequence, flat strokes over the rib cage.
- Small basic sequence, first and second sequence, ventral side.
- Small basic sequence, first and second sequence, ventral side of the body, treatment of the upper arm, flat strokes of forearm and hand.
- Small basic sequence, first, second, and third sequence, ventral side of the body, treatment of the upper arm, flat strokes on forearm and hand.
- Small basic sequence, first, second, and third sequence, facial treatment, ventral side.
- Small basic sequence, first, second, and third sequence, ventral side, treatment of face and arm.

Balancing strokes over the pectoral muscles, dorsal dispersion stroke, and flat strokes on both arms are applied at the end of each treatment session to support the venous backflow.

Additional Strokes

Small Basic Sequence

▶ **From dorsal** (▶ Fig. 2.27)
- Hooks to the sacral bone edges from caudal to cranial.
- Hooks along the course of the first pelvic stroke from caudal to cranial.
- Small, flat transverse strokes along the spine, within the area of the long extensor spinae muscles, from L5 to L12.
- Fanlike strokes in the upper respiratory angle.
- Stretching in the lumbar triangle (▶ Fig. 2.29).

▶ **From ventral** (▶ Fig. 2.35)
- Bimanual strokes starting from dorsal. At the same time, the therapist pulls on the lower edge of the rib cage toward the medioclavicular line and on the pelvic edge toward the anterior superior iliac spine. This set of strokes is performed bimanually, first on one side then on the other side of the patient in the supine position.
- Balancing strokes on the pectoral muscles and strokes on the ventral pelvis and abdomen (▶ Fig. 2.32).

First Sequence

▶ **From dorsal** (▶ Fig. 2.37, ▶ Fig. 2.39)
- The intercostal strokes are also pulled in the opposite direction, from the spinal column to the lateral chest wall to the ventral axillary line, and hooked in there gently.
- Small, flat transverse strokes along the spine, within the area of the long extensor spinae muscles, from T12 to T7.
- Flat transverse strokes over the spinal column, beginning at the level of T6 under the angle of the left scapula and ending under the angle of the right scapula, then pulled back to the starting point.

▶ **From ventral**
- In the ventral intercostal area a set of flat strokes are pulled beginning at the dorsal axillary line through the intercostal spaces. These should start at the lowest ribs.

Second Sequence

▶ **From dorsal** (▶ Fig. 2.45, ▶ Fig. 2.46, ▶ Fig. 2.48)
- Long downward stretching.
- Prolonged upward stretching.
- Axillary stretching with elevated arm.
- Small, flat transverse strokes over the spine within the area of the long extensor spinae muscles from T7 to T3.

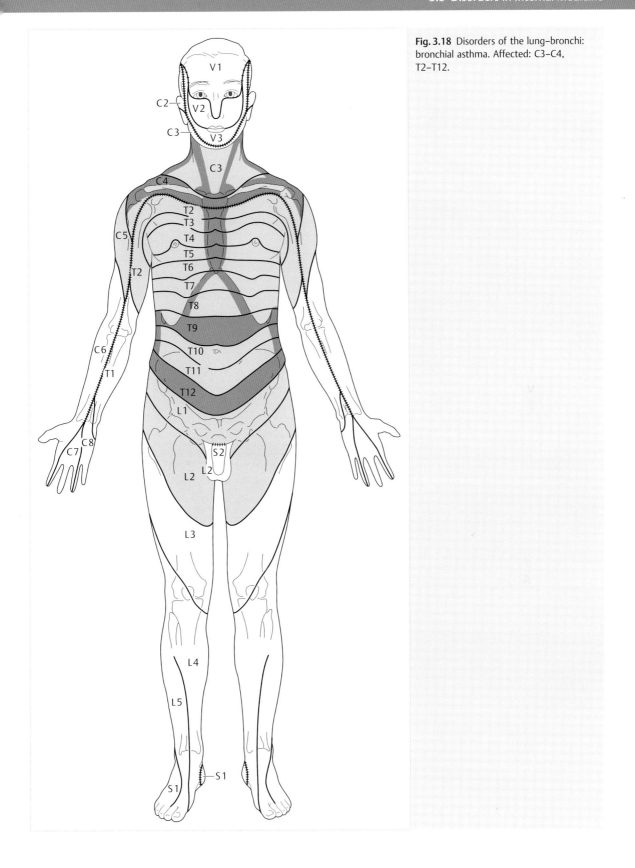

Fig. 3.18 Disorders of the lung–bronchi: bronchial asthma. Affected: C3–C4, T2–T12.

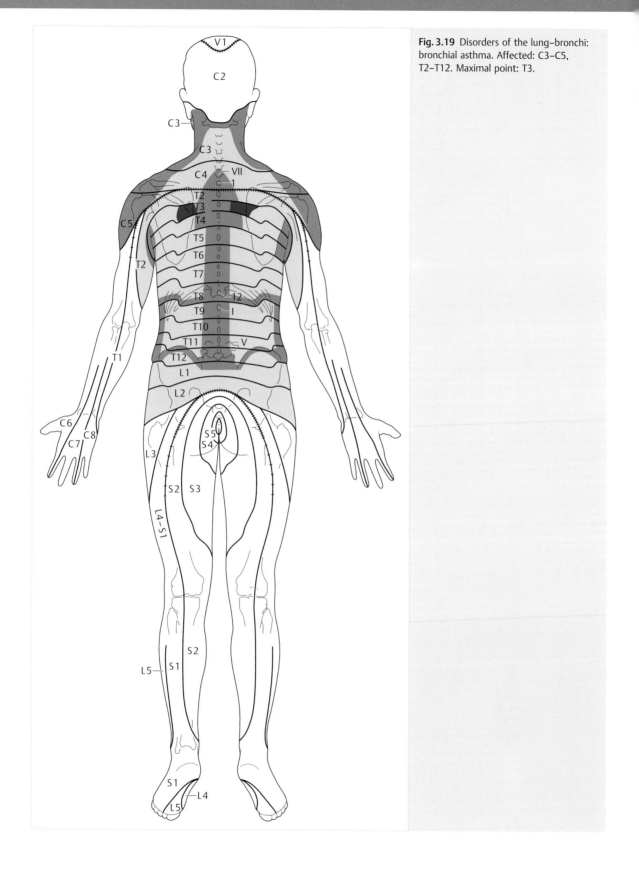

Fig. 3.19 Disorders of the lung–bronchi: bronchial asthma. Affected: C3–C5, T2–T12. Maximal point: T3.

- Set of flat strokes from the lower angle of the scapula to the spine at the level of segment T4.
- Short hooks around the angle of the scapula followed by the outline of the scapula with cutting strokes along the same course.
- Flat transverse strokes from the inner side to the lateral edge of the scapulae, starting at the level of T7 and ending at the level of the spine of the scapula.

▶ **From ventral** (▶ **Fig. 2.49**)
- The ventral edge of the trapezius muscle is pulled out starting from the cervical base, while pressing against it with the free hand.
- Strokes along the sternum, from the xiphoid process to the jugular notch.
- Short hooks on the insertion points of the ribs toward the sternum from caudal to cranial.
- Short transverse strokes along the sternum.
- Short fanlike strokes work along the medial clavicular angle toward the suprasternal notch, starting with the first stroke on the clavicle and ending with the last one on the dorsal edge of the sternocleidomastoid muscle.
- Strokes toward the interclavicular ligament.
- After the third sequence (▶ Fig. 2.47), a flat fan-shaped stroke transversely over the scapula toward the shoulder joint, starting at the outer edge of the scapula and ending at the lower edge of the spine of the scapula.

Comments

- When strokes in small basic sequences produce only a minor sensation or no cutting sensation (scratching in the deep layers; p. 24) is perceived by the patient, the therapist should prepare the tissue with the patient in supine or prone position with flat strokes until red dermographism (p. 24) signals that strokes in the small basic sequence can now be applied.
- Extensive, soothing balancing strokes are repeatedly integrated into the treatment plan.
- The rock-hard abdominal wall is treated with vibrations, and exercises for abdominal respiration are performed with emphasis on expiration. Strokes are applied along the pelvic edges to the symphysis while the patient alternately moves one of the heels downward. This should trigger respiration by loosening spasms and enabling spontaneously triggered breaths.
- In the second sequence the therapist works from lateral to medial and only applies hooks to the spinal column during the fourth or fifth treatment session. Stimuli placed close to the spinal column reach the autonomic nervous system along the shortest route and may under certain circumstances cause reactions that are too strong.
- When the tense tissue in the area of the rib cage decreases and the respiration has improved, the therapist

then works between the scapulae and their lateral edges.
- If the patient reports a blunt sensation of pressure in certain areas of the body during CTM, the therapist must return to applying the strokes in small basic sequence (see Remedies for Adverse Reactions and Abnormal Sensations, p. 25).
- Stretching strokes are applied along the axilla.
- The large balancing stroke is repeatedly integrated into the treatment.
- On the ventral side of the body, flat strokes are applied to the intercostal spaces and the lower edge of the rib cage. The area around the epigastric angle is omitted because the diaphragm can be stimulated from here, which could trigger an asthma attack.
- As the condition improves, more attention is paid to the ventral side of the body above the sternum, at the attachment spots between the ribs and the sternum up to the clavicle. Due to the strokes in the surrounding body parts, the tissue tension is loosened in the region of the sternal angle and respiration is improved.
- After the third sequence and the facial treatment, sustained and intensive balancing strokes are applied over the entire body of the supine patient.
- CTM should be administered every day during the patient's stay as an inpatient, and during outpatient care two to three times a week for several months.
- When the patient develops dyspnea during CTM the therapist can apply balancing and branching strokes and the "rake" (▶ Fig. 2.11). The window should be opened and the patient should assume a pain relief position (postural drainage). The following strokes can be applied when the patient is accustomed to CTM, that is when he or she has been in therapy for some time:
  - Large balancing strokes alternating with the branching of the lower rib cage edges
  - Flat transverse strokes between the scapulae to the spine of the scapula
  - Repeated large balancing strokes; the treatment session concludes with small and large flat branching strokes
- A rolled-up hot pack is applied to the dorsal and ventral side of the body after the tissue tension has decreased in the following areas:
  - From dorsal: on the sacral bone, on the lower edge of the rib cage, on the lateral and medial side of the scapula, on the area of the neck
  - From ventral: on the symphysis, groin, and abdominal space, on the lower edge of the rib cage, on the ribs and sternum
- The patient must rest for half an hour after treatment.
- CTM must be applied in combination with physical therapy measures that are considered long-term therapy, which should be applied twice a year as preventive therapy to support the patient's wellbeing.

Thorax Deformities

Definition

Congenital or acquired deformities of the spinal column, particularly scoliosis and kyphotic scoliosis, but also ankylosing vertebral joints due to Bekhterev disease effect changes in the statics as well as the stretchability and elasticity of the lungs and consequently their function.

Scoliotic thorax deformities cause restrictive ventilation disturbances, the severity of which depends on the extent of the deformity. There is a negative correlation between the scoliotic angle and vital capacity. If this was restricted by more than 50% of the norm, hypoxemia and pulmonary hypertension will be present (see also Orthopedic Disorders).

Respiratory insufficiency includes pathologies of various etiologies that lead to disturbances in the gas exchange, causing premature oxygen deprivation and that additionally develop hypercapnia in later and following stages. The respiratory reserves are reduced; the ventilation may be predominantly restrictive, obstructive, or mixed. There is often cyanosis depending on the absolute amount of reduced hemoglobin. The initial difficulty in respiration is often already perceived as dyspnea. Disturbances of the respiratory technique additionally increase the respiratory burden. However, there is not necessarily a relation between the extent of dyspnea and disturbances in gas exchange. The evaluation is always based on a pulmonary function test including a blood gas analysis.

In addition to physical therapy exercises, CTM should be applied to tissue structures surrounding the spinal column.

CTM shows positive results in all chronic obstructive disorders.

Findings

Increased turgor and muscle tone are located over the back.

Special attention must be paid to the segmental parts that belong to the organs, namely, C3–C8 and T1–T9.

The muscles of the torso are especially weak with osteoporosis and Bekhterev disease. The patients have often worn a brace for many years. If there is a pathological scoliosis, changes in the tension of the tissue are difficult to palpate.

The edge of the rib cage lies on the pelvic crest. The abdomen is very hard and there is no longer abdominal respiration. Due to acute respiratory tract infections and bronchial infections, the adhesions in the tissue are mainly located in the subcutaneous layers of the skin.

Treatment Plan

Starting position: sitting, supine position.
- Small basic sequence, flat strokes over the rib cage from caudal toward cranial.
- Small basic sequence, first sequence, flat strokes over the rib cage.
- Small basic sequence, first and second sequence, ventral side.
- Small basic sequence, first, second, and third sequence, ventral side.

Balancing strokes over the pectoral muscles and dorsal branching end each treatment session.

Additional Strokes

Small Basic Sequence

▶ **From dorsal** (▶ Fig. 2.27)
- Hooks to the sacral bone edges from caudal to cranial.
- Hooks along the course of the first pelvic stroke from caudal to cranial.
- Small, flat transverse strokes along the spine within the area of the long extensor spinae muscles from L5 to L12.
- Fanlike strokes in the upper respiratory angle.
- Stretching in the lumbar triangle (▶ Fig. 2.29).

▶ **From ventral** (▶ Fig. 2.35)
- Bimanual strokes starting from dorsal. At the same time, the therapist pulls on the lower edge of the rib cage toward the medioclavicular line and on the pelvic edge toward the anterior superior iliac spine. This set of strokes is performed bimanually, first on one side and then on the other side of the patient in a lying position.
- Balancing strokes on the pectoral muscles and strokes on the ventral pelvis and abdomen (▶ Fig. 2.32).

First Sequence

▶ **From dorsal** (▶ Fig. 2.37, ▶ Fig. 2.39)
- The intercostal strokes are also pulled in the opposite direction from the spinal column to the lateral chest wall to the ventral axillary line and hooked in there gently.
- Small, flat transverse strokes along the spine within the area of the long extensor spinae muscles from T12 to T7.
- Flat transverse strokes over the spinal column, beginning at the level of T6 under the angle of the left scapula and ending under the angle of the right scapula, then pulled back to the starting point.

▶ **From ventral**
- In the ventral intercostal area a set of flat strokes are pulled beginning at the dorsal axillary line through the intercostal spaces. These should start at the lowest ribs.

Second Sequence

▶ **From dorsal** (▶ Fig. 2.45, ▶ Fig. 2.46, ▶ Fig. 2.48)
- Long downward stretching.
- Prolonged upward stretching.

- Axillary stretching with elevated arm.
- Small, flat transverse strokes over the spine within the area of the long extensor spinae muscles from T7 to T3.
- A set of flat strokes from the lower angle of the scapula to the spine at the level of segment T4.
- Short hooks around the angle of the scapula followed by outlining of the scapula with cutting strokes along the same course.
- Flat transverse strokes from the inner side to the lateral edge of the scapulae, starting at the level of T7 and ending at the level of the spine of the scapula.

▶ **From ventral** (▶ Fig. 2.49)
- The ventral edge of the trapezius muscle is pulled out starting from the cervical base, while pressing against it with the free hand.
- Strokes along the sternum, beginning at the xiphoid process, to the jugular notch.
- Short hooks on the insertion points of the ribs toward the sternum from caudal to cranial.
- Short transverse strokes along the sternum. These start at the junction between the xiphoid process and the body of the sternum, along the area of the sternal angle. At the base of the second rib at the sternum, the strokes should become wider to just under the sternoclavicular joints.
- Short fanlike strokes work along the medial clavicular angle toward the suprasternal notch, starting with the first stroke on the clavicle and ending with the last one on the dorsal edge of the sternocleidomastoid muscle.
- Strokes toward the interclavicular ligament.
- After the third sequence (▶ Fig. 2.47), a flat fan-shaped stroke transversely over the scapula toward the shoulder joint, starting at the outer edge of the scapula and ending at the lower edge of the spine of the scapula.

Comments

- Respiration is positively influenced by CTM: the respiratory movements are more extensive, the involvement of costal and abdominal movements becomes more distinct; the auxiliary respiratory muscles are no longer used or are used only during exertion.
- The muscles show increased stretchability through the effects of CTM and other physical therapy measures. Blood supply and metabolic processes are activated in the muscle cell.
- A rolle-up hot pack is applied to the dorsal and ventral regions of the body once the tension in the tissue has decreased:
  ○ From dorsal: on the sacral bone, on the lower edge of the rib cage, on the lateral and medial side of the scapula, on the area of the neck
  ○ From ventral: on the symphysis, groin, and abdominal space, on the lower edge of the rib cage, on the ribs and sternum

3.5.4 Disorders of the Gastrointestinal Tract

In addition to the processing of ingested food, the gastrointestinal tract is responsible for assimilation and dissimilation, including the corresponding peristaltic, secretory, absorptive, and excretory processes (▶ Fig. 3.20, ▶ Fig. 3.21).

A generalized plan for the treatment of gastrointestinal tract disorders has been created for the application of CTM. The symptoms that can be influenced by CTM (e.g., changes in tension of the skin and muscles and influence on the autonomic nervous system [p. 7]) are closely related in these clinical pictures. The therapist is able to adapt the generalized concept to the patient's current condition, obtaining specific information that can be integrated into the treatment plan. The therapist will also check and integrate or omit the signs perceived during the additional strokes. The Comments sections contain additional information regarding the individual pathologies.

Acute Gastritis

Definition

Acute inflammatory conditions in the gastrointestinal tract are caused by food that is spoiled, bacterially infected, or contains individually aggressive allergens. These cause functional disturbances in the stomach, which spread over the whole digestive tract so that nausea, vomiting, gas, and diarrhea develop.

The term "nervous gastritis" describes an excessive irritability of the stomach. Symptoms include disturbances in motility and painful spasms followed by irritation of the gastric mucosa.

The therapeutic approach to inflammatory processes depends on their severity and cause. The minor stages usually disappear quickly under simple hydrotherapy and dietetic measures. Bacterial gastritis requires special drug therapy. If the gastritis is caused by an allergy, the triggering allergen must be identified and excluded.

The majority of cases of acute gastritis usually disappear within days and require no further treatment. Only if the complaints persist for longer is treatment with CTM beneficial during the declining stage.

Patients with acute inflammation of the gastric mucosa or current gastric or duodenal ulcers should not be treated with CTM.

Before treatment is started, a physician must check whether the complaints are caused by gastritis, a ventricular ulcer, or a duodenal ulcer.

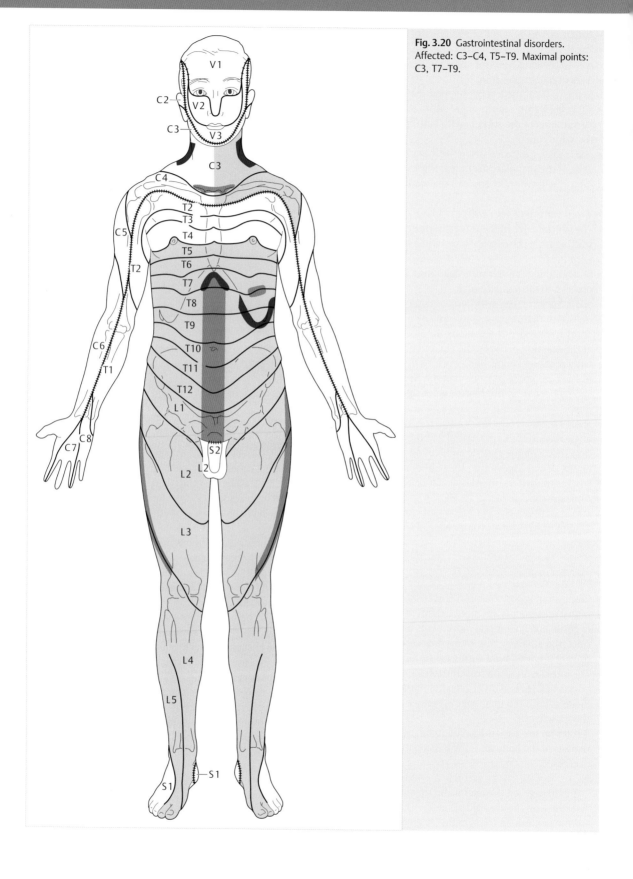

Fig. 3.20 Gastrointestinal disorders. Affected: C3–C4, T5–T9. Maximal points: C3, T7–T9.

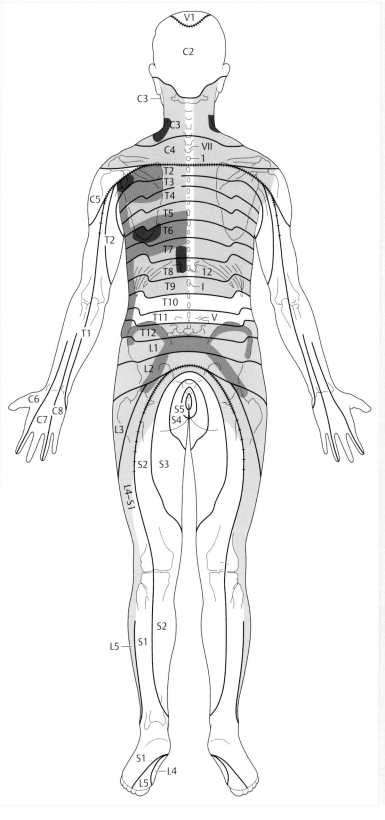

Fig. 3.21 Gastrointestinal disorders. Affected: C3–C4, T5–T9, L1–L5. Maximal points: C3, T2, T6, T7–T8.

Should pain on the xiphoid process imitate a gastric disorder, therapeutic local anesthesia (TLA) may sometimes quickly improve the situation.

Findings, Treatment Plan, Additional Strokes, Comments

See Constipation (p. 149).

Chronic Gastritis

Definition

Recurrent mucosal inflammation of the peptic digestive system (i.e., of the stomach), acute attacks, and persistent noxa can eventually turn acute gastritis into a chronic condition.

A differentiation is made between genetic factors and continuous exogenous damage of the stomach—for example, through malnutrition and especially through excessive coffee and alcohol consumption. Allergic gastritis caused by specific nutritional allergens such as fish, chocolate, or milk must also be considered. Nervous dysfunctions and mental processes also cannot be excluded. These connections become particularly obvious when certain reflexes mimic an allergy or vice versa, when symptoms of allergy persist although desensitization has been performed.

Chronic gastritis can have very little in the way of symptoms and can provoke only few complaints. In those cases cardinal symptoms include stomach pressure, belching, coated tongue, loss of appetite, malaise, and emaciation, which are accompanied by disturbances of defecation and signs of retroperistalsis. Connection with migraines is often confirmed. Gastric carcinoma must be excluded.

The primary goal of treatment with complete dystrophy should be to achieve general strengthening. Special diets, manual colon treatment, and CTM with a rolled-up hot pack are advisable. Relaxation therapy should be performed in physical therapy in addition to CTM from the very first day.

During treatment, general movement exercises are performed to boost the metabolism, and it is advisable to carry out small movements of the hands, arms, feet, and legs in which the exercise sequences are performed at a faster pace at first, while imposing sufficient pauses for recovery.

Findings, Treatment Plan, Additional Strokes, Comments

See Constipation (p. 149).

Ventricular and Duodenal Ulcer

Definition

In these conditions an ulcer primarily develops in the lower gastric sections or in the upper part of the duodenum (duodenal bulb); it causes pain that depends on the consumption of food and it can become life-threatening due to hemorrhages and perforation of the abdominal cavity. Relapses are frequent, over decades. Cancer may develop on the floor of chronic gastric ulcers.

The patient's pain history is extremely important in determining an indication for CTM. The most important pain triggers are disturbances in motility, which lead to stretching pain, spasms, and pain due to hypermotility and evacuation. Stretching pain in particular is often a sign of infiltrative inflammatory changes of the gastric wall. This gives way to penetration pain, when an ulcer penetrates the gastric wall and infiltrates the pancreas, the surrounding area of the gallbladder, or even the abdominal cavity, subsequently causing peritonitis. The pain usually stems from the inflammatory irritation of the surrounding area.

Planning of CTM is less focused on the origin of the pain in the gastric region as reported by the patient than on body surface including the skin, connective tissue, periosteum, bones, and other viscera. The Head's zones are again to be seen here as projection fields of deeper-located visceral disorders of the body surface. They present themselves as changes in the tension of the skin and hyperesthesia in this area at the slightest touch or under stronger pressure. Even a light scratch is perceived as uncomfortable. Segmental relations of the pain often concern trophic disorders in the different tissue layers.

Chronic gastritis with or without ulcers causes changes on the lower costal arch in the long run.

Of course, in these disorders, from gastritis to ulcers, infection with *Helicobacter pylori* must be excluded and, if necessary treated with antibiotics.

Findings, Treatment Plan, Additional Strokes, Comments

See Constipation (p. 149).

Disorders of the Small Intestine

Definition

Disorders of the small intestine mostly present with painful intestinal spasms and diarrhea. Such symptoms often occur once or twice in the morning after breakfast in chronic enteritis (inflammation of the small intestines). The causes are the same as in gastritis (p. 143).

When treating residual conditions, which manifest in general as diarrhea, a focus is placed on dietetic and medicinal measures, but CTM can benefit the patient as a supportive measure.

Findings, Treatment Plan, Additional Strokes, Comments

See Constipation (p. 149).

Hirschsprung Disease (Congenital Aganglionic Megacolon)

Definition

This is a congenital anomaly of the colon with an absence of ganglia cells in the wall of individual intestinal segments, which causes pencil-thin obstructions in the intestinal passage so that the parts of the colon above them can distend enormously with stool. This malformation cannot be controlled through conservative measures; the aganglionic piece of the colon must be surgically removed.

After full recovery and repositioning of the preternatural anus, normal intestinal function must be trained again. CTM in combination with physical therapy and respiratory therapy is indicated before and after surgery.

Findings

Increased turgor and muscle tone are located in the segments L1–L5, T5–T9 and C3–C4. The maximal points are:

▶ **From dorsal**
- In the region of the shoulder and neck
- On the outer edge of the spine of the scapula
- On the lower angle of the scapula
- In the angle of the spinal column and 12th rib

▶ **From ventral**
- Three fingers below the epigastric angle, at the level of the eighth/ninth/tenth rib

▶ **Tissue changes on the posterior side of the body**
- On the edges of the sacral bone
- On the sacral bone in the upper third
- Under the edges of the pelvis
- From the sacroiliac joint to the area of the trochanter over the iliotibial tract on the thigh
- In the region of the ribs on the left side of the thorax below the lower angle of the scapula
- In the region of the shoulder and neck

▶ **On the anterior side of the body**
- Retractions on the left edge of the rib cage
- Along the course of the rectus muscle to the symphysis
- In the epigastric angle
- Under the left costal arch
- On the jugular fossa
- In the region of shoulder and neck

▶ **On the leg**
- On the iliotibial tract of both legs
- The tissue of the left leg is affected more and is sensitive to traction

Treatment Plan

Starting position: sitting, supine position, lateral position.
- Small basic sequence, flat strokes from the pelvis and back from caudal to cranial.
- Small basic sequence, first sequence, flat strokes on both legs.
- Small basic sequence, first sequence, treatment of the thigh, flat strokes over lower leg and foot.
- Small basic sequence, first and second sequence, ventral side of the body, treatment of the thighs, flat strokes on lower leg and foot.
- Small basic sequence, first, second, and third sequence, ventral side, treatment of leg.

Balancing strokes over the pectoral muscles, dorsal dispersion stroke, and flat strokes of the legs are applied at the end of each treatment session to support the venous backflow.

Additional Strokes

Small Basic Sequence

▶ **From dorsal** (▶ Fig. 2.27)
- Hooks pulled to the sacral bone edges from caudal to cranial.
- Hooks pulled along the course of the first pelvic stroke from caudal to cranial
- Flat transverse strokes pulled over the sacral bone from caudal to cranial
- Small, flat transverse strokes along the spine within the area of the long extensor spinae muscles from L5 to L12.
- Fanlike strokes in the upper respiratory angle.
- Stretching in the lumbar triangle (▶ Fig. 2.29).
- Small, flat transverse strokes along the spine within the area of the long extensor spinae muscles from L5 to L12.

▶ **From ventral** (▶ Fig. 2.35)
- Bimanual strokes starting from dorsal. At the same time, the therapist pulls on the lower edge of the rib cage toward the medioclavicular line and on the pelvic edge toward the anterior superior iliac spine. The strokes are performed bimanually, first on one side then on the other side of the body.
- The liver stroke.
- Balancing strokes on the pectoral muscles and strokes on the ventral pelvis and abdomen (▶ Fig. 2.32).

First Sequence

▶ **From dorsal** (▶ Fig. 2.39)
- The intercostal strokes are also pulled in the opposite direction from the spinal column to the lateral chest wall to the ventral axillary line and hooked in there gently.

- Flat transverse strokes over the spinal column, beginning at the level of T6 under the angle of the left scapula and ending under the right scapula, then pulled back to the starting point.
- Small, flat transverse strokes along the spine within the area of the long extensor spinae muscles from T12 to T7.

▶ **From ventral**

- In the ventral intercostal area a set of flat strokes are pulled beginning at the dorsal axillary line through the intercostal spaces. These should start at the lowest ribs.

Second Sequence

▶ **From dorsal** (▶ Fig. 2.46, ▶ Fig. 2.48)

- Long downward stretching.
- Prolonged upward stretching.
- Small, flat transverse strokes over the spine within the area of the long extensor spinae muscles from T7 to T3.
- Set of flat strokes from the lower angle of the scapula to the spine at the level of segment T4.
- Flat transverse strokes from the inner side to the lateral edge of the scapulae, starting at the level of T7 and ending at the level of the spine of the scapula.

▶ **From ventral** (▶ Fig. 2.49)

- The ventral edge of the trapezius muscle is pulled out starting from the cervical base, while pressing against it with the free hand.
- Strokes along the sternum, beginning at the xiphoid process to the jugular notch.
- Short hooks on the insertion points of the ribs at the sternum from caudal to cranial.
- Short fanlike strokes work along the medial clavicular angle toward the suprasternal notch. Start with the first stroke on the clavicle, ending with the last one on the dorsal edge of the sternocleidomastoid muscle.

After the third sequence, flat fan-shaped strokes are applied transversely over the scapula toward the shoulder joint.

Comments

- When applying the small basic sequence, flat strokes are applied to the region of the pelvis and abdominal space with very sensitive patients. Only when a light reddening of the skin can be detected is the small basic sequence applied in flat technique.
- At the beginning the small basic sequence should omit the angle between the pelvic crest and spinal column if there is a severe increase in the tension of the tissue. The patient usually tolerates treatment in this area of the body after three or four sessions.
- The treatment of the ventral side of the body is started in the abdominal space and applied upward over the

costal arches in cranial direction. The lower costal arch must only be included in the treatment after five or six sessions since the stomach will quickly become upset if it is stimulated.

- It has also proven to be tolerable when flat strokes to the ventral side of the body are first applied to the right and after a couple of sessions are moved to the left side of the body.
- When applying the additional section sequences the therapist must be very careful, since the patient may respond with increased complaints and nausea. This is especially the case with relapses.
- Intercostal and scapular strokes are applied in an accentuated flat technique.
- Particular attention must be paid when applying CTM to segments T5–T9 and C3–C4. The therapist waits for the response to the strokes in the tissue and then works toward the next body area. The pressure on the stomach can decrease; the patient will recover appetite and tolerate food better.
- The application of a rolled-up hot pack in the region of the pelvis and leg, which is slowly moved closer to the area of the lumbar spine and from the ventral side to the lower abdominal area, has a curative effect.
- Physical therapy and the application of CTM must be coordinated especially well. A quiet atmosphere must be created, so as not to overburden the patient. Resting after CTM is absolutely imperative.

3.5.5 Functional Gastrointestinal Disorders

Functional syndromes of the gastrointestinal tract lack organically detectable correlations. They often develop and become chronic. A connection between psychosocial factors and disturbed gastrointestinal function is undisputed, but it remains unclear to what extent disturbances of primary motor functions can be the cause of chronic disorders.

Functional complaints of the gastrointestinal tract include loss of appetite, dysphagia, heartburn, aerophagia, functional dyspepsia, irritable bowel syndrome, meteorism, chronic constipation, and functional diarrhea. Stress situations in the broadest sense may aggravate such function-limiting syndromes.

Meteorism

Definition

Meteorism, which involves increased amounts of air in an intestinal loop, build-up of gas in greater convolutions, or a completely distended abdomen, is not in itself a disorder but rather a symptom, though one that is not trivial. An increased amount of air in the intestines often indicates a pathological factor.

Various foods, such as types of cabbage and leguminous plants, promote meteorism. Combinations of certain foods and faulty eating behavior (insufficient chewing, hasty swallowing) may also cause meteorism.

Significant meteorism develops in the colon with bacterial build-up of gas and stagnating intestinal content. Meteorism is also known with circulatory insufficiency and cirrhosis of the liver caused by venous stasis when evacuating normal amounts of gas from the intestines into the circulation of the portal vein.

Migraine is often also associated as a reflex to the inhibition of intestinal peristalsis and meteorism. If timely treatment of the colon can resolve the delayed peristalsis with its increased development of gas in individual loops, incipient or even more severe migraine symptoms frequently disappears.

Gas-reducing colonic treatment leads to astonishing results in functional cardiac pain associated with Roemheld syndrome.

The stimulation of peristalsis serves primarily to remove build-up of gas by promoting transport and excretion.

Findings, Treatment Plan, Additional Strokes, Comments

See Constipation (p. 149).

Constipation

Definition

The medical definition of constipation is evacuation of the bowels less than three times a week. There are many causes.

Constipation in early childhood may indicate a defect of the autonomic ganglia cells in the intestinal wall (Hirschsprung disease, p. 147).

Chronic constipation during adulthood is often caused by malnutrition and a low-fiber diet.

The possibility of a malignant tumor in the colon must be considered, especially in older persons.

Connective tissue massage can have an effect on the irritable bowel, also called spastic colon, with chronic constipation. This dysfunction, which presents no tangible organic changes, often affects middle-aged women.

Patients with IBS complain of abdominal pain, especially in the left lower abdomen, meteorism, back pain, and general nervous complaints such as fatigue, sleeplessness, and so on. The phases of constipation can be interrupted in the morning by predominantly thin, mucous loose stool. This disorder can significantly affect well-being and give patients reason for concern.

Triggering factors include unresolved problems, stress situations, bad eating habits, and inadequate organization of everyday activities; less frequent factors include chronic intoxication with stimulants or heavy metals. The possibility of pathological intestinal flora—that is, the settlement of the colon with unphysiological bacteria, for example after the administration of antibiotics—should also be considered. Cold legs and feet (insufficient clothing) may aggravate the pathology.

Applying CTM therapeutically involves a smooth and calm, generally elevated autonomic nervous tone to locally dissolve the spasm. Part of this involves an effect on the whole autonomic nervous system by creating an appropriate environment that conveys peace and quiet as well as the resolution of everyday problems.

A distinction between spastic and chronic constipation is purely theoretical and almost impossible to diagnose. The distinction has no consequences for CTM.

Findings

The segmental adhesions are especially located in L1–L4, T9–T12, C3–C4; dorsal, S 3.

▶ **On the anterior side of the body** (▶ Fig. 3.22)
- Region of the shoulder and neck
- Oblique abdominal muscles
- Lateral and medial side of the thighs
- Groin and around the trochanter

▶ **On the posterior side of the body** (▶ Fig. 3.23). Increased tension is predominantly found in skin and subcutaneous tissue.
- Region of the shoulder and neck
- Above the sacral bone to the pelvic crests
- Pelvis, junction to the thigh on the lateral side
- Medial side of the thighs

The tissue over the sacral bone and in the angle between the pelvic crest and spinal column often firmly adheres to the layers.

Treatment Plan

Starting position: sitting, supine position, lateral position.
- Small basic sequence, flat strokes over pelvis and back from caudal toward cranial.
- Small basic sequence, first sequence, flat strokes on the legs.
- Small basic sequence, first and second sequence, ventral side of the body, treatment of the thighs, flat strokes on lower leg and foot.
- Small basic sequence, first, second, and third sequence, ventral side, treatment of leg.

Balancing strokes over the pectoral muscles, dorsal dispersion stroke, and flat strokes are applied on the legs at the end of each treatment session to support the venous backflow.

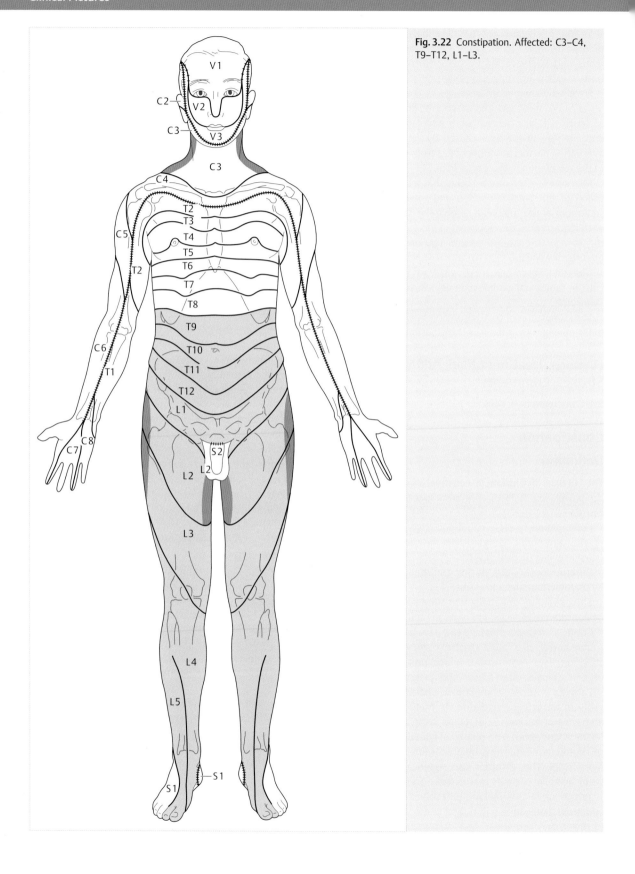

Fig. 3.22 Constipation. Affected: C3–C4, T9–T12, L1–L3.

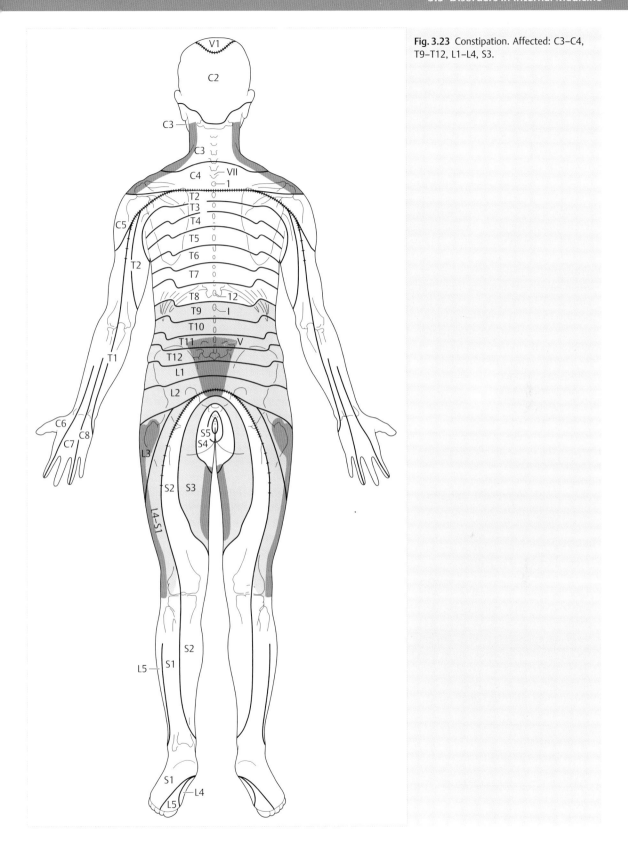

Fig. 3.23 Constipation. Affected: C3–C4, T9–T12, L1–L4, S3.

Additional Strokes

Small Basic Sequence

▶ **From dorsal** (▶ Fig. 2.27, ▶ Fig. 2.28, ▶ Fig. 2.29)
- Hooks to the sacral bone edges from caudal to cranial.
- Short hooks along the intergluteal cleft pulling up from the lateral side (▶ Fig. 2.34).
- Flat transverse strokes over the sacral bone, from caudal to cranial.
- Small, flat transverse strokes along the spine, within the area of the long extensor spinae muscles, from L5 to T12.
- Hooks and stretching stroke at the ischial tuberosity.
- Stretching stroke in the lumbar triangle.
- Fanlike strokes in the upper respiratory angle.

▶ **From ventral** (▶ Fig. 2.35)
- Bimanual strokes, starting from the dorsal side. At the same time, the therapist pulls on the lower edge of the rib cage toward the medioclavicular line and on the pelvic edge toward the anterior superior iliac spine. These strokes are performed bimanually, first on one side then on the other side of the body.
- Short hooks along the rectus sheath from the symphysis to the level of the navel.
- Short strokes, like rays, pulling toward the navel.
- Bimanual strokes crossing over the abdominal walls, starting in the dorsal region and ending at the opposite edge of the rectus abdominis muscle.
- The liver stroke.
- Balancing strokes on the pectoral muscles and strokes on the ventral pelvis and abdomen (▶ Fig. 2.32).

First Sequence

▶ **From dorsal** (▶ Fig. 2.39)
- The intercostal strokes are also pulled in the opposite direction, from the spinal column to the lateral chest wall to the ventral axillary line, and hooked in there gently.
- Small, flat transverse strokes along the spine within the area of the long extensor spinae muscles from T12 to T7.
- Flat transverse strokes over the spinal column, beginning at the level of T6 under the angle of the left scapula and ending under the right scapula, then pulled back to the starting point.

▶ **From ventral**
- In the ventral intercostal area a set of flat strokes are pulled beginning at the dorsal axillary line through the intercostal spaces. These should start at the lowest ribs.

Second Sequence

▶ **From dorsal** (▶ Fig. 2.46, ▶ Fig. 2.48)
- Long downward stretching.

- Prolonged upward stretching.
- Small, flat transverse strokes over the spine, within the area of the long extensor spinae muscles, from T7 to T3.
- Short hooks around the angle of the scapula followed by outlining the scapula with cutting strokes along the same course.
- A set of flat strokes from the lower angle of the scapula to the spine at the level of segment T4.
- Flat transverse strokes from the inner side to the lateral edge of the scapulae, starting at the level of T7 and ending at the level of the spine of the scapula.
- The large balancing stroke starts in the ventral axillary line at the level of the sixth/seventh intercostal space and is flatly pulled around the lower angle of the scapula toward C7 (▶ Fig. 2.38).

Comments

- The strokes around the trochanter to the pelvis, which were included during the first treatments, are applied to intensively work over the region of the pelvic crest and anterior superior iliac spine. This may reduce the tension of the abdominal wall.
- The adhesions in the thoracic regions are reduced by flat strokes after the small basic sequence, so that the scapula can swiftly be treated after the first sequence and during the second sequence.
- A rolled-up hot pack is applied from the tract to the adductor muscles on the area of the body above the symphysis to the pelvic crests. Heat packs can be applied between the thighs during the resting phase after treatment if the adductor muscles are very tense.
- In very stubborn cases the colonic massage can be applied in the supine position with the lower legs resting on a chair.
- The application of physical therapy and of CTM should be well coordinated. The patient must rest after therapy.

3.5.6 Disorders of the Liver and Gallbladder

Functional disturbances of the liver, the flow of bile, and the digestive processes in the stomach and small intestines often persist for some period after an inflammation of the liver (hepatitis C) and cause very characteristic complaints: bloating; fullness; a strange taste in the mouth; bad breath; absorption of intestinal gases into the circulation, the expiration of which is often the cause of bad breath; and loss of appetite.

Functional disturbances can be alleviated with CTM in disorders of the draining bile ducts and of the gallbladder. Acute inflammatory disorders of the gallbladder or the bile ducts must never be treated with CTM (▶ Fig. 3.24, ▶ Fig. 3.25).

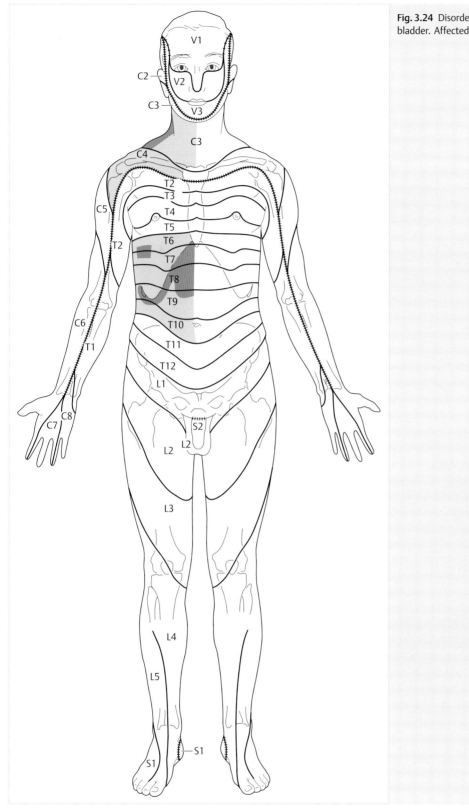

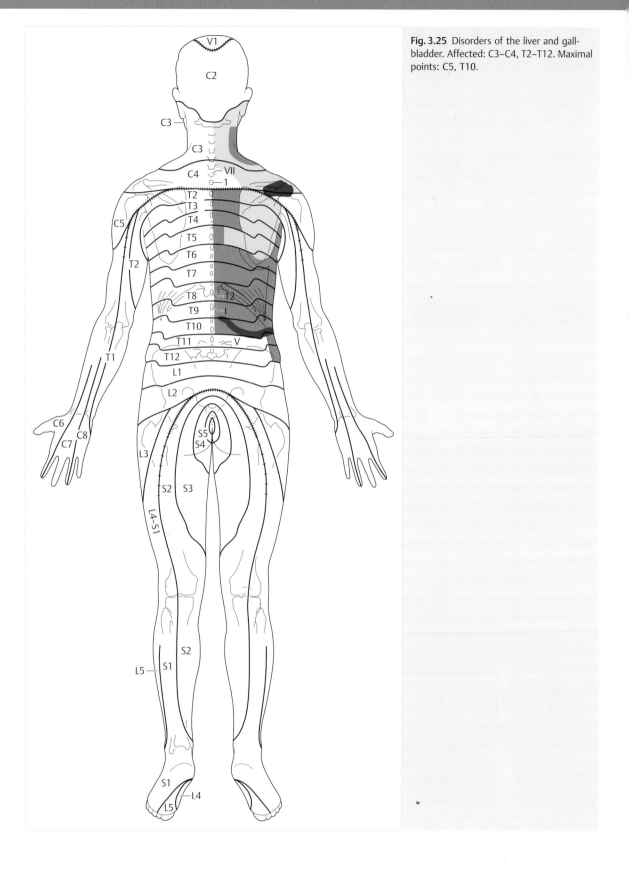

Fig. 3.25 Disorders of the liver and gall-bladder. Affected: C3–C4, T2–T12. Maximal points: C5, T10.

The majority of cases of biliary colic are caused by stones. Biliary colic usually disappears within hours or after a maximum of 2 days.

Colic attacks with gallbladder stones that are accompanied by jaundice require interventional measures because in those cases the draining bile ducts are blocked by a stone. Susceptibility to colic without the detection of stones as well as complaints after surgical removal of the gallbladder can therefore be influenced effectively with CTM, since this is a dysfunction that is also characterized by a tendency to spasms.

Findings and Treatment

Findings

Changes in turgor and muscle tone are located in the segments C3–C4 and T6–T10; dorsal, C3–C4 and T2–T12 (▶ Fig. 3.24, ▶ Fig. 3.25).

▶ **Tissue changes on the posterior side of the body** (▶ **Fig. 3.25**)
- Lower edge of the rib cage
- Lower angle of the right scapula
- On the edge of the latissimus dorsi muscle on the right side of the rib cage
- Between the right scapula and the spinal column, at the level of the upper and lower angle of the scapula
- In the triangle of the shoulder and neck on the right side of the body

▶ **On the anterior side of the body** (▶ **Fig. 3.24**)
- Lower edge of the rib cage on the right side to the epigastric angle
- Upper part of the straight abdominal muscles on the right side of the body
- The upper abdomen is bulged and tense. The major painful spots are located on the right side on the lower edge of the rib cage with increased tension on the right half of the rib cage, retractions on the right edge of the ribs, and distensions in the angle of the lowest rib and spinal column (T10).

The maximal point is located on the spine of the right scapula to the outermost area toward the acromion (C5). This is of great value to differential diagnosis since it provides distinctive signs of disturbances in the liver and gallbladder. The area is painful to pressure and in general also persists for a period during CTM treatments.

Treatment Plan

Starting position: sitting or lateral position.
- Small basic sequence, flat strokes over the rib cage from caudal toward cranial.
- Small basic sequence, first sequence, flat strokes over the rib cage.

- Small basic sequence, first and second sequence, flat strokes over the rib cage.
- Small basic sequence, first and second sequence, ventral side, flat strokes on the right arm.
- Small basic sequence, first and second sequence, ventral side of the body, treatment of the right upper arm, flat strokes of forearm and hand.
- Small basic sequence, first, second, and third sequence, ventral side, treatment of the right arm.

Balancing strokes over the pectoral muscles, dorsal dispersion stroke, and flat strokes on both arms are applied at the end of each treatment session to support the venous backflow.

Additional Strokes

Small Basic Sequence

▶ **From dorsal** (▶ **Fig. 2.27**)
- Hooks to the sacral bone edges from caudal to cranial.
- Hooks along the course of the first pelvic stroke from caudal to cranial.
- Small, flat transverse strokes along the spine within the area of the long extensor spinae muscles from L5 to T12.
- Fanlike strokes in the upper respiratory angle.
- Stretching stroke in the lumbar triangle on the left side.

▶ **From ventral** (▶ **Fig. 2.35**)
- Bimanual strokes, starting from the dorsal side. At the same time, the therapist pulls on the lower edge of the rib cage toward the medioclavicular line and on the pelvic edge toward the anterior superior iliac spine. These strokes are performed bimanually, first on one side then on the other side of the body.
- Short hooks along the rectus sheath from the symphysis to the level of the navel.
- Bimanual strokes crossing over the abdominal walls, starting in the dorsal region and ending at the opposite edge of the rectus abdominis muscle.
- The liver stroke.
- Balancing strokes on the pectoral muscles and strokes on the ventral pelvis and abdomen (▶ Fig. 2.32).

First Sequence

▶ **From dorsal** (▶ **Fig. 2.39**)
- The intercostal strokes are also pulled in the opposite direction, from the spinal column to the lateral chest wall to the ventral axillary line, and hooked in there gently.
- Small, flat transverse strokes along the spine, within the area of the long extensor spinae muscles, from T12 to T7.
- Flat transverse strokes over the spinal column, beginning at the level of T6 under the angle of the left scapula

and ending under the right scapula, then pulled back to the starting point.

▶ **From ventral**
- In the ventral intercostal area a set of flat strokes are pulled beginning at the dorsal axillary line through the intercostal spaces. These should start at the lowest ribs.

Second Sequence

▶ **From dorsal** (▶ Fig. 2.45, ▶ Fig. 2.46, ▶ Fig. 2.48)
- Long downward stretching.
- Prolonged upward stretching.
- Small, flat transverse strokes over the spine within the area of the long extensor spinae muscles from T7 to T3 and C7.
- A set of flat strokes from the lower angle of the scapula to the spine at the level of segment T4.
- Flat transverse strokes from the inner side to the lateral edge of the scapulae, starting at the level of T7 and ending at the level of the spine of the scapula.
- The large balancing stroke starts in the ventral axillary line at the level of the sixth/seventh intercostal space and is flatly pulled around the lower angle of the scapula toward C7 (▶ Fig. 2.38).

▶ **From ventral** (▶ Fig. 2.49)
- The ventral edge of the trapezius muscle is pulled out starting from the cervical base, while pressing against it with the free hand.
- Short hooks on the connection points between the ribs and sternum, pulling from caudal to cranial.
- After the third sequence (▶ Fig. 2.47) apply a flat fan-shaped stroke transversely over the scapula toward the shoulder joint, starting at the outer border of the scapula and ending at the lower border of the spine of the scapula.

Comments

- Treatment should be started about 4 to 6 weeks after the acute pathological process.
- As long as the liver is swollen, the liver stroke should not be applied. The therapist should wait until normalization develops from the segment on the back. A test point is on the abdomen under the liver at about the level of the navel. There is severe painful guarding here in the deeper tissue in all disorders of the liver.
- After conclusion of the treatment, a rolled-up hot pack is first applied to the dorsal left, then to the right side of the body. The ventral region of the body is only included in the treatment when the increased tension subsides. The liver stroke is applied only after the application of the rolled-up hot pack has significantly reduced guarding. After a series of liver strokes, the persistent spasm subsides and the patient experiences a very liberating effect.

- If the tissue on the right side of the thorax continues to show massive adhesion, second and third sequences are first applied to the left side of the body. The affected region on the right side of the rib cage is approached slowly and carefully. It may be the case that the maximal point can no longer be palpated during application of the small basic and additional sequences. In this case, the treatment starts with local treatment.
- A specific number of treatments cannot be recommended because of the individual nature of cases. During the patient's hospitalization, CTM should be applied every day and in outpatient care two or three times a week.
- Treatment of sensitive patients, especially those who respond with reactions of the autonomic nervous system, should be started with flat strokes over the dorsal and ventral parts of the body in the region of the pelvis. If these body parts respond with minor reddening, the small basic sequence may be started in flat technique.
- Physical therapy and CTM should be carefully coordinated. It must be ensured that the patient rests after treatment.

3.5.7 Disorders of the Kidneys and Draining Urinary Tracts

Sufficient blood supply, intact capillary walls, ability to absorb, and secretory performance of the tubules are principal requirements for normal kidney function. Numerous extrarenal factors regulate this system of urine preparation. The kidneys can only fulfill their task when the hemodynamics functions properly and the heart activity and vascular tone ensure adequate blood pressure. If blood pressure drops below a certain limit, the kidneys stop producing urine. If the normal limits are exceeded, the capillary blood flow and the structure of the capillary walls determine the scope and size of the permeable areas, and thus the renal function through the movement of fluids.

Numerous connections of reflexes exist between the skin and mucous membranes and the kidneys. Warmth on the skin promotes diuresis; cold, in contrast, causes oliguria because the blood supply is reduced. These extraordinarily important correlations have a special therapeutic significance (▶ Fig. 3.26, ▶ Fig. 3.27).

Diet, physical therapy, and CTM should therefore be applied as soon as possible. In general, the influence of therapy depends on the extent of the kidney dysfunction already present. All disorders may progress to kidney insufficiency in the form of acute or chronic kidney failure with different outcomes.

Acute and Chronic Glomerulonephritis
Definition

Acute and chronic glomerulonephritis occur either independently or in the context of various inflammatory general illnesses.

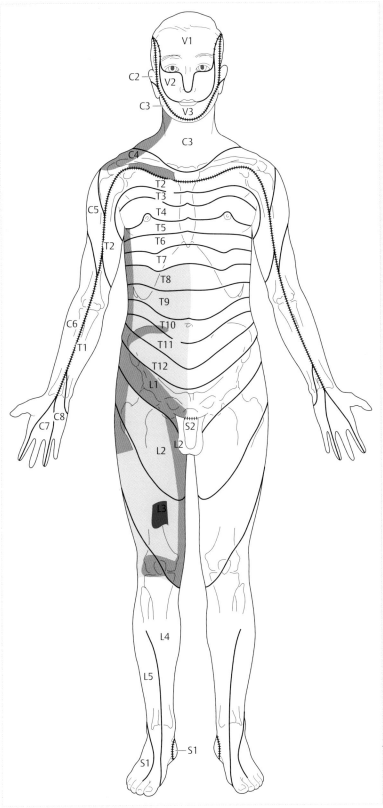

Fig. 3.26 Kidney disorders (only marked for disorders on the right side). Affected: T8–T12, L1–L3, C3–C4. Maximal point: L3.

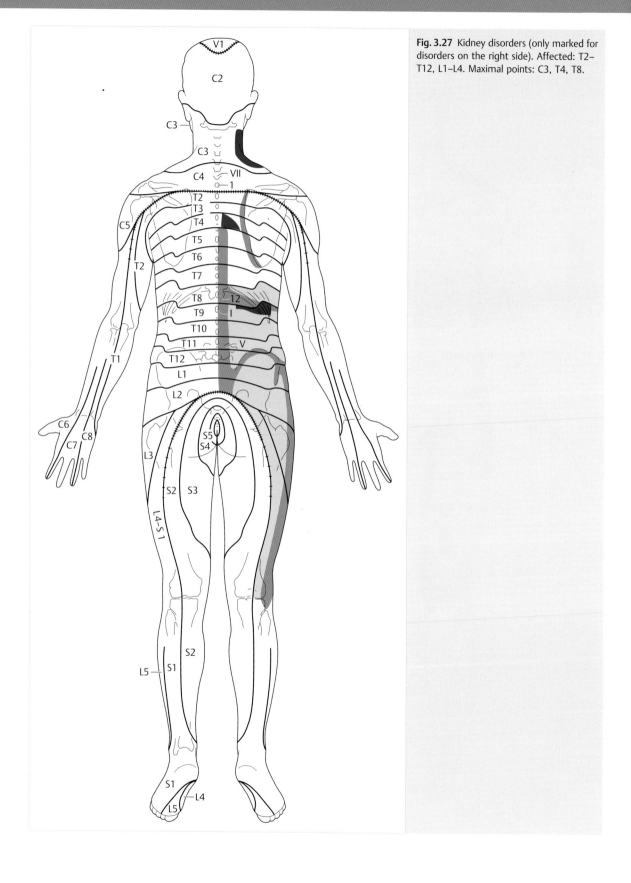

Fig. 3.27 Kidney disorders (only marked for disorders on the right side). Affected: T2–T12, L1–L4. Maximal points: C3, T4, T8.

The sooner treatment is started the better are the possibilities for successful therapy. Corticosteroids (cortisone) and antibiotics are required as medication.

Findings

Changes in turgor and muscle tone are located in segments T8–T12 and L1–L3 on the affected side of the body.

Maximal points are located between the scapulae and the spinal column, in the junction between the shoulder and neck, and on the lower edge of the ribs.

The patient complains about headaches and a tendency to having cold feet that easily swell up to the lower legs.

▶ **Tissue changes on the anterior side of the body** (▶ **Fig. 3.26**)
- In the region of the groin extending to the pelvic crests
- On the lateral side of the torso to the pelvic crest extending into the axilla
- A palm-sized tissue area, a hand's width below the groin in the adductor muscles
- Above the patella running in medial direction
- Along the course of the iliotibial tract
- In the angle between the clavicle and sternum
- Along the trapezius muscle, descending part, at the junction of the shoulder to the neck

▶ **On the posterior side of the body** (▶ **Fig. 3.27**)
- On the sacral bone
- Under the pelvic crests
- In the region of the trochanter and along the iliotibial tract extending to the popliteal cavity
- On both sides of the thoracic and lumbar spine
- On the medial edge of the scapula
- At the junction between the shoulder and neck, along the course of the trapezius muscle, descending part

The maximal point between the scapulae and the spinal column presents itself as a hard string. This change in the tissue is closely related to the tension on the lower edge of the ribs. The strokes in the second sequence around the scapula cause a spontaneous decrease of the tissue tension on the lower edge of the ribs.

Local hardening of the erector spinae muscle starting at the sacral bone to under the scapulae is palpated when there are kidney stones.

Treatment Plan

Starting position: sitting, lateral position, supine position.
- Small basic sequence, flat strokes on both legs.
- Small basic sequence, first sequence, ventral side of the body, flat strokes over both legs.
- Small basic sequence, first sequence, treatment of the thighs, ventral side, flat strokes over both legs.
- Small basic sequence, first and second sequence, treatment of thigh and knee, ventral side of the body, flat strokes over both legs.
- Small basic sequence, first, second, and third sequence, ventral side, treatment of leg.

Balancing strokes over the pectoral muscles, dorsal dispersion stroke, and flat strokes of the legs are applied at the end of each treatment session to support the venous backflow.

Additional Strokes

Small Basic Sequence

▶ **From dorsal** (▶ **Fig. 2.27**)
- Hooks to the sacral bone edges from caudal to cranial.
- Flat transverse strokes over the sacral bone from caudal to cranial.
- Hooks along the course of the first pelvic stroke from caudal to cranial.
- Small, flat transverse strokes along the spine within the area of the long extensor spinae muscles from L5 to T12.
- Fanlike strokes in the upper respiratory angle.

▶ **From ventral** (▶ **Fig. 2.35**)
- Bimanual strokes starting from dorsal. At the same time, the therapist pulls on the lower edge of the rib cage toward the medioclavicular line and on the pelvic edge toward the anterior superior iliac spine. These strokes are performed bimanually, first on one side then on the other side of the body.
- Short hooks along the rectus sheath from the symphysis to the level of the navel.
- Short strokes, like rays, pulling toward the navel.
- Bimanual strokes crossing over the abdominal walls, starting in the dorsal region and ending at the opposite edge of the rectus abdominis muscle.
- The liver stroke.
- Balancing strokes on the pectoral muscles and strokes on the ventral pelvis and abdomen (▶ **Fig. 2.32**).

First Sequence

▶ **From dorsal** (▶ **Fig. 2.39**)
- The intercostal strokes are also pulled in the opposite direction from the spinal column to the lateral chest wall to the ventral axillary line and hooked in there gently.
- Small, flat transverse strokes along the spine within the area of the long extensor spinae muscles, from T12 to T7.
- Flat transverse strokes over the spinal column, beginning at the level of T6 under the angle of the left scapula and ending under the right scapula.

▶ **From ventral**

- In the ventral intercostal area a set of flat strokes are pulled beginning at the dorsal axillary line through the intercostal spaces. These should start at the lowest ribs.

Second Sequence

▶ **From dorsal** (▶ Fig. 2.46)

- Long downward stretching.
- Prolonged upward stretching.
- The intercostal strokes are also pulled in the opposite direction from the spinal column to the lateral chest wall to the ventral axillary line and hooked in there gently.
- The large balancing stroke starts in the ventral axillary line at the level of the sixth/seventh intercostal space and is flatly pulled around the lower angle of the scapula toward C7 (▶ Fig. 2.38).

▶ **On the leg** (▶ Fig. 2.69, ▶ Fig. 2.70)

- Short strokes from the last third of the fascia lata in the shape of a fan toward the patella.
- The thigh stroke starts in the upper third of the thigh, on the lateral edge of the sartorius muscle, and ends shortly before the groin.
- Short hooks, which are pulled from the transverse intergluteal cleft to the popliteal cavity.
- Strokes from the inner side of the lower leg, starting below the patella and running around the medial malleolus.
- Bimanual stretching between the muscle bellies of the gastrocnemius muscle, from cranial to caudal, pulling in the direction of the Achilles tendon.

Comments

- The strokes in small basic sequences are applied repeatedly (except in the lower edge of the rib cage on the affected side).
- The areas of the maximal points are initially treated with vibrations and flat hooks. Treatment then swiftly proceeds to the second sequence to effect a reduction of the tension in the tissue. The initial increased tension is significantly reduced here.
- If only one kidney is affected and the adhesions in the tissue of the affected side do not permit local treatment, the unaffected side of the body is treated first.
- A rolled-up hot pack is applied to segments T5 to L2. It is perceived as particularly pleasant in the groin and adductor muscles. However, the utmost attention must be paid here, since these are obviously very sensitive regions of the body.
- Physical therapy and CTM should be coordinated with each other, and the patient must rest after CTM.

Acute and Chronic Pyelonephritis

Definition

Pyelonephritis is a bacterial inflammation of the kidneys that ascends from the renal pelvis and attacks the kidneys. The infection does not reach the renal parenchyma through the blood but rather ascends from the draining urinary tracts. This infectious pathway is promoted by chronic bladder infections, kidney stones, or other obstructions of the draining urinary tracts.

In the chronic stage, cold and dampness can cause a relapse of the bacterial infection.

The goal of physical therapy is to alleviate the complaints and to promote diuresis; in the acute stage, therapy involves targeted administration of antibiotics and removal of possible obstructions to the outflow (e.g., kidney stones).

Heat applications are indicated, which are best administered with the help of baths with a gradual increase in water temperature. The cardiac performance must be taken into account. Sufficient amounts of fluid should always be provided to promote diuresis.

It is also important here that the acute symptoms of the disorder have subsided before CTM is applied. CTM can be used afterward and after surgical procedures to normalize irritated functions. Indications are residual conditions after inflammations of the kidneys and renal pelvis, especially when the patient complains about back pain, stiffness, and also abdominal pain. Apparently there is a connection between irritations of the kidney and renal pelvis affecting the surrounding segments.

Findings, Treatment Plan, Additional Strokes, Comments

See Acute and Chronic Glomerulonephritis (p. 156)

Disorders of the Bladder

Definition

Connective tissue massage can be successfully applied after bladder infections, chronic cystitis, irritable bladder that responds to very small amounts of urine with an urge to urinate, and after surgery of the prostate with initial sphincter insufficiency.

Findings

Increased turgor and muscle tone are located in the segments T10–T12, L1–L5 and S1–S4.

Maximal points can be palpated next to the spinal column between the scapulae and above the symphysis.

▶ **Tissue changes on the anterior side of the body** (▶ Fig. 3.28):

- Above the symphysis and in the region of the groin
- Along the rectus abdominis muscle

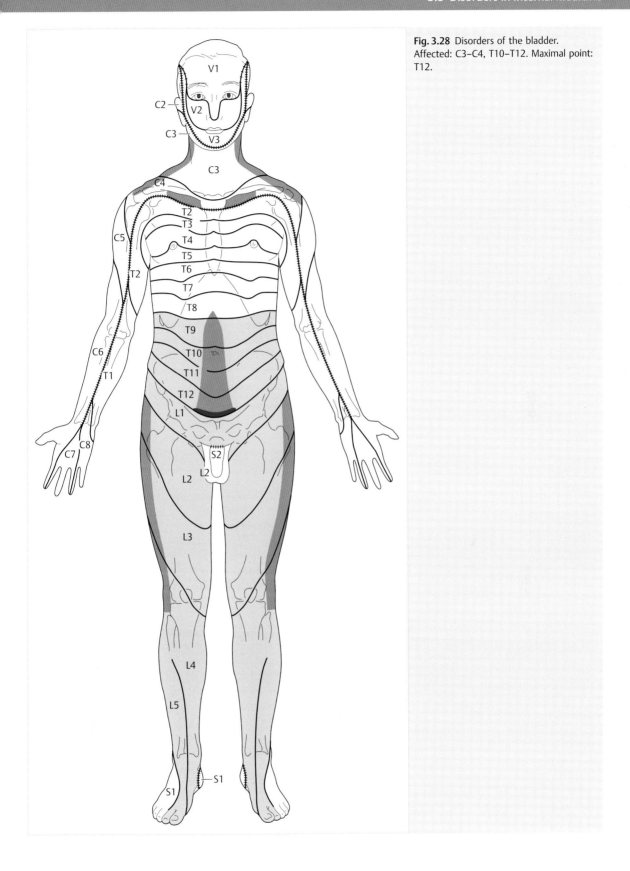

► **On the posterior side of the body** (► Fig. 3.29):
- On the sacral bone above the intergluteal cleft
- On the edges of the sacral bone to the sacroiliac joints
- Under the edges of the pelvis
- From the sacroiliac joints to the trochanter extending over the iliotibial tract to the popliteal cavity
- On both sides of the spinal column
- Between the scapulae
- At the junction of the shoulder and neck

Treatment Plan

Starting position: sitting, supine position, lateral position.
- Small basic sequence, flat strokes over the body from caudal toward cranial.
- Small basic sequence, first sequence, flat strokes on the legs.
- Small basic sequence, first and second sequence, ventral side, flat strokes on both legs.
- Small basic sequence, first, second, and third sequence, ventral side of the body, treatment of the thighs, flat strokes on lower leg and foot.
- Small basic sequence, first, second, and third sequence, ventral side, treatment of leg.

Balancing strokes over the pectoral muscles, dorsal dispersion stroke, and flat strokes of the legs are applied at the end of each treatment session to support the venous backflow.

Additional Strokes
Small Basic Sequence

► **From dorsal** (► Fig. 2.27, ► Fig. 2.29)
- Hooks to the sacral bone edges from caudal to cranial.
- Flat transverse strokes over the sacral bone from caudal to cranial.
- Hooks along the course of the first pelvic stroke from caudal to cranial.
- Small, flat transverse strokes along the spine within the area of the long extensor spinae muscles from L5 to T12.
- Stretching stroke in the lumbar triangle.
- Fanlike strokes in the upper respiratory angle.

► **From ventral** (► Fig. 2.35)
- Bimanual strokes, starting from the dorsal side. At the same time, the therapist pulls on the lower edge of the rib cage toward the medioclavicular line and on the pelvic edge toward the anterior superior iliac spine. These strokes are performed bimanually, first on one side then on the other side of the body.
- Short hooks along the rectus sheath from the symphysis to the level of the navel.

- Bimanual strokes crossing over the abdominal walls, starting in the dorsal region and ending at the opposite edge of the rectus abdominis muscle.

First Sequence

► **From dorsal** (► Fig. 2.39)
- The intercostal strokes are also pulled in the opposite direction from the spinal column to the lateral chest wall to the ventral axillary line and hooked in there gently.
- Small, flat transverse strokes along the spine within the area of the long extensor spinae muscles from T12 to T7.
- Flat transverse strokes over the spinal column, beginning at the level of T6 under the angle of the left scapula and ending under the right scapula.

► **From ventral**
- In the ventral intercostal area a set of flat strokes are pulled beginning at the dorsal axillary line through the intercostal spaces. These should start at the lowest ribs.

Second Sequence

► **From dorsal** (► Fig. 2.46)
- Long downward stretching.
- Prolonged upward stretching.
- The intercostal strokes are also pulled in opposite direction, from the spinal column to the lateral chest wall to the ventral axillary line, and hooked in there gently.
- The large balancing stroke starts in the ventral axillary line at the level of the sixth/seventh intercostal space and is flatly pulled around the lower angle of the scapula toward C7 (► Fig. 2.38).

► **From ventral** (► Fig. 2.49)
- The ventral edge of the trapezius muscle is pulled out starting from the cervical base, while pressing against it with the free hand.
- Short hooks on the connection points between the ribs and sternum, pulling from caudal to cranial.
- After the third sequence (► Fig. 2.47), a flat fan-shaped stroke is applied transversely over the scapula toward the shoulder joint, starting at the outer edge of the scapula and ending at the lower edge of the spine of the scapula.

► **On the leg** (► Fig. 2.69, ► Fig. 2.70)
- Short strokes from the last third of the fascia lata in the shape of a fan toward the patella.
- The thigh stroke starts in the upper third of the thigh, on the lateral edge of the sartorius muscle, and ends shortly before the groin.
- Short hooks, which are pulled from the transverse intergluteal cleft to the popliteal cavity.

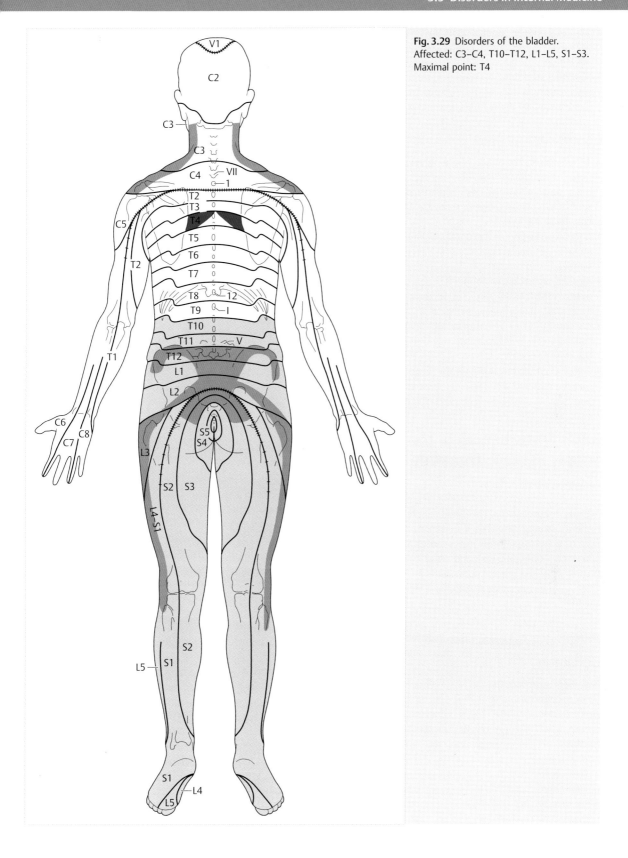

Fig. 3.29 Disorders of the bladder.
Affected: C3–C4, T10–T12, L1–L5, S1–S3.
Maximal point: T4

- Strokes from the inner side of the lower leg, starting below the patella and running around the medial malleolus.
- Bimanual stretching between the muscle bellies of the gastrocnemius muscle, from cranial to caudal, pulling in the direction of the Achilles tendon.

Comments

- If the tissue in the region of the pelvis has higher tension, the therapist works over the back with flat strokes from caudal to cranial. Only when these body parts respond with minor reddening can the small basic sequence be started.
- If the maximal point has not changed after the first sequence, the area is treated with vibrations and flat strokes.
- A rolled-up hot pack is applied to segments T9 over L3 to S1. In the further course of the treatment it can also be applied to segments C3–T4.
- A series of 10 to 15 treatment sessions, two or three times a week, is indicated to trigger improvement of the complaints.
- Before CTM the physical therapy treatment should direct the patient's attention to the lower region of the body.

3.5.8 Disturbances of the Blood Supply in the Extremities

Paul Hutzschenreuter, Elke Harms

Arterial disturbances of the blood supply (e.g., chronic peripheral arterial disease), inflammatory vascular disorders of a functional and immunological nature (thromboangiitis obliterans, Raynaud disease), and venous disturbances of the blood supply with and without venous ulcer are indications for the application of connective tissue massage.

Peripheral Arterial Disease

Definition

Peripheral arterial disease (PAD) is used as the general term for clinical pictures that lead to stenosis or occlusion of arteries in the pelvis and extremities. These disorders have in common risk factors and pathological findings in the arterial wall due to atherosclerosis (► Fig. 3.30).

Risk factors are hypertension, hypercholesterolemia, nicotine abuse, and diabetes mellitus as well as gout, obesity and a sedentary lifestyle.

Depending on the localization of the atherosclerosis we distinguish between the pelvis type, thigh type, peripheral type, and, in combined occlusions, the occlusion at multiple levels. It is commonly divided into the four Fon-

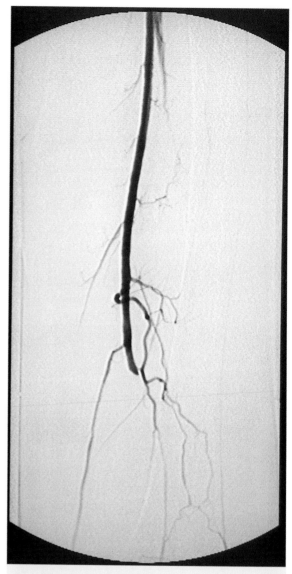

Fig. 3.30 Occlusion of the anterior femoral artery.

taine stages (1954) according to severity and clinical symptoms:
- Stage I: The patients are free of complaints.
- Stage II: Pain in the calf, since the blood supply is insufficient during exertion (intermittent claudication).
- Stage IIa: Pain in the calf only develops after a walking distance of more than 200 meters (650 feet).
- Stage IIb: Pain in the calf develops with a walking distance of less than 200 meters.
- Stage III: Pain at night during rest. Insufficient blood supply in horizontal position.
- Stage IV: Biological tissue loss and gangrene of the toes develop.

In stages II and III, CTM may be applied immediately. In stage IV, the chronic wound should first be treated conservatively with phase-adapted moist wound treatment or surgery (e.g., skin flap) and allowed to heal before CTM is administered.

To improve the arterial flow, percutaneous catheter dilatation, surgical bypass surgery, or stent implantation are carried out in stages II and III.

Infusions with alprostadil and saline solution or oral naftidrofuryl (Dusodril forte) are prescribed.

Other vasodilative medications do not influence organic stenosis or the collaterals (Mörl 1986). The combination of CTM and physical therapy with active muscle training may improve the condition, if applied in stages II and III.

Both treatment methods are applied with the goal of increasing the distance that can be walked free of pain. The application of physical therapy improves the oxygen and nutrient supply and promotes the development of collaterals. CTM reinforces the effect of both processes.

Findings

Increased turgor and muscle tone are located in the lower part of the back, in the region of the buttocks and legs (T12, L1–L5, S1–S5) (▶ Fig. 3.31, ▶ Fig. 3.32).

▶ **On the posterior side of the body** (▶ **Fig. 3.32**)
- Extremely increased tone can be detected over the whole back, which is often perceived by patients as being like wearing armor or being tied up. The diagnostic stroke shows no reddening and the skin feels cold, sweaty, or dry.
- Retractions and swelling are found in the region of the sacral bone.

▶ **On the leg** (▶ **Fig. 3.31**)
- Retractions:
  ◦ On the iliotibial tract
  ◦ Around the greater trochanter
- Painful palpations:
  ◦ Greater trochanter
  ◦ Iliotibial tract
  ◦ Tibial tuberosity
  ◦ Above the ankle joint

If the vascular disease persists over a longer period, the skin is insufficiently nourished and develops trophic changes (arterial ulcer), frequently during the transition from stage II to stage III. The arterial ulcer is located on the lateral distal area of the lower leg, the venous ulcer is usually located on the medial lower leg. The skin is dry and thin like parchment.

The palpation shows distinctive adhesions between the tissue layers and their mobility is difficult.

The palpation of arterial pulses provides information about the patency of individual arterial sections. In the region of the leg the femoral artery on the distal side of the inguinal ligament, the popliteal artery in the popliteal cavity, the posterior tibial artery on the posterior edge of the medial ankle, and the dorsal artery on the back of the foot can be palpated. The Doppler sonogram allows quantification of the patency of the affected arteries before and after a series of connective tissue massage. Ultrasound diagnostics are able to depict the localization of the arterial occlusion. Nowadays, arteriographies are performed only before surgery.

Patients with intermittent claudication often complain about cold feet. This indicates an increased sympathetic tone of the autonomic nervous system. Cold, abnormal reddening to cyanosis of the skin is a sign of dilated capillaries in the skin due to a loss of tone.

Treatment Plan

Starting position: sitting, supine position, lateral position, prone position.
- Small basic sequence, flat strokes over both legs.
- Small basic sequence, treatment of the thigh, flat strokes on lower leg and foot.
- Small basic sequence, treatment of the leg.

Balancing strokes over the pectoral muscles, dorsal dispersion stroke, and flat strokes on the legs are applied at the end of each treatment session to support the venous backflow.

Additional Strokes

Small Basic Sequence

▶ **From dorsal** (▶ **Fig. 2.27**)
- Hooks to the sacral bone edges from caudal to cranial.
- Flat transverse strokes over the sacral bone from caudal to cranial.
- Hooks along the course of the first pelvic stroke from caudal to cranial.
- Fanlike strokes in the upper respiratory angle.

▶ **From ventral** (▶ **Fig. 2.35**)
- Bimanual strokes, starting from the dorsal side. At the same time, the therapist pulls on the lower edge of the rib cage toward the medioclavicular line and on the pelvic edge toward the anterior superior iliac spine. These strokes are performed first on one side then on the other side of the body.
- Short hooks along the rectus sheath from the symphysis to the level of the navel.
- Bimanual strokes crossing over the abdominal walls, starting in the dorsal region and ending at the opposite edge of the rectus abdominis muscle.
- The liver stroke.
- Balancing strokes on the pectoral muscles and strokes on the ventral pelvis and abdomen (▶ Fig. 2.32).

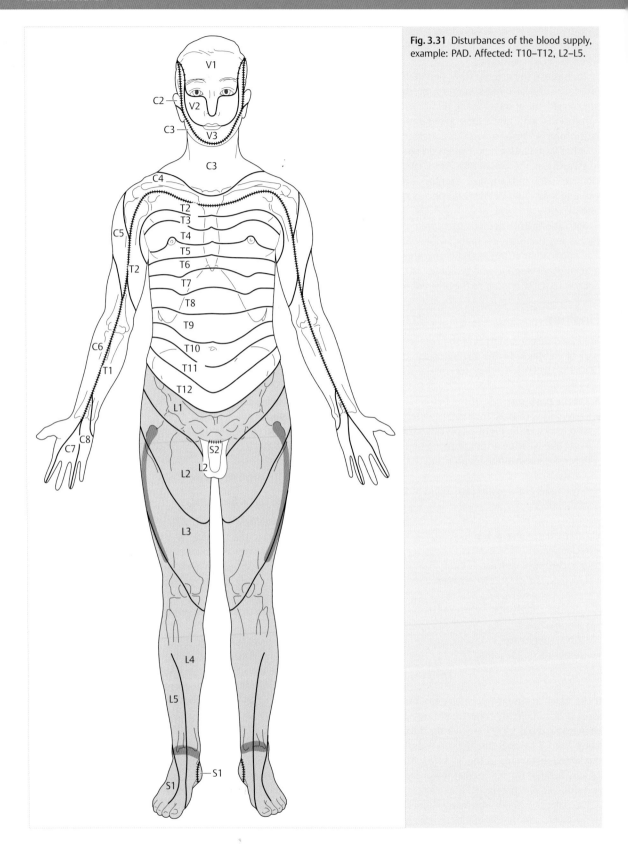

Fig. 3.31 Disturbances of the blood supply, example: PAD. Affected: T10–T12, L2–L5.

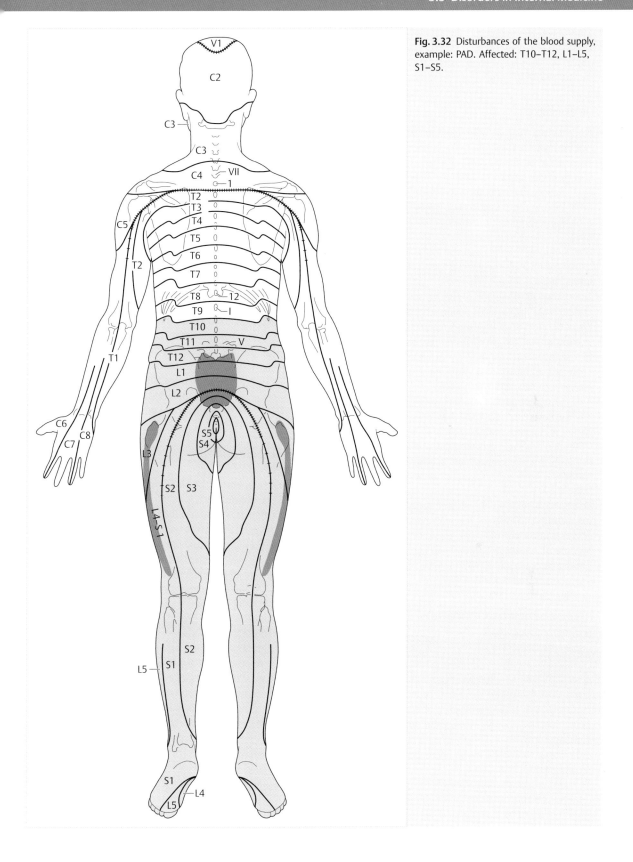

Fig. 3.32 Disturbances of the blood supply, example: PAD. Affected: T10–T12, L1–L5, S1–S5.

▶ **On the leg**
- The thigh stroke starts in the upper third of the thigh, on the lateral edge of the sartorius muscle, and ends shortly before the groin.

Comments

- The treatment can be performed in lateral and prone position with severely increased tissue tone.
- The treatment focuses on flat strokes, which is why it is very important to observe the reaction of the skin and to apply the technique in doses. Hooks are later pulled along the pelvic crest to loosen the tissue. Afterward, the small basic sequence is applied as usual.
- The rhomboid strokes and the angle between the spinal column and pelvic crest are treated especially intensively.
- The strokes in the region of the leg are initially only pulled in the proximal direction so as to avoid worsening of the flow velocity (Helmrich 1985).
- In addition to CTM, physical therapy should be added to optimize treatment of PAD with its many possible applications: for example, Ratschow test, Ratschow exercises, gait test, and gait training.
- A rolled-up hot pack is applied on the sacral bone, below the navel, in the area of the trochanter, and in the region of the neck and shoulder.
- CTM should be applied every day until the firm retractions and constrictions of connective tissue have changed. Afterward, treatment can be scheduled two or three times a week.
- Relief and alleviation of pain can be generated by massaging strokes in the lumbar region and buttocks. Massage in the region of the leg is not recommended because of a possible paradox vascular reaction.
- Physical therapy and CTM should be coordinated. It must be ensured that the patient rests after treatment.

Thromboangiitis Obliterans (Buerger Disease)

Definition

The term thromboangiitis obliterans subsumes peripheral arterial disturbances of the blood supply, which start in the intima and characteristically affect the vessel segments. Men and women acquire the disease in a ratio of 9:1 irrespective of age. The men affected are predominantly heavy smokers. Compared with sclerotic PAD this disease is rare.

In terms of the pathophysiology, a chronic productive inflammation of the arteries causes thickening of the corresponding sections of vascular wall. As soon as the inflammatory processes have reached the circular smooth muscle cells, they can no longer fulfill their vasomotor task.

The patient must not smoke during treatment, since nicotine is probably a triggering factor. Aspirin and corticoids are the medicines provided.

CTM has become indispensable in treatment of this condition and is highly effective in combination with physical therapy.

The goal of treatment is to gradually decrease pain and increase the warmth of the affected extremities by dilating arterial and venous vascular lumina.

Findings, Treatment Plan, Additional Strokes, Comments

See Peripheral Arterial Disease (p. 164).

Diabetic Vascular Diseases

Definition

Two types of vascular disease can be distinguished in diabetes, which often occur in the same patient:
- Diabetic macroangiopathy (i.e., stenosis and occlusions of larger arteries). The symptoms and the vascular changes indicate PAD without diabetes.
- Diabetic microangiopathies, which are specific to diabetes. These affect the capillaries in a systemic way, that is to say a generalized manner, which has an impact on many organs.

The clinically most relevant symptoms are disturbances of the blood supply of:
- The retina, where they lead to severe visual impairment and even blindness
- The kidneys, which may lead to renal insufficiency, disturbances in the excretion of substances in the urine, uremia, and high blood pressure (hypertension)

In the region of the extremities disturbances in the blood supply develop in the terminal vessels, which are particularly noticeable in fingers and toes, also with good function (pulsation) of the greater vessels.

Also important is diabetic microangiopathy of the vessels of the nerves, which triggers focal polyneuropathies that worsen the blood supply of the tissue due to vasoparesis. In the long term, diabetes mellitus causes regular distal symmetric polyneuropathies, which typically cause vasoparesis and anhidrosis of the feet.

Attempts to influence these pathologies with CTM are consistent with the measures described in the section Peripheral Arterial Disease (p. 164).

Findings in the Upper Extremity

Increased turgor and muscle tone can be palpated in the whole region of the sacral bone, pelvis, and back. Depending on the relief posture or malposition, the findings are seen on both sides or more accentuated on one side.

Changes in tissue and tension are located:
- Along the skull sutures
- Between and around the scapulae
- On the trapezius muscle, deltoid muscle, triceps brachii, and in the region of the forearm

The fingers are usually cold and pale; the nails may be brittle and break easily.

Treatment Plan for the Upper Extremity

Starting position: sitting, supine position.
- Small basic sequence.
- Small basic sequence, first sequence, flat strokes on the arms.
- Small basic sequence, first and second sequence (shoulder only), ventral side, flat strokes on the arms.
- Small basic sequence, first and second sequence, ventral side, flat strokes on the arms.
- Small basic sequence, first, second, and third sequence, ventral side of the body, treatment of the upper arm, flat strokes of the forearm and hand.
- Small basic sequence, first, second, and third sequence, ventral side, treatment of the arm.

Balancing strokes over the pectoral muscles, dorsal dispersion stroke, and flat strokes of the arms are applied at the end of each treatment session to support the venous backflow.

Additional Strokes in the Upper Extremity

Small Basic Sequence

▶ **From dorsal** (▶ Fig. 2.27)
- Hooks to the sacral bone edges from caudal to cranial.
- Flat transverse strokes over the sacral bone from caudal to cranial.
- Hooks along the course of the first pelvic stroke from caudal to cranial.
- Fanlike strokes in the upper respiratory angle.

▶ **From ventral** (▶ Fig. 2.35)
- Short hooks along the rectus sheath from the symphysis to the level of the navel.
- Bimanual strokes crossing over the abdominal walls, starting in the dorsal region and ending at the opposite edge of the rectus abdominis muscle.
- The liver stroke.
- Balancing pelvic strokes.
- Flat transverse strokes over the abdominal space.

First Sequence

▶ **From dorsal** (▶ Fig. 2.39)
- The intercostal strokes are also pulled in the opposite direction from the spinal column to the lateral chest wall to the ventral axillary line and hooked in there gently.

Second Sequence

▶ **From dorsal** (▶ Fig. 2.46, ▶ Fig. 2.48)
- Long downward stretching.
- Prolonged upward stretching.
- Set of flat strokes from the lower angle of the scapula to the spine at the level of segment T4.
- Flat transverse strokes from the inner side to the lateral edge of the scapulae, starting at the level of T7 and ending at the level of the spine of the scapula.

▶ **From ventral** (▶ Fig. 2.35)
- Short hooks on the insertion points of the ribs toward the sternum from caudal to cranial.
- Strokes over the sternum, beginning at the xiphoid process and ending at the suprasternal notch.
- Short transverse strokes along the sternum. These start at the junction between the xiphoid process and the body of the sternum, along the area of the sternal angle. At the base of the second rib at the sternum, the strokes should become wider to just under the sternoclavicular joints.
- Short fanlike strokes working along the medial clavicular angle toward the suprasternal notch. The first set of strokes are started on the clavicle, ending the last set of strokes on the dorsal edge of the sternocleidomastoid muscle.
- Strokes toward the interclavicular ligament.

Comments on the Upper Extremity

- At the beginning of the treatment flat strokes are increasingly applied in the region of the pelvis and back.
- As the treatment progresses, segments C3–C8 (arm segments) and T6–T12 should be focused on.
- As with all disorders of the extremities, the therapist should work contralaterally at first: when the right side is more affected, one should start with the left extremity and wait for the consensual effect.
- The arms should only be treated after the tension in the tissue on the back has significantly decreased.
- The generally reduced blood supply and the increased tension in the tissue of segments C3–T4 causes a predisposition for pain in shoulder, neck, and head so that treatment of headaches can be added (see the section Neurological Diseases, p. 101).
- A rolled-up hot pack is also applied to the region of the shoulder and neck.
- It significantly contributes to the improvement of the complaints when physical therapy and CTM are properly coordinated. The patient must rest after CTM.
- CTM must be applied as long-term therapy.

Findings in the Lower Extremity

Increased turgor and muscle tone are located in the lower part of the back, in the region of the buttocks and legs (T10–T12, L1–L5, S1–S5).

The palpation shows distinctive adhesions between the tissue layers and they are significantly difficult to move. Retractions are located on the edges of the sacral bone up to the lumbar region and along the iliotibial tract around the greater trochanter. Distensions are located on the sacral bone.

Treatment Plan for the Lower Extremity

Starting position: sitting, prone position, lateral position, supine position.
- Small basic sequence.
- Small basic sequence, flat strokes over both legs.
- Small basic sequence, first sequence, flat strokes on both legs.
- Small basic sequence, first sequence, ventral side of the body, treatment of the thighs, flat strokes over the lower leg and foot.
- Small basic sequence, first sequence, ventral side, treatment of the leg.

Balancing strokes over the pectoral muscles, dorsal dispersion stroke, and flat strokes of the legs are applied at the end of each treatment session to support the venous backflow.

Additional Strokes in the Lower Extremity

Small Basic Sequence

▶ **From dorsal** (▶ Fig. 2.27)
- Hooks to the sacral bone edges from caudal to cranial.
- Flat transverse strokes over the sacral bone from caudal to cranial.
- Hooks along the course of the first pelvic stroke from caudal to cranial.
- Fanlike strokes in the upper respiratory angle.

▶ **From ventral** (▶ Fig. 2.35)
- Bimanual strokes, starting from the dorsal side. At the same time, the therapist pulls on the lower edge of the rib cage toward the medioclavicular line and on the pelvic edge toward the anterior superior iliac spine. These strokes are performed first on one side then on the other side of the body.
- Short hooks along the rectus sheath from the symphysis to the level of the navel.
- Bimanual strokes crossing over the abdominal walls, starting in the dorsal region and ending at the opposite edge of the rectus abdominis muscle.
- The liver stroke.

First Sequence

▶ **From dorsal** (▶ Fig. 2.39)
- The intercostal strokes are also pulled in the opposite direction from the spinal column to the lateral chest wall to the ventral axillary line and hooked in there gently.

- Small, flat transverse strokes along the spine within the area of the long extensor spinae muscles from T12 to T7.
- Flat transverse strokes over the spinal column, beginning at the level of T6 under the angle of the left scapula and ending under the angle of the right scapula.

▶ **From ventral**
- In the ventral intercostal area a set of flat strokes are pulled beginning at the dorsal axillary line through the intercostal spaces; start at the lowest ribs.

▶ **On the leg**
- The thigh stroke starts in the upper third of the thigh, on the lateral edge of the sartorius muscle, and ends shortly before the groin.

Comments on the Lower Extremity

- When the tension level in the torso is increased, treatment should be applied in the lateral position or prone position, and primarily flat strokes are used.
- The strokes on the legs are only applied in proximal direction at the beginning of treatment.
- Physical therapy and CTM must be coordinated with each other. The patient must rest after treatment.

Raynaud Phenomenon

Definition

Raynaud phenomenon is a benign illness that symmetrically affects the extremities, in particular the fingers, and is associated with intermittent vasospastic attacks, the cause of which is essentially unknown. Such attacks can be the early symptoms of inflammatory or degenerative vascular diseases.

Examination of patients shows the so-called tricolor effect (Raynaud 1862): Fingers or toes suddenly turn pale and become a dark cyanotic color after a few minutes. When they warm up again, burning pain develops. Subsequently they take on their pinkish color once more.

In terms of the pathophysiology, each attack starts with arterial spastic vasoconstriction. This is followed by vasodilation after a short time (minutes).

The following causes were detected in 100 patients with Raynaud phenomenon (Vayssairat et al 1986): 50 patients with collagenosis, 7 with inflammatory arterial disease (obliterating atherosclerosis, giant-cell arteritis), 10 with atherosclerosis of the arterioles, 10 with posttraumatic disorders, 3 with paraneoplastic syndromes, 2 with cold agglutinin disease. True Raynaud, characterized by the tri-color effect, was found only in 18 patients, while pathologies that have other causes are called secondary Raynaud phenomena.

In a large number of cases appropriate medication is needed for treatment: calcium antagonists, vasodilators, and prostaglandins, especially prostacyclin and thromboxane A$_2$. Connective tissue massage has become indispensable here and is highly effective in combination with physical therapy.

In rare cases, Raynaud phenomenon also occurs in the lower extremity.

Findings in the Upper Extremity

Increased turgor and muscle tone can be palpated in the whole region of the sacral bone, pelvis, and back. Depending on relief posture or malposition, the findings are found on both sides or are more accentuated on one side.

Changes in tissue and tension are located:
- Along the spinal column
- Between and around the scapulae
- On the trapezius muscle, the deltoid muscle, and the triceps brachii and on the region of the forearm

The fingers are usually cold and pale and can turn red to cyanotic depending on the stage and severity of the illness. The nails can be brittle and break easily.

Treatment Plan, Additional Strokes, Comments on the Upper Extremity

See Diabetic Vascular Diseases (p. 168).

Findings in the Lower Extremity

See Diabetic Vascular Diseases (p. 168).

Treatment Plan, Additional Strokes in the Lower Extremity

See Diabetic Vascular Diseases (p. 168).

Comments on the Lower Extremity

See Diabetic Vascular Diseases (p. 168).
- The periodic nature of the attacks must be taken into account when treating Raynaud phenomenon.
- Treatment should be applied in the lateral position with severely increased turgor in the region of the back, buttocks, and legs.

Venous Disturbances of the Blood Supply

Definition

According to experts, chronic venous insufficiency is a common disease that affects women more often than men.

The superficial venous system is used to drain the skin and dermal fatty tissue and transports about 10% of the venous backflow; the deep leg veins cover the remaining 90% (▸ Fig. 3.33). For this reason it is also possible to remove the superficial venous system in Babcock's surgery as long as the deep venous system functions properly. The venous valve system plays a key role here. When the venous valve system is intact, the blood is transported through the veins by means of the muscle pump mechanism.

If the valvular system is insufficient, there will be a low venous return that subsequently causes bulging of the veins, which are then called varices (varicose veins).

The following localization and causes are distinguished: truncal varices (great or small saphenous vein), secondary varices, insufficient perforating veins, and starburst varices. The last are of cosmetic significance only.

Primary varices are believed to be caused by congenital weakness of the soft tissue. Secondary varices are caused by overstrained dermal veins due to previous damage of the deep vein system. The prescription of medication or physical therapy and of CTM is only considered necessary if chronic signs of congestion are present, as seen with chronic venous insufficiency.

Examination of the patient shows that "heavy legs" are reported with venous stretch pain. If this pain increases in its intensity, it is called "burst pain." Venous stretch pain intensifies with heat and is initially reversible by elevating the legs.

The medical significance of varices lies in possible complications such as acute phlebitis or varicophlebitis as well as phlebothrombosis of the leg. These complications are treated with compressive therapy. The application of CTM in the periphery is contraindicated.

The treatment of varices with CTM can only be done segmentally by applying the small basic sequence and is only advisable if combined with compressive therapy (bandages or compressive stockings) and physical therapy. Targeted physical therapy exercises activate the muscle pump and the compressive therapy increases the interstitial pressure in the tissue, thus improving the reabsorption rate of the venous capillary dispersion stroke. The segmental effect of CTM is expected to cause a tonization of veins which, according to Dicke, is achieved by working through the deeper layers of connective tissue.

Varices may lead to trophic dermal necroses, usually in the medial region of the lower leg (venous ulcer).

When the venous ulcer is in its exudative phase (yellowish white ulcer) or granulation phase (pinkish red ulcer), it should first be closed with phase-adapted (moist) treatment and simultaneous manual lymphatic drainage as well as consistently applied bandaging. CTM may be prescribed after intravascular ligature of the perforating veins (causal therapy).

Findings

Increased turgor and muscle tone are located in the segments T10–T12, L1–L4, and S1–S3. The findings in the tissue show:

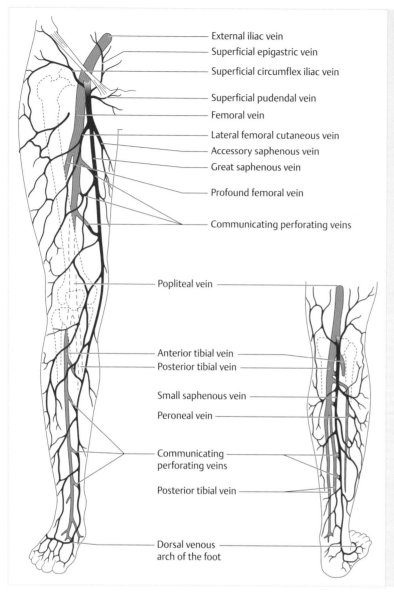

Fig. 3.33 Anatomy of leg veins. Dark vessels: superficial veins. Light vessels: deep veins (after Sigg K. Beinleiden [Leg Complaints], 2nd ed. Berlin: Springer; 1976).

- External iliac vein
- Superficial epigastric vein
- Superficial circumflex iliac vein
- Superficial pudendal vein
- Femoral vein
- Lateral femoral cutaneous vein
- Accessory saphenous vein
- Great saphenous vein
- Profound femoral vein
- Communicating perforating veins
- Popliteal vein
- Anterior tibial vein
- Posterior tibial vein
- Small saphenous vein
- Peroneal vein
- Communicating perforating veins
- Posterior tibial vein
- Dorsal venous arch of the foot

- Firm swelling on the sacral bone
- Retractions of the iliac wings, the gluteal muscles, and the sacroiliac joints
- Tenderness at the rhomboid end points, at the sacroiliac joints, along the pelvic crest, and around the greater trochanter

The skin shows gray-white to reddish-blue discoloration, is often mottled, and feels cold when there is no inflammation. Reddening is seen with inflammation and eczema, while cyanotic changes develop with obstructed venous drainage. The trophicity is disturbed: the skin is in places as thin as tissue paper and is easily injured. Brown, spot-shaped, or extensive pigmentation is caused by microbleeding.

Treatment Plan

Starting position: sitting, prone position, supine position, lateral position.
- Small basic sequence.
- Small basic sequence, flat strokes over the legs from caudal toward cranial.
- Small basic sequence, ventral balancing strokes in the abdominal space, treatment of the thighs, flat strokes on the lower leg and foot from caudal to cranial.
- Small basic sequence, ventral balancing strokes in the abdominal space, treatment of the leg.

Balancing strokes on the pectoral muscles, dorsal dispersion stroke, and flat strokes of the legs are applied at the end of each treatment session to support the venous backflow.

Additional Strokes

See Diabetic Vascular Diseases (p. 168).

Comments

- The strokes are first applied softly—with flatly positioned fingertips—then intensively with fingertips at an oblique angle.
- When treating the legs, strokes are applied only in the proximal direction at the beginning.
- Peripheral treatment is not recommended with varices, inflammations, and edemas, since the development of thrombosis cannot be excluded. Ice applications are an exception here.
- In addition to CTM and physical therapy, other supplemental measures of physical therapy are available.
- Ice applications in the form of pads, infusions, poultices, and wading.
- Swimming: the temperature should not be above 28 to 30°C (82 to 86°F) and the duration of the activity should not exceed 15 to 20 minutes.
- Massages in conjunction with elevation, intermittent pressing, and stroking should be applied here.
- Compression bandages and stockings and manual lymphatic drainage.
- The application of physical therapy and CTM should be coordinated. It must be ensured that the patient rests after therapy.

3.6 Gynecology and Obstetrics

Mahmoud Mesrogli, Elke Harms

3.6.1 Anatomical and Physiological Principles

Connective tissue massage is increasingly given for treatment of gynecological complaints and in obstetrics. Knowledge of the female physiology is fundamentally significant in the application of a therapy that particularly aims to strengthen and employ the body's own abilities of regulation and regeneration. The discussion of individual indications and measures for treatment below is preceded here by a few anatomical and physiological principles.

Compared with the male pelvis, the female pelvis is characterized by a wider pelvic space and wider trochanters as well as a more marked lordosis of the lumbar spine. The resulting difference in statics causes a more frequent occurrence of back pain in women. The significant strain and physiological wear to which the female body is subjected during pregnancies and births also contribute to this.

The subcutaneous layer of fatty tissue is generally thicker in women than in men, while the amount of muscle and bone mass in relation to the total weight is less, which must be taken into consideration when applying CTM. Obesity has a higher prevalence in women.

Certain disorders of the skeletal system, such as osteoporosis, affect women during or after menopause.

The Regular Menstrual Cycle

The menstrual cycle of women is 28 ± 3 days. The permanently repeating processes of maturation and regression in the ovary lead to cyclical fluctuations in the hormonal stimulation of genital organs. The first half of the cycle, the follicular or proliferative phase, is marked by estrogens, while the second half of the cycle, the luteal or secretory phase, is marked by progesterone.

These repetitive processes are subject to central regulation. The hypothalamus secretes the gonadotropin-releasing hormone (GnRH), which in turn effects the secretion and pulsatile excretion of the gonadotropins LH (luteinizing hormone) and FSH (follicle-stimulating hormone) from the anterior pituitary.

Under the influence of these hormones an ovarian follicle develops from a primary follicle to a so-called antral follicle, whereas the follicle increasingly produces estradiol. This increase in the ovarian estrogen production leads to an intensified excretion of LH and FSH via positive feedback, which in the end triggers ovulation.

In the following days the empty follicle develops into the corpus luteum, which produces estrogen as well as progesterone. A sufficient serum concentration of LH is the essential prerequisite for the secretion of progesterone from the luteal cells. If there is no pregnancy, the corpus luteum is not sufficiently stimulated in the long term, and regresses again over the course of about 14 days. Due to a drop in the serum progesterone level, follicular maturation starts again, while at the same time menstruation—a progesterone-withdrawal bleeding—sets in.

The central dependence of the menstrual cycle conversely simultaneously includes the possibility of influencing these processes by external stimuli through the autonomic nervous system.

The cyclical fluctuations of the hormonal status have not only an immediate impact on the reproductive organs but also effects on processes that appear at first glance to be independent of this. In general, it can be said that estrogens have a parasympathetic-mimetic effect and progesterone a sympathetic-mimetic effect. This results in dependence on the cycle of all processes that are controlled via the autonomic nervous system.

Climacteric and Menopause

The number of available follicles in the ovaries that are capable of maturing continuously decreases with time. By the age of 30 to 35 years the follicular apparatus is stimulated less due to regressive processes, so that ovulation and the development of corpora lutea become irregular and finally cease altogether. The same regressive processes cause a measurable reduction in weight of the ovaries in the premenopausal period. The ovary is therefore the endocrine organ that ages first.

Menopause—the last menstruation controlled by the ovary with a menstruation-free period of at least a year—usually occurs about the age of 50 years.

The premenopause (the period from the beginning to the middle of the fifth decade of a woman's life to the onset of menopause) is characterized by irregularities in the cycle and is often accompanied by neurovegetative complaints. These disorders, summarized under the term "climacteric complaints" or "menopausal syndrome," are ultimately caused by insufficient coordination by the hypothalamus. This is caused by the gradual decrease of ovarian hormone production, which results in a permanently increased release of GnRH by the hypothalamus and subsequently increased secretion of gonadotropins through negative feedback.

3.6.2 The Most Important Indications

Therapists face complex symptoms in gynecology that cannot be explained simply on the basis of the pathological picture alone.

Often one symptom causes another, so that the elimination of one symptom can result in weakening or elimination of another. Depending on the direction, small basic sequence, stimulating strokes, and flat transverse strokes over the sacral bone can produce relaxation and resolution or stimulation in the lumbosacral segment and therefore directly influence the organs. Ventral strokes in the abdominal space achieve relaxation of the abdominal wall: "The abdomen sinks in" according to Dicke. In order to address radiating complaints and secondary symptoms, one, two, or three additional treatment sequences, the treatment of the thighs, and additional techniques outside the pelvic/abdominal space are performed.

As with all treatments, soft, flat strokes have a soothing effect, while intensive, cutting strokes have a stimulating effect.

Strokes on the sacral bone must never be applied from caudal to cranial—that is, in the vertical direction—since these may trigger cramps in the uterine muscles. In the worst case such a spasm may last up to several hours. Relieving the spasm may be attempted with strokes over the pelvic edges.

If the sacral bone shows distensions, flatly applied transverse strokes must be omitted.

The most important indications of CTM in gynecology are:
- Hormonal disturbances, in particular menstrual disturbances, hormone-related sterility, and climacteric complaints
- Chronic salpingitis
- Complaints due to adhesions of various etiology
- Back pain

In obstetrics CTM is indicated:
- During pregnancy without problems for back pain and sciatica (from the fifth month)
- During delivery for spasmolysis and support of labor activity
- In nursing with disturbances of lactation

> Changes in turgor and muscle tone are located in the segments T11–T12, L1–L5, and S1–S5.

Contraindications

The following issues should be considered in addition to the general contraindications for CTM from the gynecological and obstetrical indications:
- In the treatment of menstrual disturbances CTM should remain limited to those indications that were explicitly stated. In particular, hypermenorrhea, metrorrhagia, menorrhagia, and polymenorrhea may worsen; this also applies if (e.g., due to a lumbar spine syndrome) CTM includes the lumbar and sacral zones. In these cases other methods should be preferred for treatment.
- For treatment of complaints during pregnancy CTM should only be given if successful treatment cannot be expected with other measures, such as special physical therapy exercises or general massage.
- CTM is contraindicated if the patient is predisposed to premature contractions, in risk pregnancies, and until the fifth month of pregnancy.
- Since CTM is used to achieve a re-adaptation of the autonomic nervous system, caution must always be applied and medical evaluation is always necessary.

3.6.3 Back Pain

Lower Back Pain

Women often complain of back pain. The causes are highly diverse and largely consistent with the statements found in the sections on orthopedics (Section 3.3, p. 63) and neurology (Section 3.4, p. 101).

Pregnancies and births also play an important role due to their hormonal influence (build-up of fluid in tissue, static loads). Disorders of the female genitals may also manifest themselves as back pain (parametritis, salpingitis, tumors, uterine retroflexion, scars after surgery, menstrual disturbances, and also the onset of menopause). Careful medical diagnosis is necessary here before an often helpful course of CTM is prescribed.

Findings

Extensive changes in the tissue can be found in T11–T12, L1–L5 and S1–S5.

Back pain caused by disruptive nervous reflexes leads to typical hypertonic strings that are palpable especially in the region of the abdomen and hip muscles.

Treatment Plan

Starting position: prone position, supine position, lateral position.
- Small basic sequence.
- Small basic sequence, treatment of the thigh, flat strokes over both legs.
- Small basic sequence, treatment of the thigh, first sequence.

Balancing strokes over the pectoral muscles, dorsal dispersion stroke, and flat strokes of the legs are applied at the end of each treatment session to support the venous backflow.

Additional Strokes

Small Basic Sequence

▶ **From dorsal**
- Flat transverse strokes over the sacral bone from caudal to cranial.
- Small, flat transverse strokes along the spine within the area of the long extensor spinae muscles from L5 to T12.

▶ **From ventral** (▶ Fig. 2.32)
- Bimanual strokes, starting from the dorsal side. At the same time, the therapist pulls on the lower edge of the rib cage toward the medioclavicular line and on the pelvic edge toward the anterior superior iliac spine. These strokes are performed bimanually, first on one side then on the other.
- Bimanual strokes crossing over the abdominal walls, starting in the dorsal region and ending at the opposite edge of the rectus abdominis muscle.
- The liver stroke.
- Balancing pelvic strokes.
- Flat transverse strokes over the abdominal space.

First Sequence

▶ **From dorsal**
- The intercostal strokes are also pulled in reverse from the spinal column to the lateral thorax wall to the ventral axillary line.

▶ **From ventral**
- In the ventral intercostal area a set of flat strokes are pulled beginning at the dorsal axillary line through the intercostal spaces. These should start at the lowest ribs.

Comments

- Treatment should be dosed gently at the beginning.
- First sequence and treatment of thighs may be applied alternately or on the same day.
- While the treatment of statically originating back pain must focus on intensive kinesiotherapy, CTM is preferred in the treatment of back pain caused by nervous reflexes based on the general findings in the connective tissue.
- Relaxation techniques support the efforts.

3.6.4 Hormonal Disturbances

Menstrual Disturbances

In general, disturbances of rhythm and anomalies in the nature of bleeding must be differentiated in menstrual disturbances. The following notations are common in accordance with rhythm, duration, and type of menstruation:
- *Eumenorrhea:* unremarkable menstruation without any considerable complaint
- *Amenorrhea:* no menstruation for at least 6 months
- *Oligomenorrhea:* too infrequent occurrence of menstruation (intervals greater than 35 days)
- *Polymenorrhea:* too frequent occurrence of menstruation (intervals less than 24 days)
- *Hypermenorrhea:* heavy menstrual bleeding (more than five sanitary napkins per day)
- *Hypomenorrhea:* light menstrual bleeding (fewer than two sanitary napkins per day)
- *Menorrhagia:* prolonged menstruation (over 6 days).
- *Metrorrhagia:* acyclic menstruation.
- *Dysmenorrhea:* painful menstruation, the cause of which is hormonal or physical, but may also often be caused by cramping of the muscles in the abdomen, pelvis, and back

Also belonging to this group is premenstrual syndrome (PMS), which may present itself with malaise during the last days before menstruation and shows irritability, depressive mood, lethargy, breast pain, and/or edemas with weight gain.

CTM can have a positive effect on oligomenorrhea, hypomenorrhea, secondary amenorrhea, and dysmenorrhea.

Depending on the findings in the tissue, the menstrual disturbances can be either atonic or spastic.

Oligomenorrhea, Hypomenorrhea, Secondary Amenorrhea

Definition

These menstrual disturbances are atonic and frequently affect women with a pyknic physique. Accompanying symptoms often include fatigue, disposition to depressive moods, and loss of appetite; there are also frequently disturbances of the bladder (▶ Fig. 3.34, ▶ Fig. 3.35).

Findings

The most important findings when examining atonic menstrual disturbances are a loose abdominal wall, bulging abdomen, and connective tissue with only little relief over the sacral bone and the sacroiliac joints as well as proneness to varices and edemas.

Treatment Plan

Starting position: sitting, lateral position, supine position, prone position.
- Apply the small basic sequence twice. Balancing strokes over the pectoral muscles, dorsal dispersion stroke, and flat strokes of the legs are applied at the end of each treatment session to support the venous backflow.

Additional Strokes

Small Basic Sequence

▶ **From dorsal** (▶ Fig. 2.27, ▶ Fig. 2.29)
- Hooks to the sacral bone edges from caudal to cranial.
- Flat transverse strokes over the sacral bone from caudal to cranial.
- Hooks along the course of the first pelvic stroke from caudal to cranial.
- Hooks and stretching stroke at the ischial tuberosity.
- Stretching stroke in the lumbar triangle.

▶ **From ventral** (▶ Fig. 2.35)
- Bimanual strokes starting from dorsal. At the same time, the therapist pulls on the lower edge of the rib cage toward the medioclavicular line and on the pelvic edge toward the anterior superior iliac spine. These strokes are performed bimanually, first on one side then on the other.
- Short hook along the rectus sheath from the symphysis to the level of the navel.
- Bimanual strokes crossing over the abdominal walls, starting in the dorsal region and ending at the opposite edge of the rectus abdominis muscle.
- The liver stroke.
- Balancing pelvic strokes.
- Flat transverse strokes over the abdominal space.

Comments

- The goal of the treatment is at first to normalize the cycle and stimulate ovarian function in addition to influencing the connective tissue.

- Soft doses should be applied initially if there is distended and painful tissue. The fan-shaped stroke, the stroke on the lower rhomboid, and the stimulating strokes must be applied using the cutting stroke technique as much as possible.
- The balancing strokes on the pectoral muscles are only applied after the stimulating strokes.
- Hydrotherapy measures such as hot compresses, rolled-up hot packs, galvanic baths, peat pulp, and sulfur baths as well as physical therapy relaxation and mobilization techniques can all support the treatment process. Physical therapy is applied before CTM to ensure that the patient is able to rest after CTM treatment.
- Treatment is started in the middle of the cycle with oligo- and hypomenorrhea. Treatment is given on 4 to 5 consecutive days, each time for 20 minutes.
- Treatment is given on 4 to 5 consecutive days with amenorrhea. If there is no menstruation after interruption of treatment for 10 days, the treatment cycle is repeated, several times if necessary.
- Vertical strokes over the sacral bone must be avoided always, since this may provoke uterine cramp under certain circumstances. The cramp can be loosened by pulling the pelvic strokes.

Dysmenorrhea

Definition

Dysmenorrhea is one of the spastic forms of menstrual disturbances, which occur mainly in the asthenic type. In addition to pain in the back and lower abdomen, spastic constipation can often be found, which normalizes once menstruation starts. Migraines, circulatory disturbances, and vomiting associated with menstruation are occasionally observed. Externally the patients show a remarkable cramped posture with tense abdominal walls. The pelvis is severely straightened.

Findings

Characteristic findings in the connective tissue include retraction and/or distensions on the upper third of the sacral bone and between the sacroiliac joints. There is also severely increased tension on the sacral bone and on the iliac crests as well as severe tenderness of the rhomboid end points.

If there are complaints such as constipation (p. 149) and migraine (p. 121), the findings can change accordingly.

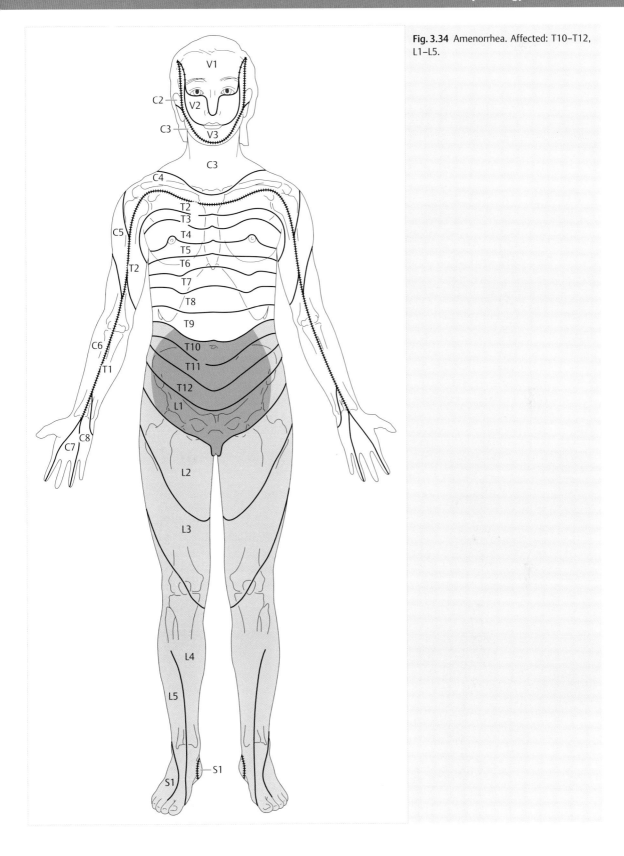

Fig. 3.34 Amenorrhea. Affected: T10–T12, L1–L5.

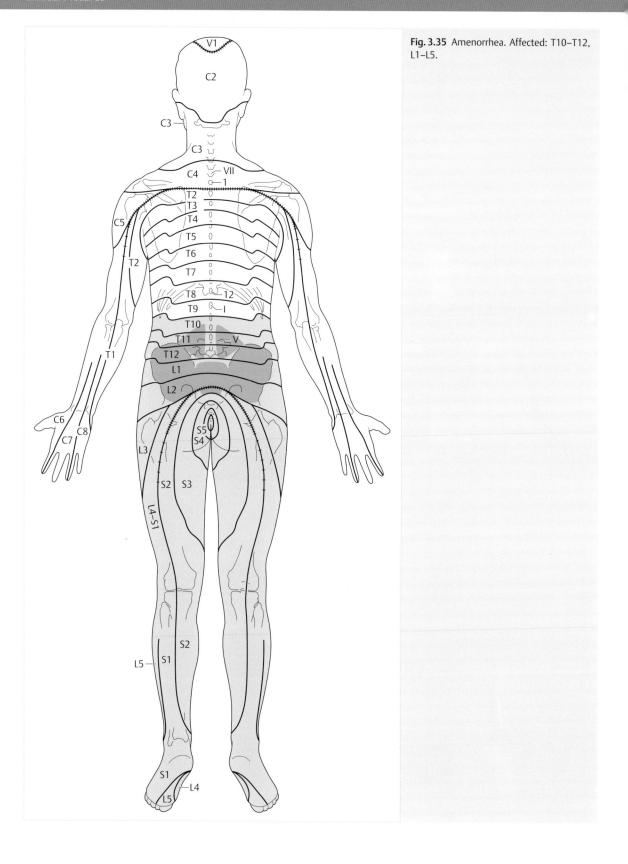

Fig. 3.35 Amenorrhea. Affected: T10–T12, L1–L5.

Treatment Plan

Starting position: sitting, lateral position, supine position, prone position.
• Apply the small basic sequence twice.

Balancing strokes over the pectoral muscles and dorsal branching end each treatment session.

Additional Strokes

Small Basic Sequence

▶ **From dorsal** (▶ Fig. 2.20)
• Flat transverse strokes over the sacral bone from caudal to cranial.
• Small, flat transverse strokes over the spinal column within the long erector spinae muscle from L5 to T12.

▶ **From ventral** (▶ Fig. 2.35)
• Bimanual strokes, starting from the dorsal side. At the same time, the therapist pulls on the lower edge of the rib cage toward the medioclavicular line and on the pelvic edge toward the anterior superior iliac spine. These strokes are performed bimanually, first on one side then on the other.
• Balancing pelvic strokes.
• Flat transverse strokes over the abdominal space.

Comments

• CTM should cause a neurohumoral reconfiguration by stimulating the autonomic nervous system with the goal of having a positive influence on the complaints and eliminating the pathological tension and connective tissue zones.
• Treatment is started in the second half of the cycle and applied three times a week.
• Women who are used to CTM can be treated on the first day of their period. During the second cycle of the small basic sequence all strokes, perceived as uncomfortable or worse than before are applied with less pressure, while all other strokes are applied with normal intensity.
• As with all menstrual disturbances, special attention should be given to pain in the region of the sacral bone and iliac bone.
• A rolled-up hot pack and physical therapy exercises may have a supportive effect.
• Physical therapy is administered before CTM to ensure that the patient can rest after treatment.

Premenstrual Syndrome

Definition

Premenstrual syndrome (PMS) is a spastic menstrual disturbance. Pain in the back, neck, abdomen, and/or chest is characteristic during the second half of the cycle.

Headaches, circulatory disturbances, constipation, and frequently occurring distended abdomen disappear as soon as menstruation starts.

Findings

Changes in the tissue can be found:
• On the sacral bone, in the region of the sacroiliac joints and on the iliac bone
• Along the spinal column and in the region of the shoulder and neck
• Ventrally in the region of the rib cage

Treatment Plan

Starting position: sitting, supine position, prone position.
• Small basic sequence.
• Small basic sequence, first sequence, ventral side.
• Small basic sequence, first and second sequence, ventral side.

Balancing strokes over the pectoral muscles and dorsal branching end each treatment session.

Additional Strokes

Small Basic Sequence

▶ **From dorsal** (▶ Fig. 2.20)
• Hooks to the sacral bone edges from caudal to cranial.
• Flat transverse strokes over the sacral bone from caudal to cranial.
• Hooks along the course of the first pelvic stroke from caudal to cranial.
• Small, flat transverse strokes along the spine within the area of the long extensor spinae muscles from L5 to T12.
• The liver stroke.

▶ **From ventral** (▶ Fig. 2.32)
• Bimanual strokes, beginning simultaneously from dorsal on the lower edge of the rib cage to the medioclavicular line and from the pelvic edge to the anterior superior iliac spine. These strokes are performed bimanually, first on one side then on the other.
• Bimanual strokes crossing over the abdominal walls, starting in the dorsal region and ending at the opposite edge of the rectus abdominis muscle.
• The liver stroke.
• Balancing pelvic strokes.
• Flat transverse strokes over the abdominal space.

First Sequence

▶ **From dorsal**
• Large balancing stroke. This starts at the level of the sixth/seventh intercostal space and is flatly pulled around the lower angle of the scapula to C7.

► **From ventral**

• In the ventral intercostal area a set of flat strokes are pulled beginning at the dorsal axillary line through the intercostal spaces; start at the lowest ribs.

Second Sequence

► **From dorsal**

• Flat fan-shaped strokes are pulled transversely over the scapula toward the shoulder joint.
• Flat transverse strokes from the inner side to the lateral edge of the scapulae, starting at the level of T7 and ending at the level of the spine of the scapula.
• Small hooks around the scapula.

Comments

• By pulling out strokes on the lower edges of the rib cage and with transverse strokes between the shoulder blades, but which are applied only to T2 due to the maximal point, symptoms of migraine and headaches should be influenced positively. If necessary, the third sequence can be added.
• Mastodynia is influenced by the large balancing strokes; lethargy and depressive mood are influenced by pulling out the lower edges of the rib cage and by the liver stroke.
• For the treatment of constipation see Constipation (p. 149).
• The additional strokes may be applied several times. If necessary, pulling out of the lower edges of the rib cage is repeated.
• Supportive measures (relaxation and mobilization techniques) of physical therapy should as usual be applied before CTM to ensure that the patient can rest after treatment.

Sterility and Infertility

CTM may be indicated in certain forms of sterility. These are primarily dysfunctions of the ovary, which are the cause of the sterility in about 40% of women patients. In these cases and in the presence of secondary amenorrhea, CTM is advisable as a first step, or in support of hormone therapy.

The treatment is consistent with CTM applied during menstrual disturbances of the atonic type, but one should aim for more intensive and more targeted effect on the organs of the lower abdomen.

Findings

See the sections Menstrual Disturbances (p. 175), and Oligomenorrhea, Hypomenorrhea, Secondary Amenorrhea (p. 176).

Treatment Plan

Starting position: sitting, prone position, lateral position, supine position.
• Small basic sequence is applied twice.
• Small basic sequence, first sequence.
• Small basic sequence, first and second sequence.
• Small basic sequence, first, second, and third sequence.

Balancing strokes over the pectoral muscles and dorsal branching end each treatment session.

Additional Strokes

Small Basic Sequence

► **From dorsal**

• Hooks to the sacral bone edges from caudal to cranial.
• Flat transverse strokes over the sacral bone from caudal to cranial.
• Hooks along the course of the first pelvic stroke from caudal to cranial.
• Hooks and stretching stroke at the ischial tuberosity. This stroke may be applied four to six times.
• Stretching stroke in the lumbar triangle. This stroke may also be applied four to six times.
• A fan-shaped stroke in the respiratory angle.

► **From ventral**

• Bimanual strokes, starting from the dorsal side. At the same time, the therapist pulls on the lower edge of the rib cage toward the medioclavicular line and on the pelvic edge toward the anterior superior iliac spine. These strokes are performed bimanually, first on one side then on the other.
• Short hooks along the rectus sheath from the symphysis to the level of the navel.
• Bimanual strokes crossing over the abdominal walls, starting in the dorsal region and ending at the opposite edge of the rectus abdominis muscle.
• The liver stroke.
• Balancing pelvic strokes.
• Flat transverse strokes over the abdominal space.

Comments

• First, second, and third sequences and liver stroke are included in the treatment to influence the general state of the autonomic nervous system and disturbances of superordinate centers.
• CTM must be applied as long-term therapy.
• Application of a rolled-up hot pack may be advisable as a supportive measure.
• Apply the rolled-up hot pack after CTM.

Climacteric Complaints

Definition

The climacteric syndrome is characterized by menstrual disturbances and three groups of symptoms: an autonomic nervous, a mental, and an organic symptom complex.

Symptoms of the vasomotor and autonomic nervous system predominantly include hot flashes, excessive sweating, cardiac complaints (e.g., tachycardia and heart palpitations) and paresthesia. Mental symptoms comprise, for instance, depressive mood, insomnia, irritability, reduced motivation, headaches, and anxiety.

The most important organic symptoms are osteoporosis, arthropathies, and atrophic changes in skin and mucous membranes.

Since climacteric complaints are essentially an estrogen deficiency syndrome, temporary (2–5 years) estrogen substitution therapy is implemented. A longer duration of therapy is proven to carry the risk of various illnesses, including breast cancer.

Many of the symptoms mentioned can be positively influenced by CTM, especially the mental ones, and to a large extent also those complaints that are caused by the vasomotor and autonomic nervous system as well as complaints in the region of the sacral bone.

Indications for CTM are
- Depressive mood
- Reduced motivation
- Headaches
- Insomnia
- Swollen legs
- Paresthesia in the hands, feet, arms, and legs
- Cramps in the feet and calves
- Digestive disorders (pressure and bloating in the upper abdomen, constipation, etc.)
- Cardiac complaints
- Back pain

Findings

Tissue changes are located in the segmental areas of T10–L1; in depressive mood they are additionally accentuated from T6 to T10. These zones should be included in CTM.

▶ **Changes in turgor and muscle tone on the posterior side of the body**
- On the sacral bone and iliac crest, and along the spinal column and the lower edge of the rib cage
- Between and on the scapulae and in the region of the shoulder and neck

▶ **On the anterior side of the body**
- In the region of the upper abdomen, along the lower edge of the rib cage, and in the region of the rib cage (pectoral muscle, sternocleidomastoid muscle, sternoclavicular angle)

Treatment Plan

Starting position: sitting, supine position, prone position.
- The small basic sequence is applied twice.
- Small basic sequence (once), first sequence.
- Small basic sequence, first and second sequence.
- Small basic sequence, first, second, and third sequence.

Balancing strokes over the pectoral muscles, dorsal dispersion stroke, and flat strokes of the legs and arms are applied at the end of each treatment session to support the venous backflow.

Additional Strokes

Small Basic Sequence

▶ **From dorsal**
- Flat transverse strokes over the sacral bone from caudal to cranial.
- Small, flat transverse strokes along the spine within the area of the long extensor spinae muscles from L5 to T12.

▶ **From ventral** (▶ Fig. 2.32)
- Bimanual strokes, starting from the dorsal side. At the same time, the therapist pulls on the lower edge of the rib cage toward the medioclavicular line and on the pelvic edge toward the anterior superior iliac spine. These strokes are performed bimanually, first on one side then on the other.
- Bimanual strokes crossing over the abdominal walls, starting in the dorsal region and ending at the opposite edge of the rectus abdominis muscle.
- The liver stroke.
- Balancing pelvic strokes.
- Flat transverse strokes over the abdomen.

First Sequence

▶ **From dorsal**
- Large balancing stroke. This starts at the level of the sixth/seventh intercostal space and is flatly pulled around the lower angle of the scapula toward C7.

▶ **From ventral**
- In the ventral intercostal area a set of flat strokes are pulled beginning at the dorsal axillary line through the intercostal spaces. These should start at the lowest ribs.

Second Sequence

▶ **From dorsal**
- Flat fan-shaped strokes are pulled transversely over the scapula toward the shoulder joint.

- Flat transverse strokes from the inner side to the lateral edge of the scapulae, starting at the level of T7 and ending at the level of the spine of the scapula.
- Small hooks around the scapula.

Comments

- Because of the complexity of the symptoms that accompany this pathological picture it is necessary to work over the entire back.
- Through the first, second, and third sequence, the fan-shaped strokes on the scapulae (arm segments T6–T12, C3–C8) can influence paresthesia.
- When treating hot flashes, pulling out the lower edges of the rib cage is an important element of treatment in addition to the treatment of the sacral bone.
- Patients with back pain during the night and subsequent morning stiffness respond particularly positively to treatment with CTM.

3.6.5 Inflammatory Diseases

Salpingitis and Parametritis

While CTM is contraindicated during acute salpingitis as with all acute inflammatory diseases, the subsequent conditions after healing of an acute inflammation of the fallopian tubes, ovaries, or pelvic connective tissue as well as complaints caused by chronic salpingitis or parametritis are essential indications for CTM. Typical subsequent consequences of acute salpingitis, which must be expected in 20% of cases, are

- Uncharacteristic lower abdominal pain, caused by adhesions
- Back pain
- Fixed retroflexed uterus
- Sterility or disposition for tubal pregnancies
- Dysmenorrhea

Back pain, dysmenorrhea, and adhesion-related complaints can be positively influenced by CTM.

Also spastic parametropathy often responds well to CTM treatment. This disorder, which is caused by a dysfunction of the autonomic nervous system, presents with severe pressing, stabbing, or pulling pain in the abdomen and the region of the sacral bone, which often persists over years, and with spastic intestinal complaints.

Psychosomatic causes can equally be found and must be taken into account for therapy.

Findings

▶ **Changes in turgor and muscle tone on the dorsal side of the body**
- On the sacral bone
- On the gluteal muscles on the affected side
- Along the lumbar spine
- In the angle between the lumbar spine and pelvic crest

▶ **On the ventral side of the body**
- In the region of the pubic bone
- In the region of the abdominal space

▶ **On the lateral side of the body**
- Between the anterior superior iliac spine and the greater trochanter
- Along the iliotibial tract

Treatment Plan

Starting position: sitting, prone position, lateral position, supine position.
- The small basic sequence is applied twice.
- Small basic sequence (once) and treatment of the thigh. Flat strokes over both legs.
- Small basic sequence (once), first sequence and treatment of the thigh. Flat strokes over both legs.

Balancing strokes over the pectoral muscles and dorsal branching end each treatment session.

Additional Strokes

Small Basic Sequence

▶ **From dorsal**
- Flat transverse strokes over the sacral bone from caudal to cranial.
- Small, flat transverse strokes along the spine within the area of the long extensor spinae muscles from L5 to T12.

▶ **From ventral (▶ Fig. 2.32)**
- Bimanual strokes, starting from the dorsal side. At the same time, the therapist pulls on the lower edge of the rib cage toward the medioclavicular line and on the pelvic edge toward the anterior superior iliac spine. These strokes are performed bimanually, first on one side then on the other.
- Bimanual strokes crossing over the abdominal walls, starting in the dorsal region and ending at the opposite edge of the rectus abdominis muscle.
- The liver stroke.
- Balancing pelvic strokes.
- Flat transverse strokes over the abdomen.

First Sequence

▶ **From dorsal**
- The intercostal strokes are also pulled in reverse from the spinal column to the lateral thorax wall to the ventral axillary line.

▶ **From ventral**
- In the ventral intercostal area a set of flat strokes are pulled, beginning at the dorsal axillary line through the intercostal spaces. These should start at the lowest ribs.

▶ **Thigh**
• Stroke between the anterior superior iliac spine and the greater trochanter.

Comments

• Treatment should be dosed gently at the beginning.
• The treatment of the thigh can be supported because of the segmental allocations.

3.6.6 Complaints after Surgical Procedures

After gynecological surgery various disturbances may develop that affect the patient's wellbeing and health.

One of the most frequent complications after surgery is the development of adhesions, which may lead to severe pain, tubal sterility, and, among other things, even to ileus. Adhesion prophylaxis, which is ideally applied during surgery, is absolutely imperative to minimize the trauma from surgery, since it is difficult to treat adhesions that have already developed. Surgical intervention can provoke new adhesions if no microsurgical techniques are applied. Improvement may be achieved, for example, by repeatedly applying absorptive measures such as balneotherapy.

CTM may have a particularly positive effect on pathological tension of the connective tissue caused by adhesions, and also on organic disorders resulting from adhesions of the uterus and the adnexa, of which bladder and rectum are especially often affected. The treatment must be based in this case on the findings determined in the connective tissue.

After gynecological surgery patients occasionally report complaints in the region of the lower extremities, especially in the ankle, and "heavy legs." CTM may alleviate the complaints in these cases. The same applies to back pain, which often develops after surgery.

See the following sections for findings, treatment plan, additional strokes, and comments:
• Scar Treatment (p. 98)
• Disorders of the Gastrointestinal Tract (p. 143)
• Constipation (p. 149)
• Disorders of the Bladder (p. 160)
• Back Pain (p. 174)
• Nerve Root Lesions (p. 110)
• Salpingitis and Parametritis (p. 182)

3.6.7 Connective Tissue Massage during Pregnancy, Birth, and Postpartum

Back Pain and Sciatica in Pregnancy

Definition

Because of pregnancy-related loosening of the tissue, which also affects the connective tissue and cartilage, and the increased static strain due to increasing body weight, pregnancy is frequently also accompanied by faulty posture (increased lordosis).

Back pain, fatigue, and cramping of muscles, intensified by reduced muscle tone and pseudoradicular complaints as well as "sciatica," sensory deficits of individual lumbar nerves, etc. are the consequence and frequent symptoms during the last trimester of pregnancy. Under certain circumstances these complaints may take on such an extent that individual physical therapy treatment becomes necessary.

Lots of exercise and training as well as swimming, if possible, is advisable for therapy. When the increased loosening of the sacroiliac joints leads to severe back pain during the last weeks of pregnancy, which cannot be improved through other measures, CTM may be indicated, and has a beneficial effect on the back pain and the sciatica that frequently develop during pregnancy.

Findings

• See Back Pain (p. 174).
• Gestagenic processes caused extensive changes in the tissue and the findings can therefore not be evaluated correctly.

Treatment Plan, Additional Strokes

See Back Pain (p. 174).

Comments

• See Back Pain (p. 174).
• All strokes should initially be applied in flat technique.
• Contraindications include risk pregnancies and the first four months of pregnancy.

Treatment in the area of the sacral bone as well as stimulating strokes in the region of the sacral or iliac bone and the region of the tract should not be applied.

Other Indications during Pregnancy

Additional indications for CTM during pregnancy include nocturnal paresthesia as well as cramps in the calves, feet, or thighs.

Findings

Changes in turgor and muscle tone are located in the region of T10–L1 and in the leg.

Tenderness and sensitivity can be found in the region of the pelvis and sacral bone.

Treatment Plan

Starting position: sitting, lateral position, supine position.
• Small basic sequence.

- Small basic sequence and treatment of the thigh.
- Small basic sequence, treatment of the thigh and lower leg.
- Small basic sequence and treatment of the leg.

Balancing strokes over the pectoral muscles, dorsal dispersion stroke, and flat strokes of the legs are applied at the end of each treatment session to support the venous backflow.

Treatment Plan, Additional Strokes, Comments

- All strokes should initially be applied in flat technique.
- Therapy must not be started before the fifth month of pregnancy.
- Risk pregnancies as well as early pregnancies are an absolute contraindication.
- All stimulating strokes must be omitted.
- Intensive strokes, such as the tract stroke, should be applied in flat technique.

Spasmolysis

The stage of dilation during which CTM can be considered includes the period between the first regular contractions and the full opening of the cervical os. It lasts between 5 and 11 hours, or 2 to 4 hours in women who have had children before. During this period the cervix is pulled up and the cervical os starts to dilate under the influence of labor.

During this phase birth spasms of the cervical os often develop, which not only intensify the pain but may also significantly prolong the delivery. In addition to medication with spasmolytics and analgesics, there is also the indication for applications of physical therapy.

Treatment Plan

Starting position: sitting, supine position, lateral position.
- Small basic sequence is applied twice, treatment of the thigh.

Balancing strokes over the pectoral muscles, dorsal dispersion stroke, and flat strokes of the legs are applied at the end of each treatment session.

Additional Strokes

Small Basic Sequence

▶ From dorsal (▶ Fig. 2.27, ▶ Fig. 2.29)
- Hooks to the sacral bone edges from caudal to cranial.
- Flat transverse strokes over the sacral bone from caudal to cranial.
- Hooks along the course of the first pelvic stroke from caudal to cranial.
- Small, flat transverse strokes along the spine within the area of the long extensor spinae muscle from L5 to T12.

Comments

- Technique (intensity and duration) and positioning must cater to the sensations and wishes of the patient giving birth. Each paresthesia may intensify or prolong the spasm and then cause cessation of labor activity.
- All strokes should initially be applied in flat technique.
- An intensive treatment applied to the region of the pelvis and sacral bone during the spasmolytic treatment does not mean an increased traction stimulus, but rather an increased duration.
- In addition to CTM, heat applications and changes in the posture support the success of treatment.

Promotion of Labor Activity

Another area of application of physical therapy during birth is primary weakness of labor. CTM may stimulate the labor activity.

Treatment Plan

See Spasmolysis (p. 184).

Additional Strokes

See Spasmolysis (p. 184).

Comments

- In contrast to spasmolysis, the traction intensity should be increased here.
- In addition to CTM, heat applications and changes in the posture may support the success of the treatment.

Lactation Disturbances

It is not possible so far to promote milk production using medication; an exception to this rule is the application of an oxytocin nose spray to treat so-called retentive breast, when milk is simply not released. There is also known medication for delayed active milk secretion.

However, CTM may be advisable with delayed milk excretion, which normally occurs on the second to fourth day after birth, and when the amount of milk suddenly declines. These symptoms often occur during the first days and weeks after the mother is discharged from the clinic. They are often caused by the sudden, massive strain on the mother caused by everyday life. If left untreated, a decrease in milk production and repeated additional feeding with a bottle may cause the child to suck less, which then leads to complete cessation of milk production.

In early nursing, especially with delayed milk secretion, CTM is applied in those connective tissue zones that belong to the breast and which are located in the region of the rib cage and scapulae as well as the sacral bone. The general findings in the connective tissue are the basis for treatment in the postpartum period.

Findings

Changes in turgor and muscle tone can be palpated:
- Between and around the scapulae
- In the region of the neck

The tissue is in general extensively changed due to pregnancy and birth.

Treatment Plan

Starting position: sitting, lateral position.
- Small basic sequence.
- Small basic sequence, first sequence, additional strokes of the second sequence.

Balancing strokes over the pectoral muscles and dorsal branching end each treatment session.

Additional Strokes

Small Basic Sequence

▶ **From dorsal**
- Hooks to the sacral bone edges from caudal to cranial.
- Flat transverse strokes over the sacral bone from caudal to cranial.
- Hooks along the course of the first pelvic stroke from caudal to cranial.
- Balancing pelvic strokes.
- Flat transverse strokes over the abdominal space.

First Sequence

▶ **From dorsal**
- Large balancing stroke = milk stroke (stimulating stroke).

Second Sequence

▶ **From dorsal**
- Border of the scapula.
- Hooks around the scapula (medial and lateral border).
- Flat strokes over the scapula.

Comments

- The dorsal branching strokes are only applied over a small area to counteract the effect of the milk stroke. The milk stroke, however, is applied flatly but faster and in an almost aggressive manner. Only use the flat technique with asthma patients.
- The treatment of the scapulae loosens complaints and tensions in the shoulder and therefore has a supportive therapeutic effect.
- After the therapist administers the treatment to the region of the sacral bone and pelvis, the hands must be washed to avoid a risk of infection to the baby by transferring pathogens from the genital area to the mammary glands.

Additional Indications

Due to the strains of pregnancy and birth there are often also complaints present during the postpartum period. These especially include:
- Sleep disorders
- Bladder disorders
- Hemorrhoids
- Constipation, back pain

In these cases CTM can significantly improve the complaints on the basis of the general findings in the connective tissue.

Index

Note: Page numbers set **bold** or *italic* indicate headings or figures, respectively.